BIOMATERIALS

A Nano Approach

BIOMATERIALS
A Nano Approach

Seeram Ramakrishna
Murugan Ramalingam
T. S. Sampath Kumar
Winston O. Soboyejo

CRC Press
Taylor & Francis Group
Boca Raton London New York

CRC Press is an imprint of the
Taylor & Francis Group, an **informa** business

CRC Press
Taylor & Francis Group
6000 Broken Sound Parkway NW, Suite 300
Boca Raton, FL 33487-2742

Printed in the United States of America on acid-free paper
10 9 8 7 6 5 4 3 2 1

International Standard Book Number: 978-1-4200-4781-3 (Hardback)

Library of Congress Cataloging-in-Publication Data

Biomaterials : a nano approach / Seeram Ramakrishna ... [et al.].
p. ; cm.
Includes bibliographical references and index.
ISBN 978-1-4200-4781-3 (hardcover : alk. paper)
1. Nanostructured materials. 2. Biomedical materials. 3. Biotechnology. I. Ramakrishna, Seeram. II. Title.
[DNLM: 1. Biocompatible Materials. 2. Nanostructures. QT 37 B5753 2010]

TP248.25.N35B557 2010
660.6--dc22
2009051865

Visit the Taylor & Francis Web site at
http://www.taylorandfrancis.com

and the CRC Press Web site at
http://www.crcpress.com

This book is dedicated to all the students, researchers, and teachers who contributed their hard work to advance this fascinating field of biomaterials.

Contents

Foreword

As we enter the era of nanotechnology, the field of biomaterials is becoming one of the most promising areas with assured novel products to alleviate the pain and suffering of mankind. Even though activity in this field is not new, there is currently fresh energy in this subject brought about by the convergence and remarkable advances in nanotechnology and biotechnology. This includes the development of the next generation of biomaterials by the so-called tissue regeneration approach. Another upcoming strategy is to design nanomaterials to encapsulate, target, and deliver from small molecules to large molecules to a specific tissue site, which could contribute immensely to the eradication of cancer morbidity or the cure of other diseases.

Although many well-known textbooks on biomaterials are currently available, some with multiple editors and editions over several decades, none of these books seem to address to a significant extent the outcome of the emerging nanotechnology. The driving force for the exploitation of nanotechnology in biomaterial applications is the similarity of the length scale in the biological structures, which range from proteins to cells and cellular structure. *Biomaterials: A Nano Approach* provides a comprehensive discussion on biomaterials and scientifically plausible extrapolation to likely occurrences of situations where nanotechnology could play a significant role. The subject matter of the book, written by experts in the field of biomaterials, is intended to stimulate new research investigations and to inspire a much greater appreciation for the need to investigate nanobiomaterials rather than just exposure. I am sure that their efforts, combined with emerging capabilities in nanotechnology, shall define an exciting new field of nanobiomaterials that not only targets repair and reconstruction of biological systems, but also science and technology in general.

Serena M. Best
Cambridge Center for Medical Materials
University of Cambridge, U.K.
Editor, Journal of Materials Science: Materials in Medicine

Preface

Biomaterials are the subject of intense and demanding development. It is well known that the microscale properties of biomaterials play a key role in their interaction with the surrounding environment and the success of their application. Recent investigations have shown that nano aspects of biomaterials also play an important role in terms of enhancing their properties, due to their smaller size, than their microscale counterparts. Future biomaterials will therefore use nanoscience and nanotechnologies to actively modulate cellular microenvironments. To this end, *Biomaterials: A Nano Approach*, a multidisciplinary theme, deals with basic concepts and various processing methodologies involved in the preparation of biomaterials at the nanoscale and their characterization techniques specifically for biomedical applications. This book begins with an overview of biomaterials from its historical development to current advances being useful for beginners learning about biomaterials. One of the most recent developments in biomaterials has been the exploitation of nanotechnology for the processing of advanced biomaterials with enhanced functional properties; thus, a basic concept of nanotechnology and how it can be applied in the processing of novel nanobiomaterials are described, which is the mainstay of this book. It provides extensive coverage and a good interpretation on nano aspects of metals and alloys, bioceramics, polymeric biomaterials and their composites, which possess a wide spectrum of properties favorable for a diverse range of biomedical applications; therefore, it intends to fill the communication gap between nanotechnology, materials sciences and biomedical sciences. Apart from conventionally processed nanomaterials, the book thoroughly examines the latest advances in biomimetic- and tissue-engineered nanomaterials for a variety of applications with illustrated examples. It also provides more details on the molecular-level events that happen at the cell-biomaterials and tissue-implant interfaces owing to the nano characteristics.

This book consists of 10 chapters. To meet varied needs, each chapter provides clear and in-depth discussions. Chapter 1 provides an overview of the historical developments to current advances in biomaterials. In Chapter 2, the essentials of anatomy and physiology of the human body for non-biologists to understand about the cell, tissue, organ, and organization of the body system are examined. This chapter also discusses biological responses to biomaterials with suitable *in vitro* and *in vivo* case studies. Chapter 3 deals with the mechanical aspects of biomaterials with particular emphasis on cell and tissue deformation. Chapter 4 addresses the failure of biomaterials and various biological systems with particular emphasis on fracture, toughness, fatigue, wear, and their tribology. Chapter 5 provides an in-depth understanding of nanoscale phenomena and state-of-the-art nanostructured biomaterials with their significance to the biomedical community. The safety and environmental aspects of nanomaterials are also briefly discussed. In Chapter 6, the various metallic materials, their classification and processing techniques specific to biomedical applications are discussed. The potential of nanostructured metallic materials, with improved biological performance, has also been indicated. Chapter 7 deals with a variety of bioceramic materials and their processing and characterization techniques. The synthesis, characterization and *in vitro* and *in vivo* results of various nanostructured bioceramics are also highlighted in this chapter. Chapter 8 examines polymeric biomaterials, biodegradable and non-biodegradable, and their processing and characterization techniques. The current scenarios of processing polymeric nanofibers are highlighted with suitably illustrated examples. This chapter also emphasizes the production of nanofibrous polymeric scaffolds suitable for biological and biomedical applications. Chapter 9 looks at composite and cellular biomaterials with their biological performances. Evolution of nanocomposite biomaterials, as a new class of nanobiomaterials, is also discussed in this chapter with their processing methodology from conventional to biomimetic approaches. Chapter 10 discusses nanobiomaterials and their suitability in tissue engineering applications. In this chapter, the basic concept of tissue engineering, its importance, cell sources, scaffolding system, and cell-scaffold interactions are discussed in detail. Overall, this textbook provides a solid framework for understanding the past, present, and future trends in biomaterials with an emphasis on nano aspects of biomaterials for use in human health care systems; therefore it may serve as a single reference textbook for students and researchers who specialize in biomaterials and nanobiomaterials. We hope you all enjoy reading this book.

Seeram Ramakrishna

Murugan Ramalingam

T.S. Sampath Kumar

Winston O. Soboyejo

Acknowledgments

The authors gratefully acknowledge the support and encouragement from the colleagues and students in the following departments: Nanobioengineering Laboratories, National University of Singapore Nanoscience and Nanotechnology Initiative, Singapore; NanoScience Technology Center, University of Central Florida, USA; Department of Metallurgy and Materials Engineering, Indian Institute of Technology Madras, India; and Princeton Institute of Science and Technology of Materials, Princeton University, USA, as well as friends and family. We wish to thank Serena M. Best, Cambridge Centre for Medical Materials, University of Cambridge, U.K.; Kam W. Leong, Duke University, USA; Alexander L. Yarin, Technion-Israel Institute of Technology, Israel; James J. Hickman, NanoScience Technology Center, University of Central Florida, USA; Peter Molnar, NanoScience Technology Center, University of Central Florida, USA; Carl G. Simon, National Institute of Standards and Technology, USA; Marcus Cicerone, National Institute of Standards and Technology, USA; Zheng-Ming Huang, Department of Engineering Mechanics, Tongji University, China; S. H. Teoh, National University of Singapore, Singapore; E. Wintermantel, Technical University of Munich, Germany; V. Renugopalakrishnan, Harvard Medical School, Harvard University, USA; K. Pandurangao Rao, Spark Biotech, USA; Suseela Rajkumar, Central Leather Research Institute, India; and Susan Liao, National University of Singapore, Singapore, who discussed different topics of the book and made valuable suggestions that greatly helped to improve the text. Other valuable suggestions were made by anonymous referees, whom the authors would like to convey our special thanks.

Our publisher, CRC Press, has been extraordinarily supportive and patient with our process. Our special thanks go to the editorial staff at CRC Press, especially Allison Taub, editor of *Materials Science and Chemical Engineering,* and Cathy Giacari, project coordinator, who greatly amended the text format, technical corrections, and presentation style. We also wish to thank and formally acknowledge all the publishers and authors indicated in the text and figures, who granted us permission to use their material in this book. This list is incomplete and we apologize to anyone we omitted.

About The Book

Book Description

Biomaterials: A Nano Approach is a textbook that provides a thorough introduction, basic concepts, several processing methodologies, well-established characterization techniques, and potential applications of a broad range of biomaterials at the nanoscale. This book is an ideal companion for students, researchers, and industrial scientists who specialize in biomaterials and nanobiomaterials.

Features

- A self-contained book for understanding past, present, and future trends in biomaterials
- Extensive coverage of a range of nanobiomaterials with their potential applications
- A series of case studies that demonstrate the vital role of nanobiomaterials
- Written in an accessible way with over 100 illustrations, aimed at novice graduates and intermediate researchers
- Incorporates useful tables with current data
- Integrates the materials science and engineering, nanotechnology, bioengineering, and biosciences in the name of nanobiomaterials

Short Table of Contents

Audience

1. Senior undergraduate and graduate students of materials science and engineering, bioengineering, biomaterials, nanotechnology, biomedical engineering, medicine, and dentistry
2. Academicians and researchers in the fields of materials science and engineering, bioengineering, biomaterials, nanotechnology, biomedical engineering, orthopedics, and dentistry
3. R&D such as biomedical, pharmaceutical, and bionanotechnology industrialists

Applicable courses

1. Biomaterials
2. Nanobiomaterials
3. Materials processing and technology
4. Nanotechnology
5. Tissue engineering
6. Bioengineering
7. Biomedical engineering
8. Orthopedics

Seeram Ramakrishna
National University of Singapore, Singapore

Murugan Ramalingam
University of Central Florida, USA

T. S. Sampath Kumar
Indian Institute of Technology Madras, India

Winston O. Soboyejo
Princeton University, USA

Authors

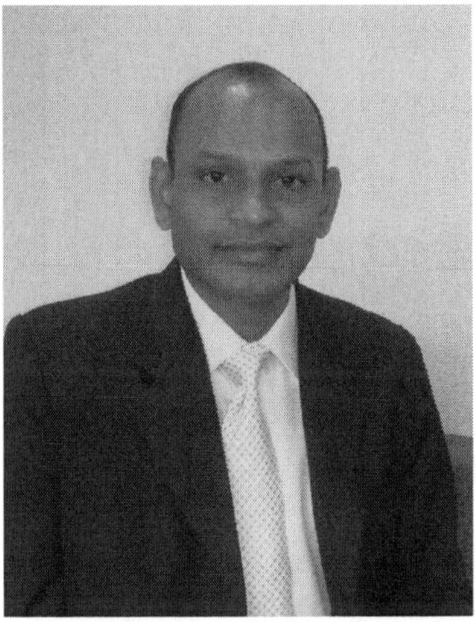

Dr. Seeram Ramakrishna is a professor of mechanical engineering and bio-engineering at the National University of Singapore (NUS). He is also vice president (Research Strategy) of NUS. He is the founding co-director of NUS Nanoscience and Nanotechnology Initiative (NUSNNI). His current research interests include biomaterials, tissue engineering, and nanotechnology. He is advancing the materials science, manufacturing technology, and design aspects of nanobiomaterials to realize their full potential in human health care. His research output has appeared in over 400 publications. The ISI Essential Science Indicators (ESI) places him among the top 110 materials scientists in the world, based on citations. These include several peer-reviewed journal publications, book chapters, books, and patents. He is a board member of 15 international journals. He is a scientific advisory board member to biomedical companies, Stem Life and Biomers International.

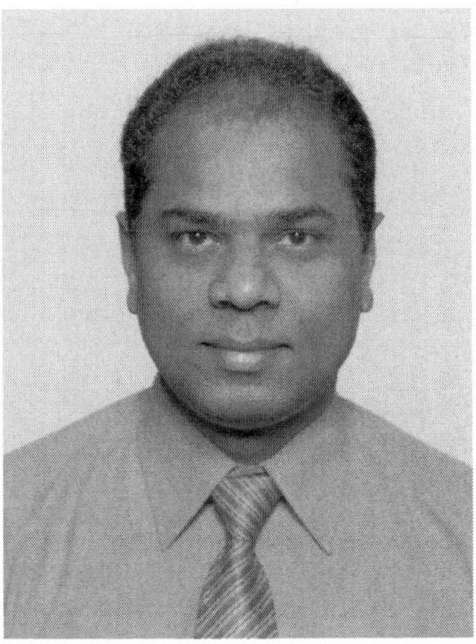

Dr. Murugan Ramalingam is an assistant professor of biomaterials and tissue engineering at the WPI Advanced Institute for Materials Research, Tohoku University, Japan. Prior to joining WPI, he worked as an NRC associate at the National Institute of Standards and Technology (NIST), Gaithersburg (USA) and at the National Institutes of Health (NIH), Bethesda (USA), under the United States National Research Council's joint NIH/NIST program. His main research interests are the development of multiphase biomaterials, through conventional to biomimetics and tissue engineering approaches. He has authored several peer-reviewed journal papers, book chapters, and patents relevant to micro/nanobiomaterials and tissue engineering.

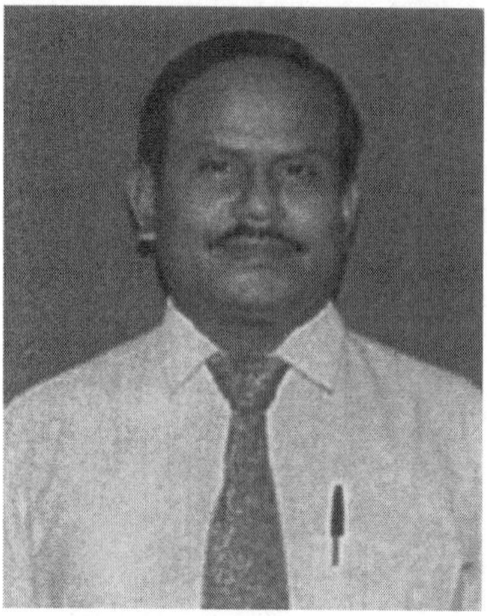

Dr. T. S. Sampath Kumar is a professor of metallurgical and materials engineering at the Indian Institute of Technology Madras, India. His research interests include nanobioceramics, functionally graded biomaterials, novel ceramic coatings, and ceramic-based drug delivery systems. He is currently the secretary of the Society for Biomaterials and Artificial Organs-India (SBAOI). He was the associate editor of the SBAOI journal *Trends in Biomaterials and Artificial Organs-India* during 2002–2005, and continues to be on its editorial board since 1991. He has published three issues of this journal and an issue of *Transactions of the Indian Institute of Metals* as a guest editor.

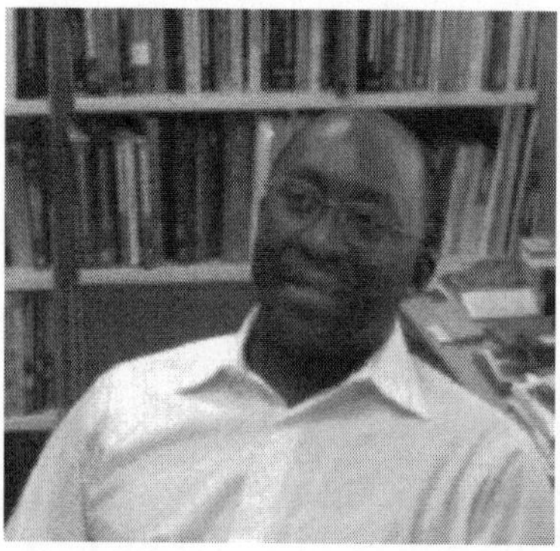

Dr. Winston O. Soboyejo received his Bachelor of Science degree in mechanical engineering from King's College London in 1985, and a PhD in materials science from Cambridge University in 1988. He then worked as a research scientist at the McDonnell Douglas Research Labs from 1988 until 1992. He worked briefly as a principal research engineer at the Edison Welding Institute before joining the faculty in the Department of Materials Science and Engineering at The Ohio State University in 1992. He was a Visiting Martin Luther King Associate Professor in the Departments of Mechanical Engineering and Materials Science and Engineering at MIT from 1997 to 1998. In 1999, he moved to Princeton University as a professor of mechanical and aerospace engineering, and a faculty member in the Princeton Institute of Science and Technology of Materials (PRISM). He is the recipient of two National Young Investigator Awards (NSF and ONR), the Lumley Research Award of the Ohio State University, and the Bradley Stoughton Award for young teachers of materials science. Professor Soboyejo is a Fellow of ASME and the Nigerian Academy of Science. He has published 250 journal papers and a textbook, *Mechanical Properties of Engineered Materials*. He has also edited a recent text on *Advanced Structural Materials* and 18 special issues of journals/conference proceedings.

1

Overview of Biomaterials

1.1 Introduction

Human life is invaluable; however, quality and survival of life is greatly affected by numerous factors, including medical complications caused by diseased, damaged, or aged tissues or organs. These circumstances often call for surgical treatments to repair, replace, maintain, or augment the functions of affected tissues or organs using some additional functional components. Traditionally, they have been treated with the help of tissues or organs procured from patients or donors. Depending on the location of reimplantation of the procured tissue (also known as graft), they are termed autograft, allograft, or xenograft (see Figure 1.1).

If the graft is implanted in the same patient, it is termed autograft and if it is placed in another individual of the same species, it is termed allograft. If the graft is placed in another species (e.g., bone from animal to human), then it is termed xenograft. Among them, autograft is considered the gold standard and has been used for a long time with good clinical results, but the supply of autograft is limited. In addition, allograft and xenograft are not much preferred because of the possibility of pathogen transfer and graft rejection. Furthermore, tissue/organ procurement is complex, expensive, and requires additional surgery. As an alternative, attention has been focused on the use of synthetic material that holds the ability to repair or restore the functions of a defective system into a normal healthy system upon implantation, which is termed alloplastic graft. The synthetic material used for this purpose is called biomaterial. The biomaterial is used either as such or to manufacture implantable devices or prostheses; some of them are illustrated in Figure 1.2.

Currently, there are many definitions for the term "biomaterial," depending on the user's own verdict. Biomaterial by definition is a substance or a combination of substances, other than drugs, derived either from natural or synthetic origin, which can be used for any period of time as a whole or as a part of the system that treats, augments, or replaces any tissue, organ, or function of the body (Williams 1987). Later, Black (1992) defined the term biomaterial

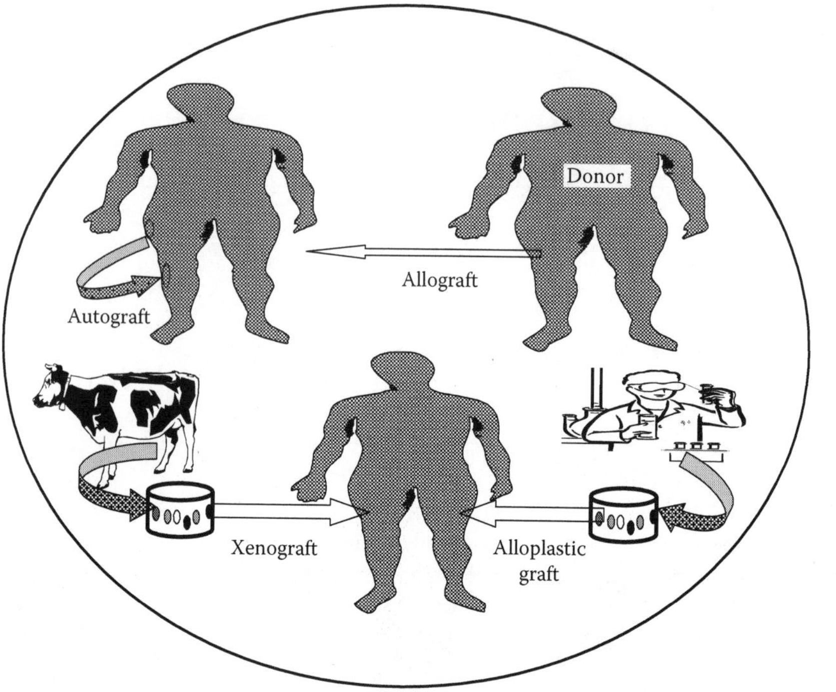

FIGURE 1.1
A schematic of tissue transplantation. (Reprinted with permission from Murugan, R. and Ramakrishna, S., *Handbook of nanostructured biomaterials and their applications in nanobiotechnology*, American Scientific Publishers, Stevenson Ranch, CA, 2005a. With permission from Copyright© American Scientific Publishers.)

as a material of natural or manmade origin that is used to direct, supplement, or replace the functions of living tissues of the human body. A biomaterial is delineated, according to authors' own description, as any material that is used for repairing or restoring the functionality of a defective biological system into a normal healthy system.

The field "biomaterials science and engineering" is a multidisciplinary theme that essentially coalesces materials science and engineering with biomedical sciences for the invention of new health-care systems. Since it is a multidisciplinary field, many experts, in particular materials scientists and engineers, mechanical engineers, physicists, chemists, biologists, and clinicians must work together for its continuous development. It has also witnessed stable growth over about half a century of existence with the major contribution from these experts. However, further research and development is directed at the design and fabrication of novel biomaterials that hold the features and properties analogous to natural tissues or organs. In the following section, some imperative successes that have come in the biomaterials field are provided.

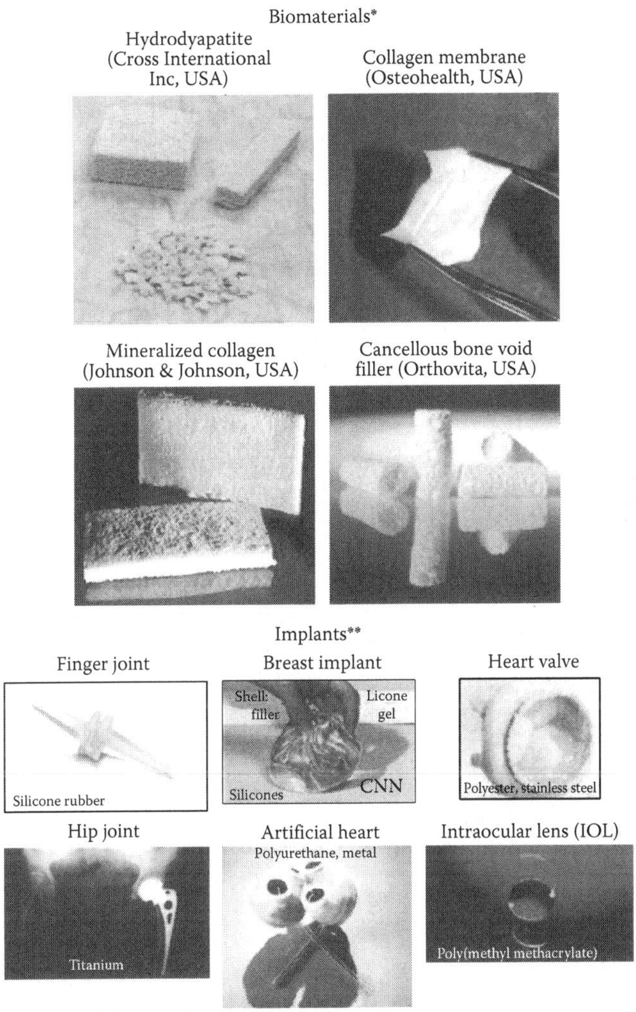

FIGURE 1.2
Prototypes of biomaterials and medical implants. (*Adapted with courtesy from the websites of respective suppliers; **Adapted from Ratner, B. D. et al., *Biomaterials science: An introduction to Materials in Medicine*, San Diego, CA: Elsevier Academic Press, 2004. With permission from Elsevier.)

1.2 Biomaterials: From Then to Now

The use of biomaterials to repair human body parts is not new, dating far back into ancient civilizations. The Egyptians used linen as a suture for wound closure in around 2000 BC. They also used elephant's tusks, walrus teeth, and some kinds of wood to replace bone or missing teeth (Williams and

Cunninghan 1979). Substitution of bone parts in the human body was also carried out at that time using copper, but the implant was not successful due to the effect of copper ion poisoning. As per historical evidence, the Indians and the Chinese used waxes, glues, and tissues in reconstructing defective parts of the human body. It was stated in the Vedic period (1800–1500 BC) of the ancient Indian literature that artificial legs, eyes, and teeth were used. In those days, Hindu surgeons performed surgery using autogeneous tissues for restoring missing parts. Around 600 BC, Sushruta repaired an injured nose with a patch of living flesh taken from the region of the cheek (Bhat 2002). Around 200 BC, the Greek literature pointed out the use of metals (e.g., gold). Hippocrates, who is known as the father of medicine, alleged that metallic wires made of gold might have been used for the treatment of bone fractures at that time. In the seventeenth century, iron and bronze were employed in human systems, but they are more corrosive than gold. Some of the major developments that have occurred in biomaterials are summarized in Table 1.1 (Park 1984, 2003; Sportnitz 1987; Friedman 1994; Greco 2005; Murugan 2005a, 2005b).

The first reported clinical application of biomaterials was carried out in the mid-eighteenth century. In 1759, Hallowell united the edges of a lacerated brachial artery using a wooden peg and twisted thread (Wesolowski 1963). The use of biomaterials has progressed much since his initial contribution. By the mid-nineteenth century, Mathijsen introduced a notable material called lint-reinforced plaster as a bandage in the treatment of bone fractures. In those days, however, infection was the most common problem of the materials that were implanted in the human body. Due to the threat of infection, clinical application of biomaterials was not very successful. In the 1860s, Lister introduced aseptic techniques, which made some significant changes in the surgical implant procedures and paved ways to realize the potential of biomaterials. In 1860, catgut was one of the first naturally occurring materials used as a suture for wound closure. In 1880, Gluck used ivory clamps and, in 1989, Jassinowsky used silk on fine curved needles to repair vessels. In this period, Lane introduced metallic implants for orthopedics.

The twentieth century was a milestone in the field of biomaterials because most of the currently used biomaterials and surgical implants were developed in this period. The practice of using metals and alloys to repair or replace human body parts was well established at that time. The first metallic bone plate made of vanadium steel was introduced in 1912 by Sherman, but it was not very successful because of mechanical failure, corrosion, and poor biocompatibility. Since this initiation, many metallic implants have been introduced into the surgical field. Bone plates are surgical tools that are used to assist in the healing of broken and fractured bones. It is worth pointing out that bone plates are designed essentially to be very strong and absorb the large stress forces generated when the bone moves. On the other hand, corrosion is also a significant concern that typically leads to the disintegration of

TABLE 1.1

Evolution of Biomaterials for Human Use

Year/Period	Materials	Applications/ Inventions	Investigators/ Introducer
~2000 BC	Elephant's tusks, walrus teeth, linen	Artificial legs, teeth, ears, and sutures	Egyptians
~1800 BC	Wood	Artificial legs	Indians, Chinese
~600 BC	Cheek flesh	Nose reconstruction	S. Sushruta
~200 BC	Gold	Wires for fractures	Greeks
Seventeenth century	Iron and bronze	Suture	–
1759	Wooden peg and thread	Brachial artery	Hallowel
1829	Silver, gold, platinum	Pins and wires for fractures	H. S. Levert
1852	Lint-reinforced plaster	Bandage for fracture fixation	Mathijsen
1860s	–	Aseptic surgical techniques	J. Lister
1860	Catgut	Suture	J. Lister
1880	Ivory clamps	Tissue vessels	Gluck
1889	Silk	Tissue vessels	Jassinowsky
1893	Carbon steel	Bone plates and screws	W. A. Lane
1912	Vanadium steel	Bone plates	W. D. Sherman
1926	18-8sMo stainless steel	Bone plates	M. Z. Lange
1931	Stainless steel	First femoral neck fixation device	M. N. Smith-Petersen
1936	Co–Cr alloy	Bone plates	C .S. Venable and W.G. Stuck
1938	–	First hip replacement prosthesis	P. Wiles
1939	Tantalum	Metal prosthesis	Burch and Carney
1939	PMMA	Denture base	–
1940s	PMMA	Corneal defects	Dorzee and Franceschetti
1944	–	First hemodialyzer	W. J. Kolff
1946	PMMA	First biomechanically designed hip prosthesis/first plastic used in joints	J. Judet and R. Judet
1947	Ti and its alloys	Bone plates and hip joints	J. Cotton
1952	Cloth	First blood vessel replacement	Voorhees et al.
1953	–	Intraortic balloon pumping	A. Kantrowitz

(Continued)

TABLE 1.1

Evolution of Biomaterials for Human Use (*Continued*)

Year/Period	Materials	Applications/ Inventions	Investigators/ Introducer
1958	–	First successful direct heart simulation	S. Furma and G. Robinson
1960	–	First commercial heart valve	A. Starr and M. I. Edwards
1960	Hydrogels	Ophthalmology	O. Wichterle and D. Lim
1961	Silicone	Breast prosthesis	Cronin and Gerow
1962	–	Total hip replacement	J. Charnley
1963	Alumina	Orthopedic implants	L. Smith
1964	Alumina	Dental restoration	S. Sandhaus
1969	Carbon	Heart valve disc	J. C. Bokros
1970s	HA	Bone substitute and dental restoration	Aoki
1970s	Nitinol	Shape memory alloys for orthodontics	Beuhler
1970s	Glass–ceramics	Bioactive bone grafts	L. L. Hench
1980s	HA-coated Ti-6Al-4V	Total hip joints	–
1980s	–	Total artificial heart	W. J. Kolff
1980s	HA–PE composite	Hip and middle ear implants	W. Bonfield
1986	Zirconia	Hip ball	G. Lord
1991	Nitinol	Vascular stent	–
1997	TransCyte®	First FDA-approved synthetic skin	Advanced Tissue Sciences, USA
1997	Carticel®	First FDA-approved product for cartilage repair	Genzyme Tissue Repair, USA
2002	InFUSE™	First FDA-approved bone growth factor, rhBMP-2	Medtronic Sofamor Danek, USA
2006	AbioCor®	First FDA-approved totally implanted artificial heart	Abiomed, Inc., USA

Source: Adapted from Park, J. B., *Biomaterials science and engineering*, Plenum Press, New York, 1984; Spotnitz, H. M., *Handbook of biochemistry*, McGraw-Hill, New York, 1987; Park, J. B. and Bronzino, J. D., *Biomaterials principles and applications*, CRC Press, Boca Raton, FL, 2003; Friedman, D. W., Orland, P. J., and Greco, R. S., *Implantation biology*, CRC Press, Boca Raton, FL, 1994; Bhat, S. V., *Biomaterials*, Alpha Science International, Pangbourne, 2002; Greco, R. S., Prinz, F. B., and Smith, R. L. *Nanoscale technology in biological systems*, CRC Press, Boca Raton, FL, 2005; Murugan, R. and S. Ramakrishna, *Handbook of nanostructured biomaterials and their applications in Nanobiotechnology*, American Scientific Publishers, Stevenson Ranch, CA, 2005a; Murugan, R. and S. Ramakrishna, *Comp. Sci. Tech.*, 65, 2385, 2005b.

Revolutions in biomaterials may be as simple as introducing a new alloy.

implants and the release of toxic or harmful products into the living system, severely damaging healthy tissues. In this regard, in the 1920s, several stainless steel alloys were developed with superior strength and notable corrosion resistance. In 1926, 18-8 stainless steel (18% chromium, 8% nickel stainless steel) was introduced into surgical applications because its strength and corrosion resistance is better than vanadium steel. Later in 1926, 18-8sMo stainless steel, which contains a small percentage of molybdenum, was introduced with improved corrosion resistance; it is also known as 316 stainless steel. In 1936, cobalt chromium (Co-Cr) alloy was introduced into surgical applications; it is also known as Vitallium®. This alloy was widely used at the time because of its superior strength and improved corrosion resistance provided by the passivity associated with chromium content. In 1939, Burch and Carney introduced a new metal prosthesis called tantalum, which is noncorrosive and almost bioinert, but expensive. In 1947, Cotton introduced titanium (Ti) and its alloys into surgical applications with great success owing to its excellent biocompatibility, strength, corrosion resistance, and wear resistance. Nowadays, these metal alloys are widely used either as such or in combination with some polymers (e.g., Ti-6Al-4V/polyethylene).

The use of polymer as a biomaterial was fortuitous. It was noticed that World War II pilots who were injured by fragments of polymethyl methacrylate (PMMA) did not suffer any adverse chronic reactions from the presence of the plastic fragments. Since then, PMMA is used for various medical applications. It is worth mentioning that PMMA was the first synthetic polymer used as a denture base in 1939, followed by corneal replacement in the 1940s. In 1946, Judet introduced PMMA for joint replacements. Extracorporeal devices were also developed in this period. The first dialysis machine (rotary drum dialyzer) was introduced for humans by Kolff in 1944, followed by Schriber in 1960 with some modifications. In the 1950s, vascular prosthesis made of woven polyester was introduced. A major advancement was made in vascular prosthesis by Voorhees in 1952, in which a porous vascular graft made of Vinyon N (a copolymer of vinyl chloride and acrylonitrile) was used. In 1962, total hip replacement was carried out by Charnley; the femoral head and stem of the joints was made of stainless steel that was immobilized in bone by PMMA cement. Later, polyethylene was introduced in manufacturing acetabular components for hip joints. In the early 1960s, an artificial heart valve was made from flexible leaftlets, but failed to withstand the fatigue for long-term performance. An artificial heart valve is used to replace a damaged valve that is no longer functioning to regulate blood flowing in an appropriate direction. At the same time, silicon rubber suitable for use as an implant in breast reconstruction was developed, followed by polyurethane implants in the 1970s.

In the 1960s, ceramics were introduced into human systems as a class of biomaterials. In 1963, alumina (Al_2O_3) was the first clinically used ceramic material, owing to its excellent biocompatibility, hardness, strength to resist fatigue, and corrosion resistance. Alumina is mainly used for orthopedic and dental implants, in particular as a good coating material for femoral stems, a bone spacer in revision surgery (porous alumina), and tooth replacements. In the 1980s, zirconia (ZrO_2) was introduced into human systems for similar applications as alumina. Both these ceramics are known for their general chemical inertness, thus there is no chance of tissue–implant interaction, which leads to implant loosening within a short period. To improve the tissue bonding, a new concept was developed in the 1970s whereby the biomaterials interact chemically with living tissues upon implantation; they are called bioactive ceramics (e.g., hydroxyapatite (HA), $Ca_{10}(PO_4)_6(OH)_2$). HA is one of the most widely used ceramic materials in dentistry and orthopedics because of its structural and compositional similarity to minerals of calcified tissues.

Shape memory alloys were introduced in the medical field in the 1970s. They are typically metals that can be deformed and then returned to their original shape by heating. Nitinol (Ni-Ti alloy) is among the widely used shape memory alloys in manufacturing bone plates and orthodontic wires. In the 1990s, intravascular stent was developed using Nitinol alloys. In the 1980s, Bonfield introduced a bioactive composite based on HA and PE for use in middle ear implantation with a notable result. Later, research was focused on surface-modified biomaterials as a relatively new class of biomaterials with improved properties. In the 1980s, ceramic-coated metallic implants were developed for orthopedic applications. HA-coated Ti-6Al-4V is a typical example, which shows a good response to host tissues upon implantation. It was also reported that bonding strength and bone volume were found to increase for HA-coated metals compared to uncoated metals (Ducheyne et al. 1980). In the 1990s, much attention was focused on injectable bone cements (e.g., Norian SRS), since they can be used for the purpose of minimally invasive surgical procedures.

It is worth mentioning that although biomaterials have been used throughout history, the word "biomaterial" was coined some 50 years ago. Most of the biomaterials prior to the 1950s had a low probability of success because of the poor understanding of safety and biocompatibility issues, surgical techniques, storage and sterilization methods. It is also evident from the above facts that various experts in the fields of science, engineering, and medicine introduced most of the new processing methodologies, design principles, and surgical techniques only in the late 1940s. As a result, today we have some excellent biomaterials and surgical implants that improve the quality of life of many people each year. Although the twentieth century witnessed many breakthroughs in the development of biomaterials with different characteristics, to date, no single material can exactly match the composition, structure, and property of any particular human body part. In recent years, nanotechnology, biomimetics, and tissue engineering concepts are becoming new frontiers in the development of biomaterials at nanoscale (also called nanobiomaterials) as a new generation biomaterial. Nanobiomaterials possess superior properties over their microscale counterparts. For example, nanocrystalline HA promotes osteoblast cell adhesion, differentiation, and proliferation, osteointegration and deposition of calcium-containing minerals on its surface better than microcrystalline HA, which leads to the formation of new bone tissue

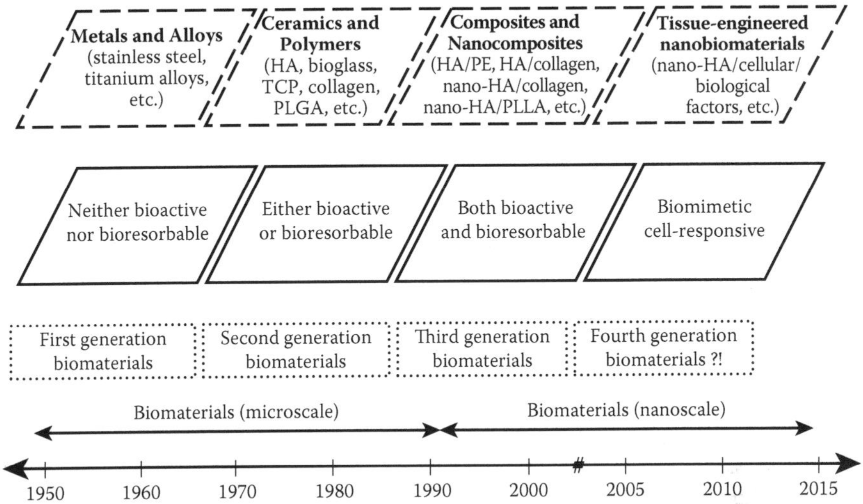

FIGURE 1.3
Evolution of biomaterials.

within a short period (Webster 2000). As per the literature survey, each year we witness an increasing number of published reports on nanobiomaterials intended for hard- and soft-tissue reconstructions. Some of the developments of biomaterials over the last few decades are illustrated in Figure 1.3. This trend clearly indicates the potentiality of nanobiomaterials to address the medical challenges that are facing day-to-day life. The twenty-first century is therefore an exciting period to realize biomaterials that mimic human tissues or organs. Based on these facts, this book addresses various aspects of nanobiomaterials with their processing methodologies, characterizations, and applications.

1.3 Impact of Biomaterials

Biomaterials greatly improve the quality and survival of life for an ever-increasing number of people each year. The range of biomaterial applications is vast and includes joint and limb replacements, dental implants, vascular grafts, corneal replacements, and skin augmentation. The biomaterials used for some of these applications are given in Figure 1.4.

The benefits of biomaterials compared to traditional grafts include availability, sterility, safety, reproducibility, cost-effectiveness, and reduced morbidity. Invention of novel biomaterials, with the help of advancements in biomedical science and technology, has dramatically changed the patient's lifestyle in the past few years. The invention of biomaterials significantly improves the health of the patients. In addition, it opens many industrial positions. Since biomaterials is a multidisciplinary field of applied research,

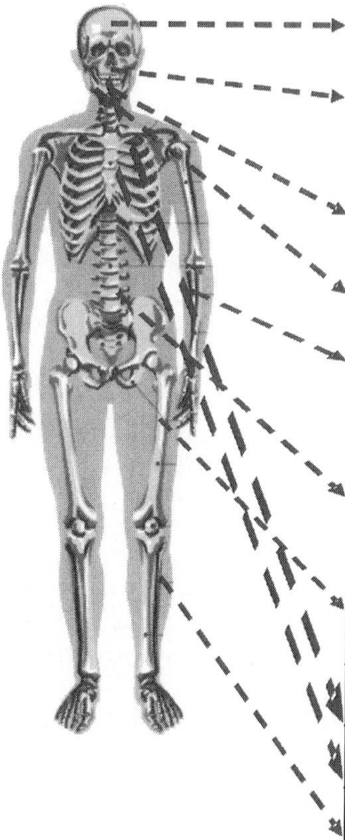

Clinical uses	Biomaterials
Cranial bone defects	Bioactive glass, alumina, HA, HA-collagen
Maxillofacial reconstruction	HA, bioactive glass, alumina, zirconia, HA-PE, bioglass-PE, PTFE-carbon
Alveolar ride augmentation	HA, TCP, bioglass, alumina, HA-PLA, HA-collagen, HA-PLGA
Periodontal defects	HA, TCP, bioactive glass, HA-PLA , HA-PLGA, HA-collagen
Bone void fillers	HA, TCP, biocoral, calcium sulfate, PMMA, HA-collagen, bioactive glass-ceramic composite
Spinal surgery	HA, bioactive glass, HA-collagen, PET-silicon, bioglass-PU
Orthopedic prostheses	Alumina, zirconia, stainless steel, Ti, Ti-6Al-4V, Co-Cr-Mo-Ni, A-W glass ceramics, HA-PE, HA-collagen, bioactive glass-coated biometals, HA-coated biometals, carbon fibers-PE
Dental implants	Ti, Ti-6Al-4V, stainless steel, PE, alumina, HA
Cardiovascular systems	PU, silicon rubber, carbon, PTFE, PE
Skin subtitutes	Collagen, collagen-glycosaminoglycan, collagen-silicon

FIGURE 1.4
Some of the uses of biomaterials in human systems. HA: Hydroxyapatite; TCP: Tricalcium phosphate; Ti: Titanium; PE: Polyethylene; PTFE: Polytetrafluoroethylene; PLA: Polylactic acid; PLGA: Poly(lactic-co-glycolic)acid; PMMA: Polymethylmethacrylate; PET: Polyethylene terephthalate; PU: Polyurethane.

it is industry oriented. Worldwide, the biomaterials market in 2000 is valued at close to US$30 billion, with a predicted growth rate of 12% per year (BHWE 2000). The US biomaterials market represents about US$13 billion and is growing at the staggering rate of 20% per year, followed by Europe and Japan. Orthopedic and dental implants represent approximately 55% of the total biomaterials market, which has occurred in response to the growing number of patients afflicted with traumatic or nontraumatic destructions. According to a recent market survey conducted by Medtech Insight (OBMR 2005), biomaterials sales, in particular bone grafts, was found to exceed US$980 million in 2001 in the USA itself and about US$1.16 billion in 2002, which is also expected to double by 2006. Table 1.2 lists the estimates of the number of medical devices containing biomaterials that are implanted

TABLE 1.2

Estimated Market for Biomaterials in the United States; Total Global Market Is Typically Two to Three Times the U.S. Market

Total U.S. health-care expenditure (2000)	US$1,400,000,000,000
Total U.S. health research development (2001)	US$82,000,000,000
Number of employees in the medical device industry (2003)	300,000
Registered U.S. medical device manufactures (2003)	13,000
Total U.S. medical device market (2002)	US$79,000,000,000
U.S. market for disposable medical supplies (2003)	US$48,600,000,000
U.S. market for biomaterials (2000)	US$9,000,000,000
Individual market device sales	
Diabetes management products (1999)	US$4,000,000,000
Cardiovascular devices (2002)	US$6,000,000,000
Orthopedic-musculoskeletal surgery (1998)	US$4,700,000,000
Wound care market (1998)	US$3,700,000,000
In vitro diagnosis (1995)	US$10,000,000,000
Numbers of devices (USA)	
Intraocular lenses (2003)	2,500,000
Contact lenses (2000)	30,000,000
Vascular grafts	300,000
Heart valves	100,000
Pacemakers	400,000
Blood bags	40,000,000
Breast prostheses	250,000
Catheters	200,000,000
Heart–lung (oxygenators)	300,000
Coronary stents	1,500,000
Renal dialysis (No. of patients, 2001)	320,000
Hip prostheses (2002)	250,000
Knee prostheses (2002)	250,000
Dental implants (2000)	910,000

Source: Reproduced from Ratner, B. D. et al., *Biomaterials science: An introduction to materials in medicine,* Elsevier Academic Press, San Diego, CA, 2004. With permission from Elsevier.

in humans each year and the size of the commercial market for biomaterials. These data, however, indicate the impact and growing need of biomaterials.

1.4 Characteristics of Biomaterials

Biomaterials have some specific characteristics that may be distinguished from other materials in that they possess a combination of properties,

TABLE 1.3
Basic Characteristics of Biomaterials

Characteristics	General Remarks
Biocompatible	Biologically compatible to host tissue, i.e., should not provoke any rejection, inflammation, or immune responses.
Vascular supportive	Should provide channels for blood supply for fast and healthy tissue regeneration.
Nontoxic	Should not evoke toxicity to tissues.
Nonimmunogenic	Should not evoke immunogenic response to tissues.
Noncorrosive	Should not corrode at physiological pH and at body temperature.
High surface area	To accommodate high density cells.
Surface modifiable	To functionalize chemical or biomolecular groups to improve tissue adhesion.
Adequate mechanical strength	To withstand *in vivo* stimuli.
Sterilizable	To avoid toxic contamination.

including physical, mechanical, chemical, and biological, which render them suitable for safe, effective, and reliable use within the physiological environment. The characteristics of biomaterials differ from one material to another, depending on their types and uses. For example, characteristics of metallic or ceramic materials are not similar to polymers; on the other hand, orthopedic uses of biomaterials need not have characteristics similar to that of skin substitutes. The biomaterials implanted within the human body must, however, satisfy a few basic characteristics (see Table 1.3). First of all, the biomaterial should be biocompatible. A perfect biomaterial should not only be biocompatible, but also have the ability to withstand corrosion in the biological environment without compromising mechanical consistency and should possess satisfactory physical and structural properties quite similar to native tissue or other biological systems being repaired. Furthermore, the biomaterial should be able to facilitate the several biochemical and biological processes needed for tissue growth in the bodily environment. Before implantation, the biomaterial should be stable during storage, and must be sterilizable without compromising any factors, in particular, mechanical. Although these characteristics are common prerequisites of a perfect biomaterial, it typically varies depending on the site of application. Furthermore, it should be noted that the success of a biomaterial depends on many other factors, such as implant design, surgical techniques, health conditions, and activities of the patient. Selection of a biomaterial is therefore of great importance and several factors are to be considered before implantation for its success. Table 1.4 summarizes various factors involved in the selection of material for biomedical applications (Seeram et al. 2001). These are some of the key points that must be keep in mind when developing and selecting the biomaterial for use in human systems.

TABLE 1.4

Various Factors of Importance in Material Selection for Biomedical Applications

Factors	Description		
First level material properties	Chemical/biological characteristics	Physical characteristics	Mechanical/structural characteristics
	Chemical composition (bulk and surface)	Density	Elastic modulus
			Poisson's ratio
			Yield strength
			Tensile strength
			Compressive strength
Second level material properties	Adhesion	Surface topology (texture and roughness)	Hardness
			Shear modulus
			Shear strength
			Flexural modulus
			Flexural strength
Specific functional requirements (based on application)	Biofunctionality (nonthrombogenic, cell adhesion, etc.)	Form (solid, porous, coating, film, fiber, mesh, powder)	Stiffness or rigidity
			Fracture toughness
	Bioinert (nontoxic, nonirritant, nonallergic, noncarcinogenic, etc.)	Geometry	Fatigue strength
		Coefficient of thermal expansion	Creep resistance
		Electrical conductivity	Friction and wear resistance
	Bioactive	Color, aesthetics	Adhesion strength
	Biostability (resistant to corrosion, hydrolysis, oxidation, etc.)	Refractive index	Impact strength
	Biogradation	Opacity or translucency	Proof stress
			Abrasion resistance
Processing and fabrication	Reproducibility, quality, sterilizability, packaging, secondary processability		
Characteristics of host: tissue, organ, species, age, sex, race, health condition, activity, systemic response			
Medical/surgical procedure, period of application/usage			
Cost			

Source: Reprinted from Ramakrishna, S. et al., *Comp. Sci. Tech.*, 61, 1189, 2001. With permission from Elsevier.

1.5 Classification of Biomaterials

Materials used in medicine are generally grouped into three classes. Class I materials are those that do not directly contact with the tissues. Elastic bandages, bedpans, and enema kits are a few notable examples. Class II materials are those that occasionally contact with the tissues. Kidney dialysis machines, heart–lung machines, and pregnancy test kits are a few notable examples. Most of the currently available medical devices are considered Class II type. Class III materials are those that have permanent contact with the tissues. Orthopedic, dental, and breast implants are a few notable examples. Nowadays, Class III materials are widely used in a variety of biomedical applications. They are commonly called biomaterials. As these biomaterials have direct contact with the tissues in many situations, they tend to elicit certain responses depending on their characteristics. Upon implantation, the biomaterials have direct contact with body fluids, blood, proteins, and cellular elements and do initiate biointegration with surrounding tissues (Suh 1998). A good biointegration, i.e., tissue–biomaterial interaction, is the key to success of any biomaterial because it determines the healing process of the defective system. According to the biointegration governed by tissue response, a biomaterial can be classified into nearly bioinert, bioactive, and bioresorbable. Nearly bioinert material refers to any material that has very minimal interaction with the host tissue. Stainless steel, titanium, alumina, partially stabilized zirconia, and ultrahigh molecular weight polyethylene are notable examples. Bioactive material refers to any material that has the ability to interact with the host tissue. HA and bioglass are notable examples. Bioresorbable material refers to any material that has the ability to provide a framework for new tissue to grow while being resorbed, leaving only the new tissue behind after complete resorption. Tricalcium phosphate and poly(lactic-co-glycolic) acid are notable examples of bioresorbable materials.

Biomaterials, on the other hand, can be broadly classified into metals, ceramics, polymers, and their composites with regard to materials aspects based on their structure and properties. Table 1.5 shows an overview of biomaterials with a broad classification. It is worth mentioning that, in most of the cases, metals and ceramics are used in hard-tissue applications; whilst polymers are used in soft-tissue applications because of their mechanical properties (see Table 1.6). A typical stress–strain comparison of various widely used biomaterials is also illustrated in Figure 1.5, to further appreciate their mechanical characteristics. These data help the clinicians to choose the right material for a particular application. Biomaterials can also be classified based on their applications, such as dental materials, orthopedic materials, skin substitute materials, and vascular graft materials. As each group consists of materials from metals, ceramics, polymers, or composites, a brief account of metallic biomaterials, ceramic biomaterials, polymeric biomaterials, and composite biomaterials are addressed in the subsequent sections. This type of classification is well accepted and practiced in academic and health-care practice.

TABLE 1.5

A Broad Classification of Biomaterials

Biomaterials	Advantages*	Disadvantages	Applications	Examples
Metals and alloys	Too strong, tough, ductile	Dense, may corrode, difficult to make	Bone plates, pins, screws, load-bearing bone implants, dental arch wire, and dental brackets	Titanium, stainless steel, Co-Cr and Ti-6Al-4V alloys
Ceramics	Bioinert	Brittle, low toughness, not resilient	Hip joints, bone defect filler, coatings on bio-implants, orbital implant, alveolar ridge augmentation, maxillofacial reconstruction, bone tissue engineering, and drug delivery	Alumina, zirconia
	Bioactive			HA, bioglass
	Bioresorbable			TCP
	High resistance to wear, corrosion resistance			
Polymers	Flexible, low density, resilient, surface modifiable, chemical functional groups	Low stiffness, may degrade	Tissue scaffolds, bone screws, pins, plates, hip joints, denture base, drug delivery, breast implant, sutures, skin augmentation, blood vessels, and heart valves	Collagen, silicone, PLGA, and PE

(Continued)

TABLE 1.5

A Broad Classification of Biomaterials (*Continued*)

Biomaterials	Advantages*	Disadvantages	Applications	Examples
Composites	Strong, design flexibility, enhanced mechanical reliability than monolithic	Properties might be varied with respect to fabrication methodology	Bone graft substitutes, hip joints, bone plates, dental restoration, maxillofacial, periodontal implants, spinal surgery, skin substitutes, middle ear implants, tissue scaffolds, and drug delivery	HA/collagen, HA/PLGA, and HA/PE
Nanobiomaterials (new generation biomaterials)	Large surface area to volume ratio, high surface reactivity, strong cell-implant interfacial-bonding, enhanced cellular adhesion, improved mechanical strength	Poor control over size uniformity	Major areas of orthopedics, dental restoration, tissue engineering, and drug delivery	Nano-HA, nano-alumina, collagen nanofibers, PLLA nanofibers

*Common characteristics of biomaterials like biocompatibility are not highlighted.

TABLE 1.6

Mechanical Properties of Biological Tissues and Biomaterials

Materials	Young's Modulus (GPa)	Tensile Strength (MPa)
Soft tissues		
Articular cartilage	10.5	27.5
Fibrocartilage	159.1	10.4
Ligament	303.0	29.5
Tendon	401.5	46.5
Skin	0.1–0.2	7.6
Hard tissues		
Cortical bone	7–30	50–150
Cancellous bone	1–14	7.4
Dentine	11–17	21–53
Enamel	84–131	10
Metals		
Ti	110	300–740
Stainless steel	190	500–950
Ti-6Al-4V alloy	120	860–1140
Co-Cr alloy	210	665–1200
Ceramics		
Alumina	380	310
Zirconia, partially stabilized	200	420
HA	30–100	50–190
Polymers		
Biodegradable		
Poly(L-lactic acid)	2.7	50
Poly(D,L-lactic acid)	1.9	29
Poly(caprolactone)	0.4	16
Nonbiodegradable		
Poly(ethylene)	0.88	35
Poly(urethane)	0.02	35
Poly(methylmethacrylate)	2.55	59
Poly(ethylene terephthalate)	2.85	61
Composites		
HA/PE (40/60)	4.29	20.67
Bioglass/PE (40/60)	2.54	10.15
Glass-ceramic/PE (40/60)	2.84	14.87

Source: Black, J. and Hastings, G. W., *Handbook of biomaterials properties*, Chapman and Hall, London, 1998; Thompson, I. and Hench, L. L., *Comprehensive composite materials*, with permission of Elsevier Science, Amsterdam, 2000; Murugan, R. and Ramakrishna, S., *Encyclopedia of nanoscience and nanotechnology*, American Scientific Publishers, Stevenson Ranch, CA, 2004; Murugan, R. and Ramakrishna, S., *Handbook of nanostructured biomaterials and their applications in nanobiotechnology*, American Scientific Publishers, Stevenson Ranch, CA, 2005a.

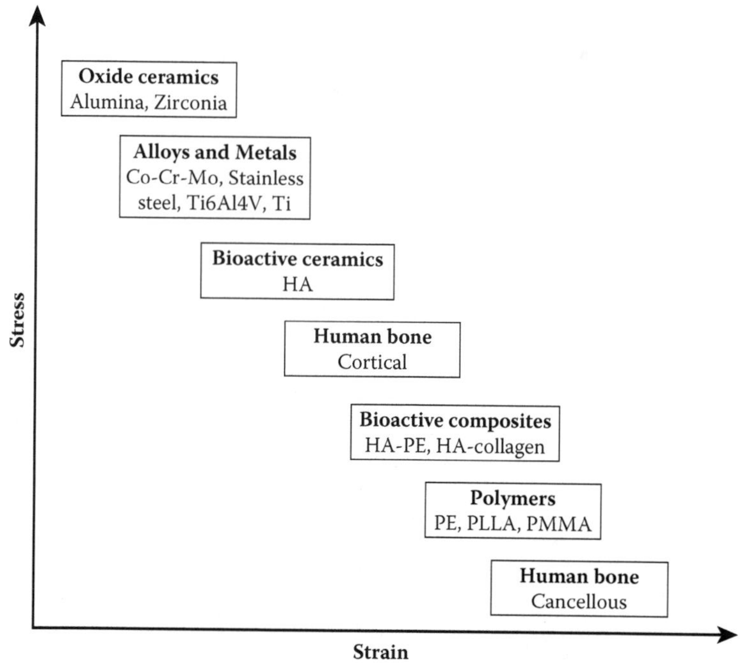

FIGURE 1.5
Mechanical consistency of various biomaterials. (From Murugan, R. and Ramakrishna, S., *Comp. Sci. Tech.*, 65, 2385, 2005b. With permission.)

1.5.1 Metallic Biomaterials

Since the early 1900s, metallic biomaterials have been widely used for replacing failed hard tissues. Stainless steel, Co-based alloys, Ti and its alloys are notable examples. Stainless steel was the first successfully used metallic implant in the surgical field. Among the above metallic implants, the elastic modulus of stainless steel and Co-Cr alloy is higher than that of natural bone, i.e., about 10 times greater, which gives somewhat complications of mechanical and structural incompatibility between implant and host tissue (Murugan and Ramakrishna 2005b). Nowadays, Ti and its alloys (e.g., Ti-6Al-4V) are often used, owing to their excellent biocompatibility, ductility, and corrosion resistance. The elastic modulus of these implants is found to be about five times greater than natural bone (Murugan 2005b). Although these metallic implants are successfully used for hard-tissue applications, there remains a mismatch of mechanical consistency with natural bone. According to Wolff's law, if a stiffer implant is placed into a hard tissue (e.g., bone), the bone will be subjected to reduced mechanical stress that gradually leads to bone resorption. This phenomenon is known as stress shielding. It has been recognized that matching the stiffness of the implant with that of the host tissue limits the stress-shielding effect. On the other hand, metallic biomaterials are bioinert, i.e., they do not have the ability to interact with the host tissue, either chemically or biologically. Owing to insufficient interfacial bonding between metallic implant and host tissue, there is limited osteointegration. To improve osteointegration, HA-coated metallic implants are introduced into orthopedics, which are extensively discussed in Chapter 6 with illustrated examples.

1.5.2 Ceramic Biomaterials

Since the 1960s, ceramics have been widely used as biomaterials, having a variety of functional properties suitable for biomedical applications. Ceramics are typically inorganic and nonmetallic materials, which are thermally and chemically stable. Ceramics, in general, have seen wide-scale use in hard-tissue reconstructions rather than soft tissue because of their high strength, wear resistance, and durability. Ceramics also possess many advantages, including biocompatibility, hemocompatibility, easy availability, shapeability, sterilizability, nontoxicity, and nonimmunogenic. The ceramics that are used for biomedical applications are commonly called bioceramics. Bioceramics, governed by tissue response, can be subcategorized into three types; (i) nearly bioinert (e.g., alumina and zirconia), (ii) bioactive (e.g., HA and bioglass), and (iii) bioresorbable (e.g., tricalcium phosphate (TCP), $Ca_3(PO_4)_2$). Alumina and zirconia are typically used in orthopedics and dental implants. They do not cause any noticeable response from host tissues upon implantation because they do not chemically or biologically react with them. HA was introduced into medical applications as a representative class of bioceramics, owing to its exceptional bioactivity (Aoki 1991). Bioactive refers to a material that, when placed within the human body, interacts with the surrounding tissues. Accordingly, HA elicits a strong interfacial interaction with host tissue; therefore, it is considered to provide osteointegrative stimuli, but it has low toughness and less bioresorption. TCP is a widely used bioresorbable material in hard-tissue replacements, which provides a framework for new bone tissue to grow while being resorbed, leaving only the new bone behind after complete resorption. The state of the art of those bioceramics is addressed in Chapter 7 with illustrated examples.

1.5.3 Polymeric Biomaterials

Polymers represent the largest class of biomaterials, which are made up of repeated small and simple chemical units called monomers. The term "polymer" was derived from the Greek words, polys meaning many and meros meaning units. Currently, a variety of polymers are available for manufacturing human health-care systems. They can be processed from natural source (e.g., collagen) or from synthetic organic process (e.g., polylactic acid). A polymer typically falls into two categories; biodegradable and nonbiodegradable. Collagen, gelatin, poly(lactic acid) (PLA), and poly(lactic-co-glycolic acid) (PLGA) are a few notable examples of biodegradable polymers. It is worth mentioning that degraded products from the biodegradable polymers must be nontoxic and should not elicit any foreign body reaction. Poly(ethylene) (PE), poly(ethylene terephthalate) (PET), and PMMA are notable examples of nonbiodegradable polymers. They are widely used in a wide range of biomedical applications, owing to their biocompatibility, design flexibility, surface modifiability, light weight, and ductile nature. Although polymers have many desirable characteristics, they tend to possess low mechanical strength (e.g., low stiffness) as compared to metals and ceramics; therefore, they are often used for soft-tissue reconstruction. Nowadays, polymers are widely used in tissue engineering applications as scaffolding material. In most circumstances, biodegradable polymers, either natural or synthetic, are considered a good choice for tissue engineering rather than nonbiodegradable polymers. All these aspects are dealt with in Chapter 8 with illustrated examples.

1.5.4 Composite Biomaterials

Composite biomaterials are a better choice than single-phase or monolithic biomaterials because they do not always provide all the properties necessary for a given application. The composite can be defined as a heterogeneous combination of two or more materials, differing in morphology or composition. Using the composite approach, it can be possible to manipulate the mechanical and other structural properties. For example, the HA-polymer composite possesses elastic modulus near to that of bone and is more mechanically reliable than its monolithic constituents. It is also well known that composites implanted into the human body tend to elicit a biochemical and/or biological response by the host tissue, depending on their surface characteristics. In this regard, composite biomaterials can be subclassified into three types: (i) nearly bioinert, (ii) bioactive, and (iii) bioresorbable. The interface of the bioinert composites is neither chemically nor biologically bonded to the host tissue. Alumina-coated biometals, carbon/carbon, and carbon/PEEK are a few notable examples. The bioactive composites are essentially designed to facilitate an interfacial bonding between implant and host tissues. HA/collagen, HA/PE, and HA/Ti-6Al-4V are a few notable examples. The bioresorbable composites are designed to degrade over time and are gradually replaced with a new tissue. TCP/collagen, TCP/PLA, and TCP/PCL are notable examples of bioresorbable composites. The state of the art of composite biomaterials is extensively discussed in Chapter 9 with illustrated examples.

1.6 Surface Modification of Biomaterials

As previously mentioned, a biomaterial that is to be clinically used must meet all the requirements for a given application. Importantly, it should possess excellent bulk and surface properties for better performance. Upon implantation, the biomaterial first comes into contact with ionic species of the body fluids, blood, plasma, cells, and tissues. The initial response of the living tissue to the biomaterial mainly depends on its surface characteristics. A good biointegration, i.e., tissue–biomaterial integration, is the ideal outcome expected of a perfect biomaterial. To facilitate this, the biomaterial should be highly biocompatible, should not elicit any adverse tissue response or foreign body reaction, and should not corrode in the body fluid. These properties are primarily influenced by the surface of the biomaterial rather than its bulk properties. Therefore, designing a biomaterial with superior surface properties, without altering its key bulk properties, favorable for biochemical and/or biological functions required for defect healing is of greater importance. The surface modification typically improves bonding strength, wear resistance, corrosion resistance, biocompatibility, hemocompatibility, protein adsorption, cell adhesion, and host–tissue interaction. Surface modification, therefore, seems to be an essential criterion in the development of a new generation of biomaterials.

Surface modification is a process that considerably changes the surface composition, structure, and morphology of the biomaterials. Surface modification of any biomaterial typically falls into two categories; (i) altering the atoms or molecules on the surface of biomaterials either chemically or physically and (ii) coating the surface of biomaterials with biocompatible and/or bioactive agents favorable for tissue integration. Multiple approaches exist to modify the surface properties of biomaterials. Figure 1.6 shows some of the available techniques.

Among them, plasma surface modification seems to be an effective and economical approach that offers excellent surface characteristics with the bulk properties remaining unchanged; therefore, it is gaining much recognition in the biomaterials field. This method can be applied to modify the surface properties of metals, ceramics, and polymers. Numerous researches have been conducted on the surface modification of biomaterials (e.g., metals) using plasma technique. A typical hip implant fabricated from such a surface-modified metal is shown in Figure 1.7. As previously mentioned,

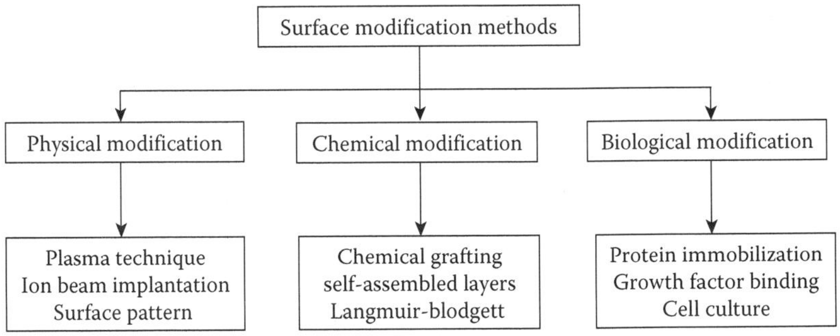

FIGURE 1.6
Various surface modification techniques for biomaterials.

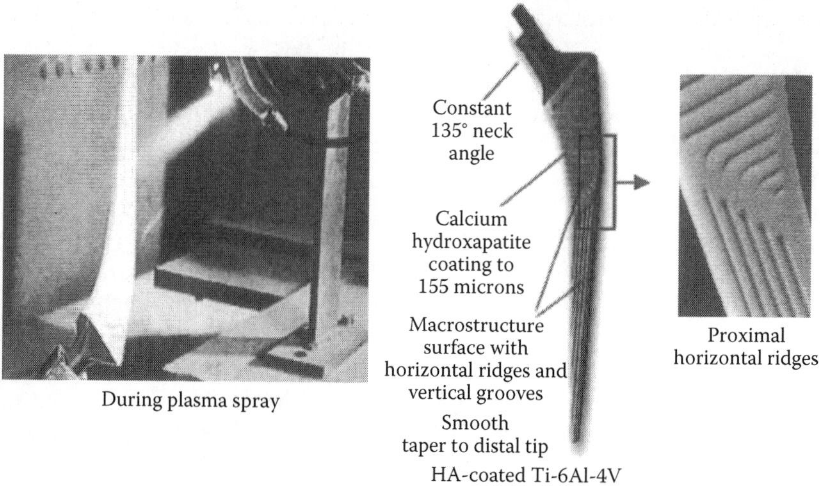

FIGURE 1.7
A typical surface-modified metallic implant; HA-coated Ti-6Al-4V. (Adapted from Johnson & Johnson Gateway © with courtesy: http://www.jnjgateway.com/home.jhtml?page=viewContent&contentId=edea000100002265&loc=USENG.)

plasma-sprayed HA onto Ti-6Al-4V implant allows a strong interfacial bonding between the implant and the host tissue, resulting in better fixation and improved long-term performance. It is worth pointing out that this type of coating process not only promotes tissue integration, but also reduces the risk of postoperative infection. The surface modification technique, therefore, typically improves the performance of biomaterials.

1.7 Recent Trends in Biomaterials

1.7.1 Nanobiomaterials: A New Generation Biomaterial

Nanobiomaterials generally refers to biomaterials with a basic structural unit less than 100 nm (nanostructured), crystalline solids with a grain size less than 100 nm (nanocrystals), ultrafine powders with an average particle size less than 100 nm (nanopowders), and extremely small fibers with a diameter less than 100 nm (nanofibers). A nanometer is a billionth of a meter (10^{-9} m). For easy understanding, the scale of some natural and manmade things is illustrated in Figure 1.11, with highlights of nanoscale items. It is worth mentioning that all hard and soft tissues of our body contain plenty of cells living in extracellular matrix (ECM) at the nanoscale hierarchical structure elegantly designed by Mother Nature. For example, bone tissue can be considered as an assembly of various levels of hierarchical structural units designed on many length scales, ranging from macro to nano, using essential organic and inorganic components, to facilitate multiple functions required for tissue formation. The nano- or micro-featured environment of the ECM is critical for the proper functions of cells and tissues. It is also recognized that the cells can attach and organize well around the nanobiomaterials than their microscale counterparts because of their typical surface properties. The fact is that nanobiomaterials have an increased number of atoms and crystal grains at their surfaces, and possess higher surface area to volume ratio compared to conventional microscale biomaterials, which makes the surface of the nanobiomaterials more reactive to cultured cells (during *in vitro*) and to host tissue (during *in vivo*), and thus greatly enhance the cell–matrix interactions, leading to faster tissue regeneration. In this regard, the rate of tissue regeneration will be greater for nanobiomaterials compared to conventional biomaterials. Nanobiomaterials are therefore perceived to be beneficial for biomedical applications, which are much discussed in the following chapters with respect to their material classifications.

1.7.2 Processing of Nanobiomaterials

1.7.2.1 Sol-Gel Processing

The sol-gel process is a remarkably versatile approach for preparing bioactive nanomaterials in different forms, such as powders, films, and fibers. The process begins with a nanometer-sized unit and undergoes reactions on the nanometer length scale, resulting in a nanophase material. In general, the sol-gel process, as the name implies, involves the evolution of inorganic networks through the formation of a colloidal suspension (sol) and gelation of the sol to form a network in a continuous liquid phase (gel). In this process, various simple molecular precursors, which contain all the elements to be present in the final product, are converted into nanometer-sized particles to form a colloidal suspension. The colloidal nanoparticles are then linked with one another in a three-dimensional fashion and form a liquid-filled rigid network (gel) with pores of submicrometer dimensions. This transformation to a gel can be initiated in several ways, but the most convenient and simple way is to change the pH of the reaction solution. The general processing steps involved in making sol-gel-derived nanomaterials include (i) mixing, (ii) gelation, (iii) aging, (iv) drying, (v) dehydration or chemical stabilization, and (vi) densification. This process allows tailoring the composition and structure of nanomaterials to a specific need by manipulating the processing variables. This process has many inherent advantages. These include simplicity, flexibility, low processing temperature, control of high-phase purity, greater homogeneity, controllable chemical composition, and can produce high quality and thin surface coatings. On the other hand, this process has its own limitations too; weak bonding, low wear resistance, high permeability, and control over porosity are notable examples.

The sol-gel process shows great potential for preparing various bioactive nanomaterials, e.g., HA. The sol-gel-derived HA powders have fine particle size, resulting in low densification temperature, and a good microstructure suitable for host tissue recognition upon implantation. Low temperature formation and fusion of the HA particles have been the contributions of the sol-gel process, in comparison to conventional methods. For instance, temperatures higher than 1000°C are usually required to sinter the fine HA crystals synthesized from wet chemical precipitation, whilst temperatures lower than the above are required to densify sol-gel-derived HA. Recently, Bigi et al. (2004) reported the synthesis of HA gels and nanocrystals through a sol-gel process and their structural and morphological properties were studied. In detail, the precursors, $Ca(NO_3)_2{\cdot}4H_2O$ and $(NH_4)_2HPO_4{\cdot}Ca(NO_3)_2{\cdot}4H_2O$, were dissolved in 50 mL of deionized water at 37°C and rapidly added to a 50-mL solution containing $(NH_4)_2HPO_4$ at 37°C under stirring. The concentrations of the reactants were varied in order to obtain a Ca/P molar ratio in solution of 1.00, 1.67, and 2.55. Before mixing, the pH value of the solutions was adjusted above 9 with NH_4OH. The syntheses in alcoholic medium were carried out following the same procedure as for aqueous medium, but dissolving $Ca(NO_3)_2{\cdot}4H_2O$, as well as $(NH_4)_2HPO_4$, in 25 mL of deionized water and 25 mL of ethanol. The powder products were obtained by filtering the solutions after 3 min of stirring at 37°C. The filtered products were repeatedly washed, and dried at 37°C overnight. Gels were obtained by drying the sols after 3 min of stirring at 37°C. A part of the sol was dried at 37°C, whereas a second part was oven-dried at 80°C overnight. The authors found that heat treatment at temperatures as low as 300°C is enough to obtain pure HA from the gels with a Ca/P molar ratio of 1.00 and 1.67. At variance, heat treatment of the gels with a Ca/P of 2.55 always produces secondary phases. The degree of crystallinity of HA increases with the Ca/P molar ratio of the sols, and it is slightly affected by the presence of ethanol in the precipitation medium. Filtering of the sols provides powders constituted of nanocrystalline HA that exhibit a degree of crystallinity, crystal morphology, and thermal stability closely related to the sols composition. The HA powders obtained by filtering the sols prepared in aqueous medium are constituted of ultrafine crystals, which are about 20–40 nm long, and less than 10 nm wide, but the crystal size varies with respect to the Ca/P molar ratios of the sol. The ability to produce nanophase HA combined with the low processing temperature, renders the sol-gel process very favorable for the preparation of nanocrystalline HA powders as well as for generating high purity HA surface coatings on metal substrates for various biomedical applications.

1.7.2.2 Biomimetic Processing

Biomimetic processing is one of the recent developments in the field of biomaterials. A novel way of fabricating biomaterials using design strategies found in nature has recently received much attention and is perceived to be beneficial over conventional methods. The term "biomimetic" can be defined as a microstructural processing technique that either mimics or inspires the biological mechanism, in part or whole. It was derived from the Greek words, bios meaning life and mimesis meaning imitation. It is also called several distinct names, such as bionics, biognosis, bioinspired, and biomimicry. The biomimetic process typically involves a bottom-up approach, which begins by designing and synthesizing molecules that have the ability to self-assemble or self-organize spontaneously into a higher order of micro- or macro-scale structure. Biomineralization is a good example of the biomimetic processing of biomaterials. HA and collagen are typically involved in this process. A key step involved in the biomineralization process is to achieve a controlled nucleation and crystal growth of the apatite phase onto the collagen matrix, as illustrated in Figure 1.8. The unique characteristic of this biomineralized system is the spatial orientation between HA and collagen macromolecules, which seems to be the source of mechanical strength. This process

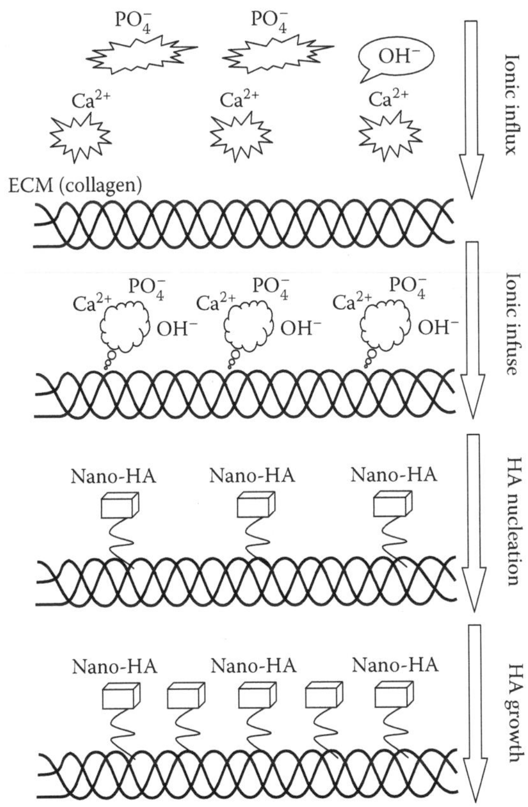

FIGURE 1.8
A schematic of biomineralization; partly mimics a biological self-assembly of HA onto collagen. (Reprinted from Murugan, R. and Ramakrishna, S., *Comp. Sci. Tech.*, 65, 2385, 2005b. With permission from Elsevier.)

partly mimics the biological phenomenon, and the biomineralized system facilitates enhanced osteoconductivity than a pure HA and a pure collagen, which implies the impact of biomimetic processing. The biomimetic process generates highly ordered molecular materials with hybrid composition and complex texture through hierarchical self-assembly. So, it is believed that developing biomaterials with certain features of biological tissues either compositionally or structurally using the biomimetic approach may replicate the process as nature does, which are much discussed in Chapter 9.

1.7.2.3 Tissue Engineering Approach

Tissue engineering is fast becoming a new research frontier in the field of biomaterials that applies the principles of engineering and biosciences for the development of novel biological substitutes capable of restoring, maintaining, or improving a tissue function that fails to regenerate or heal spontaneously with minimal surgical intervention. Although biomaterials without living cells, as previously mentioned, are considered good systems for tissue regeneration, some of them fail to stimulate several complex biological functions required for tissue ingrowth. Since only living cells ultimately generate a new tissue with all the essential features, a unique approach is to develop biomaterials that are cell-responsive upon implantation through a tissue engineering approach.

The prime concept of tissue engineering is to isolate a small biopsy of specific cells from a patient, to allow them to culture on scaffold, to transplant the cell-engineered scaffold into the defective site of the patient's body that needs tissue regeneration, and to guide or direct new tissue formation into the scaffold. In this regard, three key factors have to be considered for the success of tissue engineering; cells, scaffold, and cell–matrix (scaffold) interaction and subsequent function to organize and assemble into a functional tissue (see Figure 1.9). The scaffold, also called an artificial ECM, plays a pivotal role

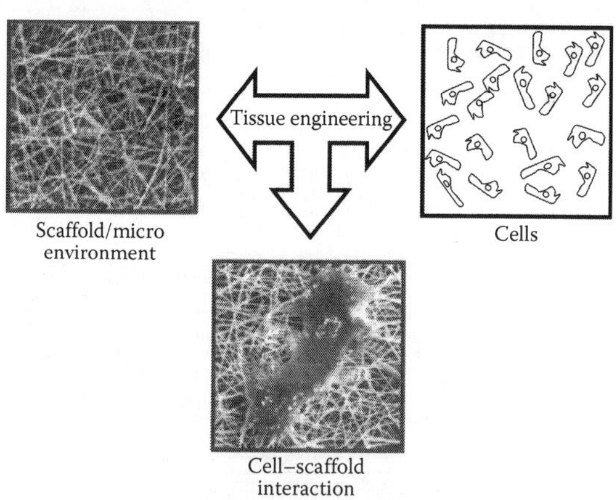

FIGURE 1.9
Factors contributing to the success of tissue engineering.

in accommodating the cells. These cells then undergo proliferation, migration, and differentiation, leading to the formation of a specific tissue. Direct delivery of cell suspension has been carried out in some cases without using a scaffold (Murugan and Ramakrishna 2006b), but this process encountered difficulties in having poor control over the localization of transplanted cells. It is worth mentioning that most of the cells are anchorage-dependent and will not survive if delivered without a suitable scaffold. Designing scaffold suitable for cell/tissue functions is therefore of great importance, and is extensively discussed in Chapter 8 and 10.

The key applications of tissue engineering in human systems are orthopedic, skin, neural, and vascular. A design strategy of tissue-engineered biomaterial suitable for orthopedic applications is schematically illustrated in Figure 1.10. A tissue engineering approach for the development of bone grafts to treat bone defects must involve the use of osteoconductive scaffold with osteogenic cells and osteoinductive growth factors. As HA is an osteoconductive agent, it can be used as a scaffold matrix for bone tissue engineering. However, it does not possess osteoinduction ability and its biodegradation is also relatively slow. To circumvent these drawbacks, biodegradable polymers (e.g., collagen) can be employed to make a composite in conjunction with HA and osteogenic cells. This tissue-engineered HA/collagen system

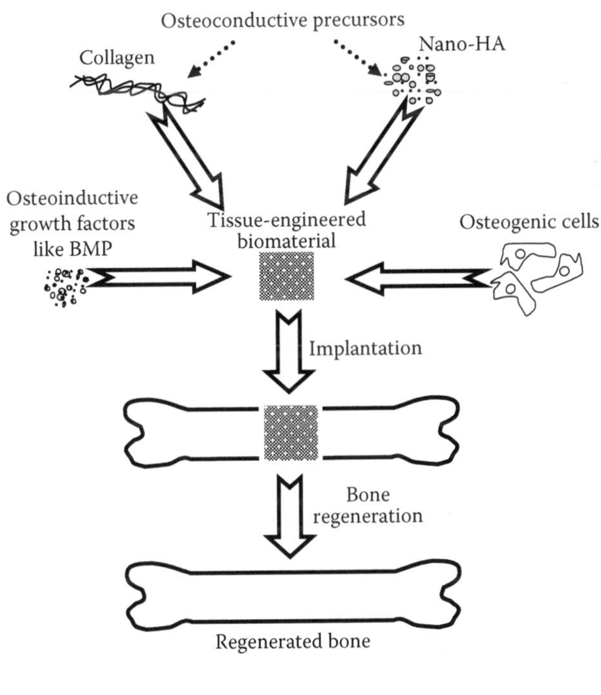

FIGURE 1.10
A design strategy of tissue-engineered biomaterial. (Reprinted from Murugan, R. and Ramakrishna, S., *Comp. Sci. Tech.*, 65, 2385, 2005b. With permission from Elsevier.)

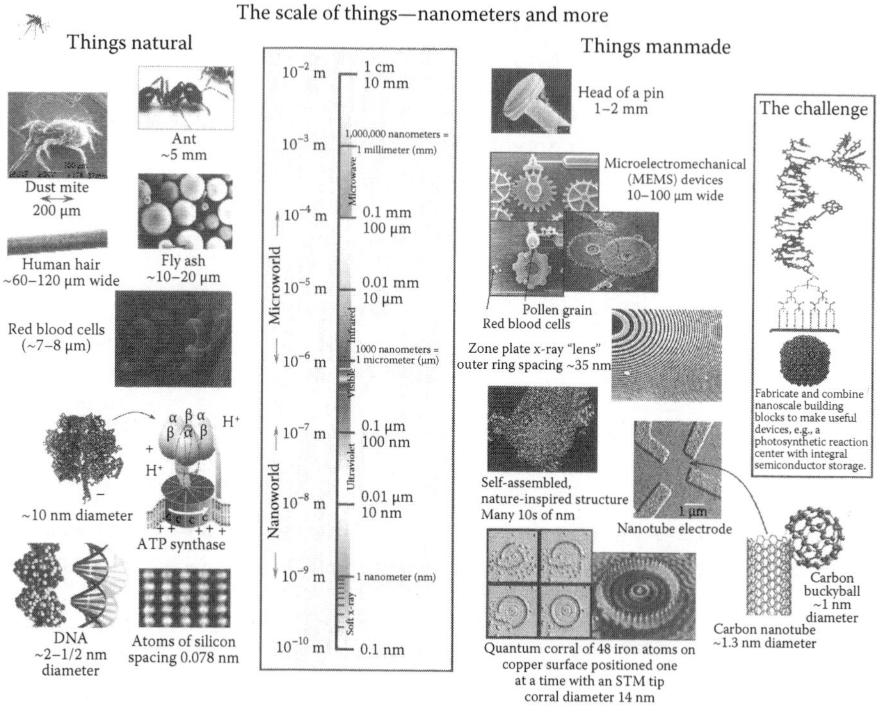

FIGURE 1.11
The scale of various natural and manmade things. (Courtesy of Dehmer, P. M., Office of Basic Energy Sciences, U.S. Department of Energy, USA.)

seems to be a very promising system for bone reconstructive or regenerative surgery. The current advances and impacts of tissue-engineered biomaterials intended for soft- and hard-tissue reconstructions are addressed in Chapter 10 with illustrated examples.

1.8 Summary

This chapter provides an overview of biomaterials, from historical perspectives to recent advances. There is a growing need for biomaterials, owing to the several limitations of traditional tissue or organ transplantation. A variety of biomaterials, including metals, ceramics, polymers, and their composites, are widely used for various biomedical applications and have played a major role in reducing the morbidity and mortality of disease and injury. Prior to the 1950s, most of the biomaterials had a low probability of success because of the poor understanding of safety and biocompatibility issues, surgical techniques, storage, and sterilization methods. Today, we have a few excellent biomaterial systems; technological advancements have allowed not only for the development of new biomaterials, but also for new techniques in the manufacturing of existing materials. Currently, the emerging themes of nanotechnology, biomimetics, and tissue engineering are promising to revolutionize the biomaterials field, which certainly plays a significant role in the development of a future generation of biomaterials, the so-called nanobiomaterials. The introduction of nanotechnology into biomaterials science has created ample opportunity for enhancing material properties and improving biological interactions. For the continuous success of biomaterials and nanobiomaterials, several experts in the fields of materials science and engineering, nanotechnology, physical sciences, biological sciences, and medicine need to work together.

Glossary

Allograft: Tissue or organ transplanted from one individual to another of the same species.

Alloplast graft: Any synthetic material substituted to repair or replace defective parts of the body.

Artificial organ: A medical device or implant intended to replace the body organs.

Autograft: Tissue or organ transplanted within the same body.

Bioactivity: Ability of the implant to play a vital role in the metabolic processes of the living body.

Bioceramics: The inorganic and nonmetallic materials that are compatible with biological tissues.

Biocompatibility: Ability of the implant to perform with an appropriate host response in a specific application.

Biodegradability: Susceptibility of implant to be decomposed by a living organism.

Bioinert: No host response to the material.

Biomaterial: Any synthetic material that is biocompatible with the tissues and the body upon implantation. It can be metal, ceramic, polymer, and a composite of each.

Biomimetics: The development of synthetic systems based on information gained from biological systems (e.g., biomineralization).

Biopsy: Removal of a small portion of tissue, usually for the purpose of making a diagnosis.

Bone: A rigid, yet dynamic connective tissue consisting of calcium phosphate-based minerals embedded with collagen fibers in conjunction with osteogenic cellular elements.

Cell: Fundamental, structural, and functional unit of all living beings that is composed of an outer membrane enclosing protoplasm and nucleus.
Cellular biomaterials: The biomaterials that are intact living cells.
Collagen: A fibrous structural protein that functions to hold tissues together.
Composite: A heterogeneous combination of two or more materials.
Compressive modulus: Ratio of compressive stress to compressive strain below the proportional limit.
Compressive strength: Maximum load sustained by a test specimen in a compressive test divided by the original area of the specimen.
Corrosion: A chemical or electrochemical degradation of metals due to surrounding environmental factors.
Fracture: Broken bones.
Graft: A transplant.
Growth factors: A heterogeneous group of substances capable of enhancing tissue growth.
Hard tissue: The general term for calcified structures of the body (e.g., bone and tooth).
Hydroxyapatite: A calcium phosphate-based material with chemical composition $Ca_{10}(PO_4)_6(OH)_2$, rich in bone minerals.
Immunogenic: Capable of stimulating an immune response.
Implant: Any medical device or prosthesis inserted or grafted in the human body.
Implantation: A surgical procedure by which a medical device or prosthesis is placed in the human body, either temporarily or permanently.
***In vitro*:** A biological study performed in the laboratory. In other words, outside the living body.
***In vivo*:** A biological study performed inside the living body.
Metabolism: A general term used to designate all biochemical changes that occur to substances within the body either by anabolism or catabolism.
Micro: A unit prefix meaning one millionth (1/1,000,000).
Modulus: One of several measures of strain vs. applied stress (e.g., Young's modulus).
Monolithic: Made from a single material.
Nano: A unit prefix meaning one billionth (1/1,000,000,000).
Nanobiomaterials: Biomaterials composed of particles or grains having nanometric tolerances; a nanometer is equal to 10^{-9} m.
Nontrauma: Any injury or wound caused by disease.
Organ: A differentiated part of an organism adapted for a definite function.
Orthopedics: The medical specialty concerned with skeletal system.
Osteoconduction: An action associated with ingrowth of capillaries and migration of bone-forming cells from the host into 3D matrix.
Osteogenesis: A process of development of the bone tissue.

Osteoinduction: A biochemical process of promoting or accelerating a new bone.
Pathogen: Any organism that is capable of producing disease.
Polymer: Long-chain high molecular weight material consisting of repeated monomer units.
Porosity: A ratio of void volume to total volume expressed in terms of percentage.
Prosthesis: A medical device that is capable of replacing organs or tissues.
Protein: A large biomolecule composed of one or more chains of amino acids in a specific sequence.
Resorption: Dissolution of a substance.
Scaffold: A temporary structural construct or matrix used to support cells for accommodation during tissue fabrication.
Strain: The change in size or shape of a body as a result of applied force.
Stress: An internal force that resists a load, expressed in force per unit area.
Stress-shield effect: Prolonged reduction of stress on a bone, which may weaken and make it prone to fracture. This process can be reversed if the natural state of stress can be restored to its original state.
Surface area: The total area of exposed surface of an object.
Tissue: A collection of similar cells and their surrounding intercellular substances.
Tissue engineering: Development of human tissues or organs in the laboratory from cells removed from the patient or other sources.
Toughness: The amount of energy absorbed by a material before breakage.
Transplantation: Surgical transfer of tissue or organ from one place to another.
Trauma: Any injury or wound caused by an external force.
Vascular: A medical term pertaining to blood vessel.
Xenograft: Tissue or organ transplanted from one species onto a different species.

EXERCISES

1.1 What are the traditional methods for the treatment of tissue or organ defects?
1.2 Define and explain autografting, allografting, and xenografting.
1.3 What is a biomaterial and what are its characteristics?
1.4 Classify various types of biomaterials with suitable examples.
1.5 Differentiate between monolithic and composite biomaterials.
1.6 What are the advantages of composite biomaterials?
1.7 What is the need of surface modification of biomaterials?
1.8 What are the techniques applied for surface modification?
1.9 What is the biomimetic process? Give an example.
1.10 Explain the concept of tissue engineering and describe its key applications in human systems.
1.11 What is a nanobiomaterial? Give some examples.
1.12 What are the impacts of nanobiomaterials over conventional biomaterials?

References

Aoki, H. 1991. *Science and medical applications of hydroxyapatite*. Tokyo: Takayama Press.

Bhat, S. V. 2002. *Biomaterials*. Pangbourne: Alpha Science International.

BHWE. 2000. Biomaterials for health, wealth and employment. http://europa.eu.int/comm/research/growth/gcc/projects/in-action-biomat03.html.

Bigi, A., E. Boanini, and K. Rubini. 2004. Hydroxyapatite gels and nanocrystals prepared through a sol–gel process. *J. Solid State Chem.* 177:3092.

Black, J., ed. 1992. *Biological performance of materials: Fundamentals of biocompatibility*. 2nd ed. New York: Marcel Dekker.

Black, J. and G. W. Hastings. 1998. *Handbook of biomaterials properties*. London: Chapman & Hall.

Chu, P. K. et al. 2002. Plasma surface modification of biomaterials. *Mater. Sci. Eng.* R36:143.

Cowin, S. C., W. C. V. Buskirt, and R. B. Ashman. 1987. Properties of bone. In *Handbook of bioengineering*, ed. R. Skalak and S. Chien, 2.1–2.27. New York: McGraw-Hill.

Dehmer, P. M., Office of Basic Energy Sciences, Office of Science, U.S. Department of Energy. http://www.sc.doe.gov/production/bes/scale_of_things.html.

Ducheyne, P. et al. 1980. Effect of hydroxyapatite impregnation on skeleton bonding of porous coated implants. *J. Biomed. Mater. Res.* 14:225.

Friedman, D. W., P. J. Orland, and R. S. Greco. 1994. Biomaterials: An historical perspective. In *Implantation biology*, ed. R. S. Greco, 1–12. Boca Raton, FL: CRC Press.

Goh, J. C. H. 2000. New challenges beyond computer-aided prosthetic socket design and manufacturing. In *Proc. 10th International Conference on Biomedical Engineering*, ed. J. C. H. Goh, 61. Singapore: National University of Singapore.

Greco, R. S., F. B. Prinz, and R. L. Smith. 2005. *Nanoscale technology in biological systems*. Boca Raton, FL: CRC Press.

Murugan, R., and S. Ramakrishna. 2004. Nanostructured biomaterials. In *Encyclopedia of nanoscience and nanotechnology*, ed. H. S. Nalwa, 595. Stevenson Ranch, CA: American Scientific Publishers.

———. 2005a. Bioactive nanomaterials in bone grafting and tissue engineering. In *Handbook of nanostructured biomaterials and their applications in nanobiotechnology*, ed. H. S. Nalwa, 141. Stevenson Ranch, CA: American Scientific Publishers.

———. 2005b. Development of nanocomposites for bone grafting. *Comp. Sci. Tech.* 65:2385.

———. 2006a. Nanoengineered biomimetic bone-building blocks. In *Handbook of molecular building blocks for nanotechnology*, ed. G. A. Mansoori, T. F. George, L. Assoufid, and G. Zhang, 301. Germany: Springer-Verlag.

———. 2006b. Nano-featured scaffolds for tissue engineering: Spinning methodologies. *Tissue Eng.* 12:435.

OBMR. 2005. Orthopedic Biomaterials market review. http://www.azom.com/details.asp?ArticleID=1361.

Park, J. B. 1984. *Biomaterials science and engineering*. New York: Plenum Press.

Park, J. B. and J. D. Bronzino. 2003. *Biomaterials principles and applications*. Boca Raton, FL: CRC Press.

Ramakrishna, S. et al. 2001. Biomedical applications of polymer-composite materials: A review. *Comp. Sci. Tech.* 61:1189.

Ratner, B. D. et al. 2004. *Biomaterials science: An introduction to materials in medicine.* San Diego, CA: Elsevier Academic Press.

Silver, F. H. 1994. *Biomaterials, medical devices and tissue engineering.* London: Chapman & Hall.

Spotnitz, H. M. 1987. Circulatory assist devices. In *Handbook of biochemistry*, ed. R. Skalak and S. Chein, 38.1–38.18. New York: McGraw-Hill.

Suh, H. 1998. Recent advances in biomaterials. *Yonsei Med. J.* 39:87.

Thompson, I. and L. L. Hench. 2000. Medical applications of composites. In *Comprehensive composite materials*, ed. A. Kelly and C. Zweben, 727. Amsterdam: Elsevier Science.

Webster, T. J., R. W. Siegel, and R. Bizios. 2000. Enhanced functions of osteoblasts on nanophase ceramics. *Biomaterials* 21:1803.

Wesolowski, S. A. and C. Dennis. 1963. *Fundamentals of vascular grafting.* New York: McGraw-Hill.

Williams, D. F. ed. 1987. Definitions in biomaterials. In *Proceedings of a Consensus Conference of the European Society for Biomaterials.* Amsterdam: Elsevier.

Williams, D. F. and J. Cunninghan. 1979. *Materials in clinical dentistry.* Oxford: Oxford University Press.

2

Basics of Human Biology

2.1 Introduction

Biomaterials intended for human applications undergo cellular/tissue responses upon implantation. Therefore, the person dealing with biomaterials must be at least familiar with the basics of the structure and function of the human body and fundamental aspects of biological responses to biomaterials. This chapter provides the *in vitro* and *in vivo* assessment of tissue responses to biomaterials to determine the intended performance characteristics and biocompatibility considerations. Biocompatibility is generally defined as the ability of biomaterial to perform with an appropriate host response in a specific application, and biocompatibility assessment is a measure of the magnitude and duration of the adverse changes in homeostatic mechanisms that determine the host response. Thus, the goal of biological response evaluation is to predict the quality of biomaterial, whether it has the potential to harm the patient or not, by evaluating conditions that simulate clinical use. To understand the key aspects of biological responses to any biomaterial in the body, it is necessary to acquire sufficient knowledge of the basic components of the human body, how they are put together in a systematic way, and how they function in the bodily environment. In the following sections, we focus our attention on the essentials of anatomy and physiology of the human body.

2.2 Structure and Function of the Human Body

The study that describes the structure of the human body, which makes up the human organism, is called anatomy, whereas the study that describes how the body functions and survives in continuously changing environments is called physiology. The human body is basically a well-organized single structure with several complex levels. They are, from smallest to largest, chemical, cellular, tissue, organ, system, and organismal. All these levels are associated with building such an amazing human body. The following sections deal with different levels of structural organization of the body.

2.3 Chemical Level

At the chemical level, the human body has many chemical substances composed of countless atoms (e.g., oxygen) and molecules (e.g., DNA), which are essential for its structure, function, and maintenance. An atom consists of a nucleus and an electron. The nucleus contains protons (p^+) and neutrons (n^0). The electron has a negative charge (e^-) that moves around the nucleus in a well-defined orbit called the electron shell. The number of electrons in an atom is equal to the number of protons. The combined total number of protons and neutrons in an atom is called the mass number, while the total number of protons is called the atomic number. The atomic number distinguishes the atoms of one chemical element from another element.

The human body has 26 different types of elements, which are essential for maintaining life, among which four elements—oxygen (O) (65.0%), carbon (C) (18.5%), hydrogen (H) (9.5%), and nitrogen (N) (3%)—are the most abundant, making up 96% of body weight. Proteins, lipids, sugars, and DNA are typical examples that comprise these four elements. The structure (at chemical level) of adenine and guanine (bases found in the DNA) is shown in Figure 2.1. In addition, body fluid, water (H_2O), and carbon dioxide (CO_2) are also composed of these elements.

Elements such as calcium (Ca) (1.5%), phosphorous (P) (1.0%), potassium (K) (0.4%), sulfur (S) (0.3%), sodium (Na) (0.2%), chloride (Cl) (0.2%), magnesium (Mg) (0.1%), and iron (Fe) (0.1%) make up 3.8% of body weight. Although these elements are present in low quantities in the body, they are very important for the maintenance of homeostasis function, a natural regulatory mechanism of the organism. Apart from this, Ca is a major element of hard tissues such as bones and teeth, Fe is a major element necessary for oxygen transport by red blood cells, S is a major element present in most proteins that maintains the strength of various tissues by forming sulfur "tie-bars" (also called sulfhydryl bonds) between connective tissue proteins and also helps maintain the pliancy of tissues and cell membranes, and K is a major element that keeps the heart beat at a normal rhythm. The remaining 14 elements—aluminum (Al), boron (Br), chromium (Cr), cobalt (Co), copper (Cu), fluorine (F), manganese (Mn), iodine (I), molybdenum (Mo), selenium (Se), silicon (Si), tin (Sn), vanadium (V), and zinc (Zn)—make up 0.2% of body weight. These elements are often called trace elements and they are essential for homeostasis, hormone secretion, and enzyme activity.

A molecule is a substance that consists of two or more atoms combined by means of chemical bonding. The force that holds or binds the atoms of

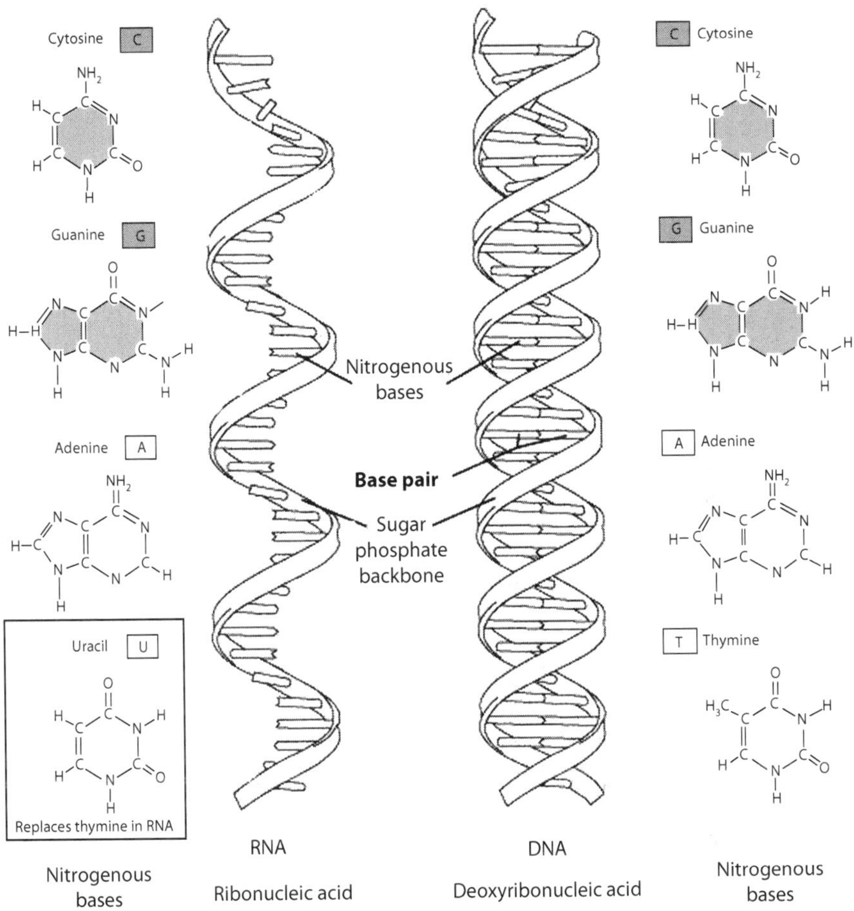

FIGURE 2.1
Structure of adenine and guanine (bases found in the DNA) at chemical level. (Obtained with courtesy from: http://en.wikivisual.com/index.php/Ribonucleic_acid.)

molecules and compounds together is called a chemical bond. Three types of chemical bonds occur in the chemical reactions in the bodily environment, namely, covalent, ionic, and hydrogen bonds. The bond in which one or more pairs of electrons are shared by two atoms is called a covalent bond. The bond in which one or more electrons from one atom are removed and attached to another atom, resulting in positive and negative ions that attract each other, is called an ionic bond. A hydrogen bond is a force of attraction between a hydrogen atom in one molecule and a small atom of high electronegativity in another molecule, meaning that it is an intermolecular force, not an intramolecular force as in the ionic and covalent bonds; therefore, it is considered as weak bonding. The human body contains several chemical molecules and compounds that can be broadly grouped into two types, namely, inorganic and organic compounds. The compound that lacks the carbon element is called an inorganic compound (e.g., water, calcium phosphates), whereas the compound with the carbon element is called an organic compound (e.g., proteins, carbohydrates).

2.4 Cellular Level

At the cellular level, the next level of structural organization, molecules combine together to form the basic functional structures of the body, called cells. It is the smallest unit capable of independent existence that can renew itself, divide, and multiply. The human body consists of billions of different types of cells (e.g., blood, nerve, and muscle cells), each responsible for carrying out specific functions. Although cells may vary greatly in size, appearance, and function, their essential features are almost similar. A schematic representation of a generalized cell structure is shown in Figure 2.2. The cells in the human body essentially consist of three components, namely, (i) the nucleus, (ii) the cytoplasm, and (iii) the cell membrane.

2.4.1 Nucleus

The nucleus, the most important part of a cell, essentially controls the cell function. It consists of nucleoli, chromosomes, and a porous nuclear membrane,

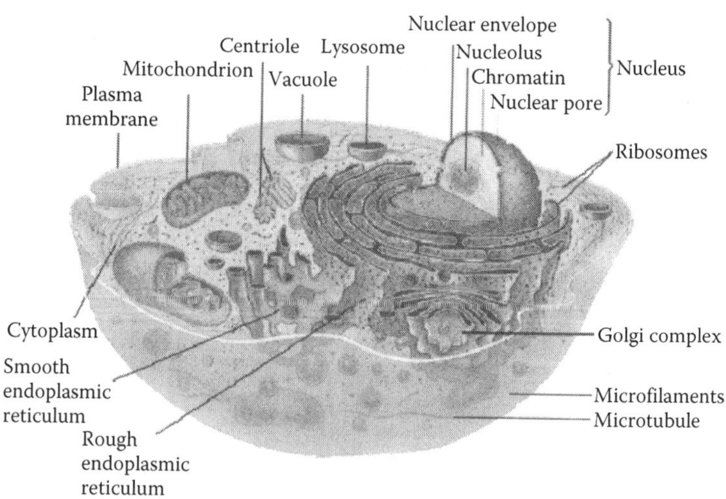

FIGURE 2.2
Schematic representation of a generalized cell structure. (From http://www.people.eku.edu/ritchisong/301notes1.htm.)

in a spherical or oval shape as a whole. Cells generally have a single nucleus, but there are some exceptional cases. For example, mature red blood cells have no nucleus and, by contrast, skeletal muscle cells have several nucleuses. The nucleus is enclosed by a porous double layer called nuclear membrane that separates the nucleus from the cytoplasm. The nucleus contains two nucleic acids, namely, deoxyribonucleic acid (DNA) and ribonucleic acid (RNA). Both the nucleic acids consist of nitrogenous bases, five carbon sugars, and phosphate groups. DNA is a unique, helical molecule that contains chains of paired nucleotides that run in opposite directions, resulting in a double helix. Each nucleotide contains either a pyrimidine base, thymine (T) or cytosine (C), with a single ring structure, or a purine base, adenine (A) or guanine (G), with a double ring. In the double helix of DNA, thymine always pairs with adenine (T-A) and cytosine always pairs with guanine (C-G). The main function of DNA is to provide instructions to synthesize proteins to perform specific functions. RNA is also a nucleic acid similar to DNA expect that it consists of a single helical strand, contains ribose instead of deoxyribose, and has uracil (U) instead of thymine. The main function of RNA is to carry out the instructions encoded in the DNA. To do this, the RNA attaches to a ribosome, where the encoded information is transformed into a specific sequence of amino acids to synthesize a new protein. Thus, the nucleic acids play a key role in synthesizing proteins in the cells.

2.4.2 Cytoplasm

Cytoplasm, a jelly-like substance between the cell membrane and the nucleus, consists of most of the cellular elements, including cytosol and organelles. Cytosol (also called intracellular fluid) is the ionic fluid portion of the cytoplasm that surrounds the organelles and accounts for about 55% of the total cell volume, in which water occupies about 75–90% and various ions (Na^+, K^+, Cl^+, etc.), proteins, amino acids, glucose, lipids, and fatty acids occupy the rest. The cytosol is the site of many chemical reactions that maintain cell structures and allow cell growth; therefore, cytosol is an important part of the cell required for its existence. Organelles are specialized cellular structures with characteristic shapes and specific functions, suspended in the cytoplasm of the cell. Each type of organelle has a typical functional component where specific processes take place. There are two types of organelles, namely, membranous and nonmembranous organelles. Membranous organelles include the nucleus, endoplasmic reticulum, Golgi complex, lysosome, and mitochondria. Nonmembranous organelles include nucleoli, ribosome, and cytoskeleton. The cytoskeleton is a network of several kinds of protein filaments that extend throughout the cytoplasm, which provide a structural framework for the cells. There are three types of protein filaments found in the cytoskeleton, namely, microfilaments, intermediate filaments, and microtubules. The microfilament is responsible for the strength and shape of the cell. Intermediate filaments are thicker than microfilaments and thinner than microtubules. These filaments help to hold organelles in place. Microtubules are the thickest components of the cytoskeleton, and are typically long and hollow tubes that help to determine the cell shape and resiliency. The cytoskeleton network also permits the distribution of biomechanical force between surrounding cells and allows the anchoring of cells to each other. The cytoskeleton is also actively involved in cell motility, cell division, and the movement of intracellular organelles. The cytoplasm also has several other components, such as the centrosome, cilia, and flagella. All these components together are responsible for the cell's existence.

2.4.3 Cell Membrane

Cell membrane, also called plasma membrane, consists mainly of lipids (phospholipids and glycolipids) and proteins (glycoproteins) that provide a layered structural support to the cells by enclosing them (see Figure 2.2). Other substances present in the membrane include cholesterol. The membrane separates the cell's internal environment (intracellular) from its external environment (extracellular). It plays a pivotal role in cell–cell and cell–matrix interactions. It controls the movement of substances into (e.g., nutrients) and out (e.g., cellular waste products) of a cell, but restricts the movement of other substances that are not required for the metabolic cell functions. This property of the cell membrane is called selective permeability. It should be noted that most of the functions of the cell membrane depend on the type of proteins that are present in the membrane and these may vary quantitatively and qualitatively among membranes with respect to cell type and even within the same cell. The proteins associated with the lipid bilayer are either stuck in it (called integral proteins) or stuck on it (called peripheral proteins). Integral proteins, called receptors, recognize and bind a specific molecule that governs some of the cellular functions. These proteins associate with the nonpolar core of the lipid bilayer either directly or indirectly. Peripheral proteins are loosely attached to the external or internal surface of the membrane. These proteins associate with either integral proteins or other peripheral proteins by ionic bonding. The integral and peripheral proteins function together as linkers, which anchor proteins in the cell membranes of adjacent cells to one another or structures inside and outside of the cell. Glycoproteins and glycolipids, often called cell identity markers, enable a cell to recognize other cells of its own kind during tissue formation or to recognize and respond against disease-carrying microorganisms, such as bacteria and viruses.

2.4.3.1 Transport across the Cell Membrane

Transport or movement of substances into and out of the cell membrane is essential for the existence of a cell, subsequent tissue formation, and continued function. Metabolic substances, such as oxygen, ions, and nutrients, must be moved into the cell and, similarly, cellular waste products and carbon dioxide must be moved out of the cell to regulate the metabolic function. All of these balanced exchanges take place across the cell membrane by a variety of processes, which can be broadly grouped into passive and active processes.

In passive processes, metabolic substances move from an area of higher concentration to an area of lower concentration through the membrane. Two types of passive processes take place: (i) diffusion, and (ii) osmosis. In the diffusion process, substances move due to their kinetic energy from an area of lower to higher concentration. The substances that are transported in diffusion processes include oxygen, carbon dioxide, various ions, such as Na^+, K^+, and Ca^{2+}, and fatty acids. In osmosis, movement of a substance (water) takes place through a selectively permeable membrane from an area of higher to lower concentration until equilibrium is attained.

In active transport, substances move through the membrane from an area of lower concentration to an area of higher concentration. Two types of active transport take place: (i) primary active transport, and (ii) secondary active transport. As active transport requires energy for the movement of substances, two types of energy sources are used: (i) energy from splitting of adenosine triphosphate (ATP) is used in primary active transport, and (ii) energy stored in a Na^+ concentration gradient is used in secondary active transport. In primary transport, substances move through a membrane by transporter proteins (called pumps) from an area of lower to higher concentration. The substances that are moved by primary transport include Na^+, K^+, Ca^{2+}, H^+, I^-, and Cl^-. The most important primary transport pump expels Na^+ from cells and brings in K^+. The pump protein also acts as an enzyme to split ATP. Due to ions it moves, this pump is called Na^+/K^+ pump (also called sodium pump). All cells have several sodium pumps in their cell membrane, which chiefly maintain a low concentration of Na^+ in the cytosol by pumping Na^+ into the extracellular fluid against the Na^+ concentration gradient. At the same time, the sodium pump moves K^+ into cells against the K^+ concentration gradient. The sodium pump must function continuously in order to maintain a low concentration of Na^+ and a high concentration of K^+ in the cytosol and extracellular fluid for the maintenance of cell functions. In secondary active transport, simultaneous movement of Na^+ and another substance cross the membrane using the energy stored in the Na^+ concentration gradient maintained by the primary transport pumps. The movement of Na^+ and the second substance in the opposite direction across the membrane is called antiporters, while in the same direction it is called symporters. There are several antiporters and symporters in the cell membrane to regulate the metabolic cycle. The substances that move through the cell membrane by the secondary active transport include ions, glucose, fructose, and various amino acids.

2.5 Tissue Level

At the tissue level, a group of similar cells and surrounding substances are organized together to perform a specific function. Tissues are somewhat more complex than cells. From an engineering point of view, tissues can be broadly classified into soft and hard, depending on their mechanical and structural properties. For example, bone and tooth pertain to a hard kind of tissue, which is stiffer (elastic modules) and stronger (tensile strength) than soft tissue. Skin and cartilage are a few notable examples of the latter type. The major differences between soft and hard tissues in terms of mechanical properties are shown in Table 1.6, in comparison with some of the widely used biomaterials, which may help the readers to assess what kind of material could be selected or used for a specific application. There are four primary tissues in the human body: epithelial tissue, connective tissue, muscle tissue, and nerve tissue (see Figure 2.3), which are briefly discussed below.

2.5.1 Epithelial Tissue

Epithelium is a tissue that serves as a protective layer for body organs and systems and keeps them separate. It covers the whole surface of the body (e.g., skin). Some examples of epithelial tissue are the outer layer of the skin, the inside of the mouth and stomach, and the tissue surrounding the body's organs. Epithelial tissue that occurs on the interior surface of the body is known as endothelium. Depending on the number of tissue layers, epithelial tissue can be divided into two groups. The epithelial tissue, which is only one cell thick, is known as simple epithelium. If it is two or more cells thick, such as the skin, it is known as stratified epithelium (also called compound epithelium). Simple epithelium can be subdivided according to the shape and function of its cells, namely, squamous, cuboidal, and columnar. Epithelium has specific functions, including protection, secretion, absorption, excretion, sensory reception, and it reduces friction.

2.5.2 Connective Tissue

Connective tissue is a tissue that supports the body and binds or connects together all types of tissues. It provides a mechanical framework (the skeleton) that plays an important role in locomotion. It is considered the most abundant body tissue. It consists of cells and a matrix material (also called ECM), which is composed of ground substances (e.g., chondroitin sulfate) and fibrous matters. The fibers provide structural framework and strength to cell adhesion. There are three types of fibrous matters, namely, collagen fibers, elastic fibers, and reticular fibers. The cells in connective tissue include fibroblasts that secrete matrix, macrophages that perform phagocytosis, plasma cells that secrete antibodies, mast cells that produce histamine,

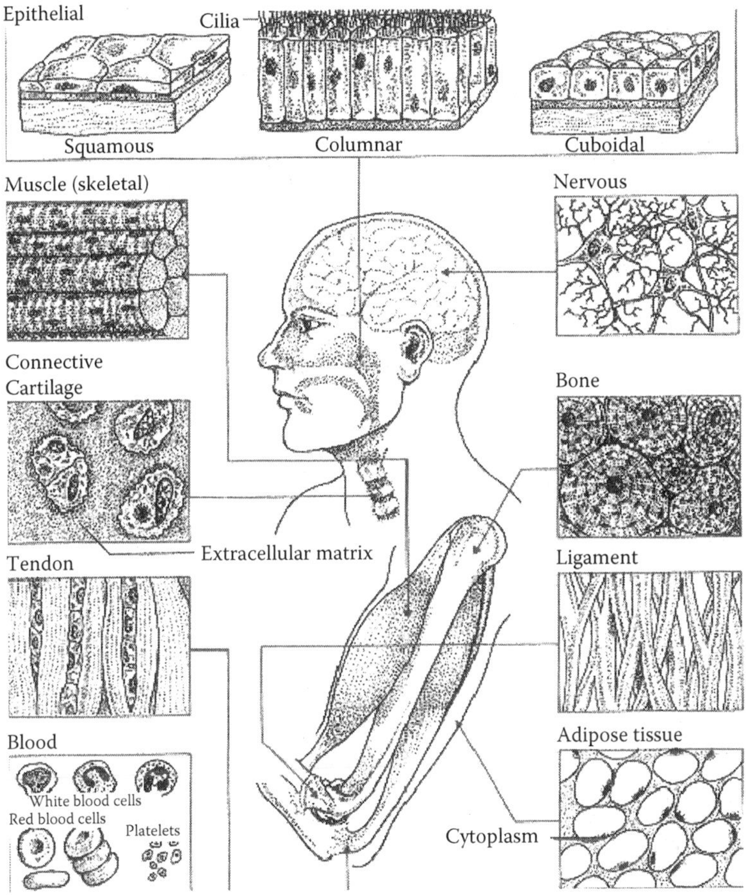

FIGURE 2.3
A schematic of various types of human tissues. (From http://biology-pages.info. With permission.)

adipocytes that help to store fat, and white blood cells that provide immunity to the body. In contrast to epithelial tissue, where cells tightly adhere to one another, connective tissue has dispersed or loosely packed cells that typically lack intercellular contact. Also, most connective tissue is vascularized (with the single exception of cartilage) and has a nerve supply. Examples of connective tissue include blood, cartilage, and bone. Connective tissues can be classified into loose connective tissue (e.g., adipose tissue), which mainly provides a natural scaffold for cell function, and dense (fibrous) connective tissue (e.g., bone), which mainly performs a mechanical function. The most abundant tissue in the vertebrates is the loose connective tissue, which acts with the underlying tissue and functions as packaging material, holding the body organs in place. Loose connective tissue includes areolar connective tissue, adipose connective tissue, and reticular connective tissue. Dense connective tissue contains more densely packed and thicker fibers than loose connective tissue. There are three types of dense connective tissues: dense regular connective tissue, dense irregular connective tissue, and elastic connective tissue.

2.5.3 Muscle Tissue

Muscle tissue is a tissue characterized by muscle cells that are highly specialized to maintain posture. The primary purpose of muscle tissue is to produce contraction and relaxation, and thus help in the movement of various parts of the body. There are other movements in the body too, which are necessary for the survival of the organism, such as the heart beat and the movements of the alimentary canal. The muscle cells contain the contractile proteins, actin and myosin, in varying amounts and configurations, depending on cell function. There are three types of muscle tissue: (i) skeletal muscle, which is normally responsible for the voluntary movement in the body; (ii) cardiac muscle, which forms the wall of the heart and relays signals from cell to cell during a heartbeat; and (iii) smooth muscle, which is found in the digestive track, bladder, arteries, and other internal organs. The functions of muscles in our bodies include support and movement, propulsion of blood through vessels, movement of food or body secretions through tracts, and thermoregulation; therefore, it is considered one of the most important tissues in humans.

2.5.4 Nerve Tissue

Nerve tissue is a highly specialized tissue that has the ability to generate and conduct electrical signals, called nerve impulses, in the body. These electrical messages are managed by nerve tissue in the brain and transmitted down the spinal cord to the body. The brain and spinal cord are typical examples of nerve tissue. Basically, nerve tissue consists of two types of cells: neurons and glia cells. Neurons are the primary cells of the nerve tissue, and specialize in transmitting signals, the so-called nerve impulses. There are three main types of neurons, which are classified according to their function. The cells that conduct impulses from the sensory organs to the central nervous system (brain and spinal cord) are called sensory neurons. The cells that conduct impulses from the central nervous system to the effector organs (e.g., muscles and glands) are called motor neurons. The cells that connect sensory neurons to motor neurons as well as different parts of the central nervous system are called connector neurons (also called interneurons). Glia cells (also called neuroglia) are secondary cells involved in nourishment and structural support. They do not have the ability to generate or conduct nerve impulses. Nerve cells consist of the cell body and two or more extensions, called dendrites and axons. The dendrites transmit an impulse that is sent toward the cell body, and the axons transmit impulses away from the cell body.

2.6 Organ Level

At the organ level, different types of tissues are organized together to form the body structure and to perform a common function. Organs are more complex than tissues in terms of structure and function. There are many different organs in the body. Examples include the skin, bone, liver, kidneys, lungs, brain, eye, stomach, and heart. Skin is the largest organ of the human body followed by bone. In the following section, we focus our attention on the structure and function of the skin and the bone in detail.

2.6.1 Skin

The skin is the largest organ of the body. It is highly complex and helps mainly in the protection of organism from the external environment. The skin serves many important functions, including regulating body temperature, maintaining water and electrolyte balance, protecting the body from disease-causing microorganisms, such as bacteria and viruses that invade the skin, shielding the body from UV radiation, stimulating synthesis of vitamin D (essential for the absorption of calcium to build and maintain bone), and sensing painful and pleasant stimuli. The skin is organized into four types of tissues, namely, epidermis, dermis, basement membrane, and subcutis (see Figure 2.4). The outer layer (~0.1 mm thick), called the epidermis, provides a barrier against infection and loss of water and electrolytes

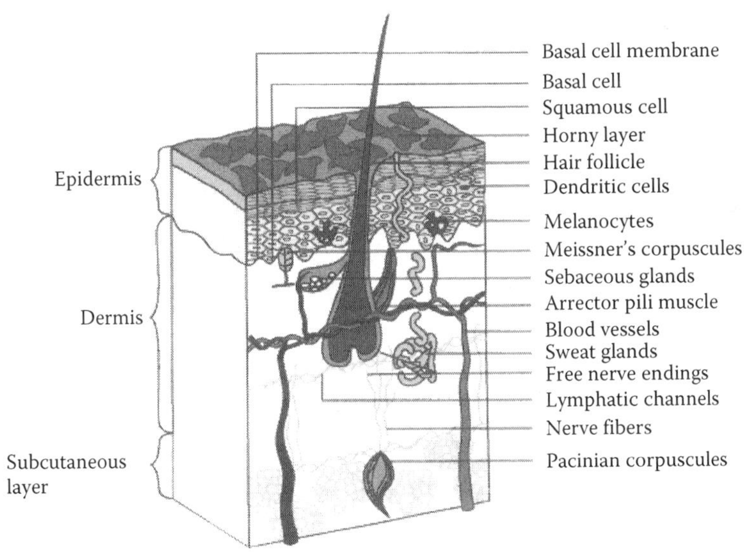

FIGURE 2.4
A schematic of skin structure. (From http://skincare.dermis.net. With permission.)

from the body. It is made up of cells called keratinocytes (about 90%), which are stacked on top of each other, forming different sublayers.

The keratinocytes develop at the bottom and rise to the top, where they are shed from the surface as dead cells. Thus, this layer is constantly renewing itself, the live cells changing into dead, hard, flattened cells. Melanocytes, Langerhans, and Markel cells are other important cells found in the epidermis, which have special functions. Melanocytes are responsible for the production of pigment called melanin that contributes to skin color and helps in shielding nuclear DNA from UV radiation. Langerhans cells are responsible for immunity against microbes that invade the skin. Markel cells are responsible for sensation and these cells are available in less number and located on the sensory neuron in deep epidermis. The inner layer (~2–5 mm thick), called the dermis, is responsible for the structural integrity of the skin. The dermis consists mostly of connective tissue (collagen and elastic fibers) with fibroblast cells and is much thicker than the epidermis. The combination of collagen and elastic fibers gives the skin its strength and elasticity, respectively. It is responsible for the skin's pliability and mechanical resistance and is also involved in the regulation of body temperature. The dermis supplies the avascular epidermis with nutrients by means of its vascular network. It contains sense organs for touch, pressure, pain, and temperature, as well as blood vessels, nerve fibers, sebaceous and sweat glands, and hair follicles. A multilayer (~20 nm thick) in between the epidermis and the dermis is called basement membrane, which is highly responsible for the mechanical support of the epidermis. Finally, the subcutis is a 0.4–4 mm thick tissue mainly composed of loose connective tissues and fat cells (adipocytes) underneath the dermis. The properties of the skin, in particular physical and mechanical, significantly vary with the body region, age, sex, and other factors. Since the skin serves as a protective barrier against the external environment, any damage in the skin must be treated very carefully. There are many techniques for the treatment of skin defects. The most recent advances in tissue-engineered skin and their potential for clinical applications are discussed in detail in Chapter 10.

2.6.2 Bone

Bone is a hard and rigid form of connective tissue pertaining to the formation of the skeletal system; therefore, it is considered a main supportive organ. Bone not only provides mechanical support for the organism, but also serves as a reservoir for minerals, particularly calcium and phosphate. Bone is considered as an assemblage of various levels of hierarchical structural units elegantly designed over many length scales (see Figure 2.5) (Murugan and Ramakrishna 2005).

At the macrostructural level, the matured lamellar bone can be distinguished into two types, namely, spongy bone and compact bone. As their names imply, they radically vary in density. They are organized with

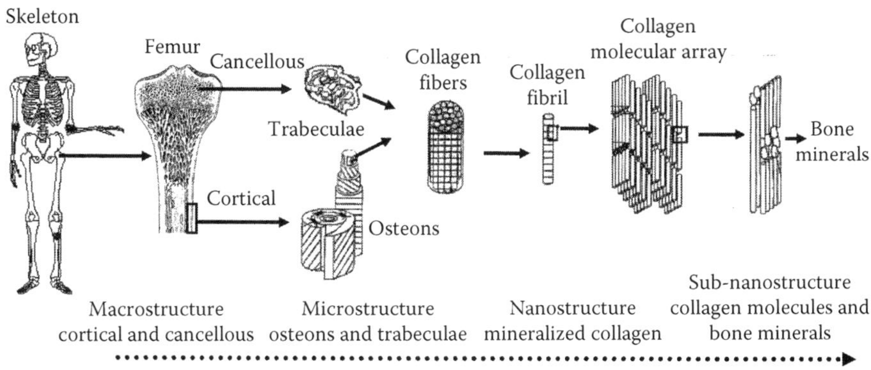

FIGURE 2.5
Hierarchical assembly of bone. (Reprinted from Murugan, R. and Ramakrishna, S., *Comp. Sci. Tech.*, 65, 2385, 2005. With permission from Elsevier.)

multilevel pores, macro to nano, for the establishment of multiple functions, including transportation of nutrients, oxygen, and body fluids. The spongy bone occupies about 20% of the total bone. It is also often called trabecular or cancellous bone. It is lighter and less dense than compact bone. It has high porosity and a higher concentration of blood vessels compared to compact bone. The porous architecture is easily visible under the lower power microscopes and/or even to the naked eye if the pores are very large. The diameter of the pores may be from a few micrometers to millimeters. On the other hand, compact bone is much denser than spongy bone. It is also known as cortical or dense bone. It occupies about 80% of the total bone. It has less porosity and thus less concentration of blood vessels. Its porous architecture is not visible to the naked eye, owing to less porosity. The pores may be perhaps 10–20 μm in diameter and mostly separated at intervals of 200–300 μm. The compact bone functions mechanically in tension, compression, and torsion, whereas spongy bone functions mainly in compression.

At the microstructural level, the repeated structural unit of compact bone is mostly of osteon or Harversian system, which act as weight-bearing pillars. By contrast, spongy bone contains no such osteon units, but they are made of an interconnecting framework of trabeculae. The trabeculae have three types of cellular structures: plate/plate-like, plate/bar-like, and bar/bar-like.

At the nanostructural level, bone is comprised mainly of collagen fibers and nanocrystals of bone minerals, particularly hydroxyapatite (HA). Although several structural levels of bone have been identified, a complete understanding of how the mineral–matrix interactions are related to their mechanical reliability at the so far identified seven hierarchical levels of the bone tissue is still needed.

Bone mainly consists of, in decreasing proportions, minerals, collagen, water, noncollagenous proteins, lipids, vascular elements, and cells. The overall

TABLE 2.1

The Composition of Bone

Inorganic Phase (wt.%)	Organic Phase (wt.%)
Hydroxyapatite ~60	Collagen ~20
Carbonate ~4	Water ~9
Citrate ~0.9	Noncollagenous proteins ~3 (osteocalcin, osteonectin, osteopontin, thrombospondin, morphogenetic proteins, sialoprotein, serum proteins)
Sodium ~0.7	Other traces: polysaccharides, lipids, cytokines
Magnesium ~0.5	Primary bone cells: osteoblasts, osteocytes, osteoclasts
Other traces: Cl^-, F^-, K^+ Sr^{2+}, Pb^{2+}, Zn^{2+}, Cu^{2+}, Fe^{2+}	

Source: Reprinted from Murugan, R. and Ramakrishna, S., *Comp. Sci. Tech.*, 65, 2385, 2005. With permission from Elsevier.

composition of bone is given in Table 2.1 (Murugan and Ramakrishna 2005). Bone mineral is mainly comprised of HA, and bone protein is mainly composed of collagen. Collagen acts as a structural framework in which plate-like tiny crystals of HA are embedded to strengthen the bone. The bone collagen has a typical fibrous structure, whose diameter varies from 100 to 2000 nm. Similarly, HA in the bone mineral is in the form of nanocrystals, with dimensions of about $4 \times 50 \times 50$ nm. The bone minerals are also enriched with a few trace elements for various metabolic functions, which include carbonate, citrate, sodium, magnesium, fluoride, chloride, and potassium. The prime role of minerals is to provide toughness and rigidity to the bone, whereas collagen provides tensile strength and flexibility. It is really amazing how nature built extremely hard and tough bone using such soft (collagen) and brittle (HA) ingredients. It is believed that key to the strength of bone is the complex structural hierarchy into which it is organized in a self-assembling mode. It is important to note that the minerals are not directly bound to collagen, but bound through noncollagenous proteins. The noncollagenous proteins make up approximately 3–5% of bone, which provide active sites for biomineralization and cellular attachment. Water is also found in sufficient quantity in all bones. It is one of the most essential substances of the body because no cells survive without water. The amount of water present in bone is an important determinant of its mechanical behavior as well. Lipids are also necessary for the cellular functions, which account for about 2% of bone. They play an important role in the process of biomineralization.

Bone consists of five distinct types of living cells: osteoprogenitor cells, osteoblasts, osteocytes, osteoclasts, and bone-lining cells (see Figure 2.6). Bone, like other connective tissues in the embryo, is derived from mesenchymal cells. These cells have the ability to divide and differentiate into bone cells,

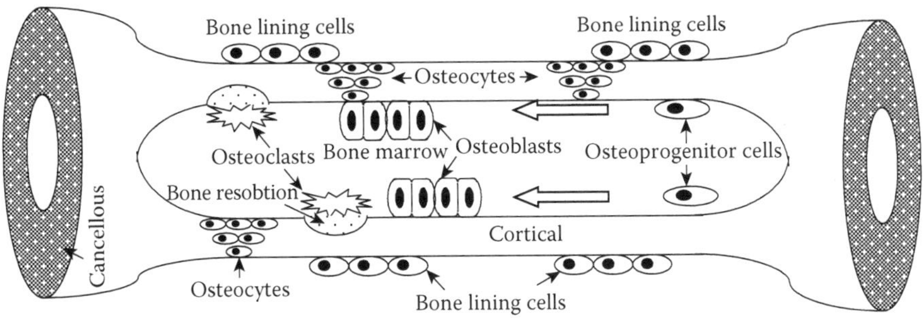

FIGURE 2.6
Schematic of bone cells that are influencing bone remodeling. (From Murugan, R. and Ramakrishna, S., Reproduced from *Handbook of molecular building blocks for nanotechnology*, Springer-Verlag, Germany, 2006a; Reproduced from Murugan, R. and Ramakrishna, S., *Tissue, cell, and organ engineering*, Wiley-VCH, Weinheim, 2006b. With permission from Copyright© Wiley-VCH Verlag GmbH & Co., KGaA.)

which are known as osteoprogenitor cells, also known as bone-precursor cells. Osteoblasts are the cells responsible for the formation of new bone. They start with secreting collagen and then coat with noncollagenous proteins, which is similar to glue, that has the ability to hold the minerals, mostly calcium and phosphate, from the bloodstream, leading to new bone formation. Osteocytes are mature cells derived from osteoblasts, which are responsible for the maintenance of bone. They function as transporting agents of minerals between bone and blood. Osteoclasts are the large cells found at the surface of the bone mineral next to the resorbing bone. They are responsible for the resorbtion of the bone. They use acids or enzymes to dissolve the minerals as well as collagen from the matured bone. The dissolved minerals then re-enter the bloodstream and are carried to different parts of the body. Bone-lining cells are found along the surface of the matured bone, which are responsible for regulating the transportation of minerals in and out of the bone tissue. They also respond to hormones by making some exclusive proteins that activate the osteoclasts. These five types of cells are responsible for building the bone matrix with hierarchical self-assembly, maintenance, and remodeling as required. All these processes must be in equilibrium to ensure a healthy bone.

2.7 System Level

At system level, the highest level of structural organization, several organs are joined together to perform complex functions for the body. Twelve major organ systems compose the human body (see Table 2.2). They are integumentary, skeletal, muscular, circulatory, respiratory, immune, digestive, urinary,

TABLE 2.2

Major Organ Systems of the Human Body

Organ Systems	Associated Organs	Major Functions
Integumentary	Skin, hair, nails	Protects against pathogens, helps regulate body temperature
Skeletal	Bones, cartilage, tendons, ligaments, joints	Provides structure, supports, and protects internal organs
Muscular	Skeletal, cardiac, and smooth muscles	Provides posture, supports, and moves trunk and limbs, moves substances through body
Circulatory	Heart, blood vessels, blood	Transports nutrients and wastes to and from all body tissues
Respiratory	Lungs, nasal	Carries air into and out of lungs, where oxygen and carbon dioxide are exchanged
Immune	Lymph nodes and vessels, white blood cells	Provides protection against infection and disease
Digestive	Esophagus, stomach, liver, pancreas, intestines	Stores and digests food, absorbs nutrients, eliminates waste
Urinary	Kidneys, ureters, bladder, urethra	Eliminate urine, maintains water and salt balance
Nervous	Brain, spinal cord, nerves, sense organs	Controls and coordinates body movements and senses, helps monitor and maintain other body systems
Endocrine	Thyroid, adrenal	Maintain homeostasis, regulates metabolism, water and mineral balance, growth and sexual development, and reproduction
Lymphatic	Lymph nodes, glands, spleen	Cleans and returns tissue fluid to the blood and destroys pathogens that enter the body
Reproductive	Ovaries, uterus, testes	Produce egg (in female) and sperm (in male)

nervous, endocrine, lymphatic, and reproductive. All these organ systems are essential to ensure a healthy body.

The integumentary system provides sensory receptors and protects the body. Examples include skin, hair, nail, and various glands. This system makes up most of the external surface of the body and is always in direct contact with the external environment. Therefore, this system plays a major biological role in maintaining homeostasis. The major functions of the integumentary system are serving as a barrier between the body and its surroundings, providing information about the external environment, regulating body temperature, helping the process of vitamin D production, and actively defending the body from outside harmful physical and biological stimuli. The skeletal system, mainly constituted by bones and cartilages, provides a structural framework for the body. It is also responsible for several functions: protects all internal organs from external stimuli, assists in movement of the body in conjunction with muscles, and stores essential minerals, such as calcium and phosphorous, needed for bone metabolism. The muscular system (e.g., skeletal muscle) provides the body with movement and maintains posture. The circulatory system (also called cardiovascular system) provides an environment for the distribution of blood, nutrients, and oxygen to all parts of the body. It also helps in carrying body waste products from the body. Heart, blood, and blood vessels are typical examples of this system. The respiratory system (e.g., lungs, nasal, and alveoli) carries oxygen to the body from the air and it carries carbon dioxide from the body to the air, for the existence of life. The inhaled oxygen is broken down in the alveoli and then passed into the capillaries where it travels into the blood. Similarly, carbon dioxide from the blood is passed back into the alveoli and exhaled from the body through the nose. The immune system (e.g., lymph nodes and vessels) helps the body to fight against disease and infection. White blood cells are another important part of the immune system that helps defend the body. The lymphatic system (e.g., lymph and glands) is the main defense system that cleans and returns excess tissue fluid called lymph and some proteins to the blood and destroys pathogens that enter the body, preventing tissue damage. The digestive system ingests food and water, breaking them down into small molecules, and absorbing their nutrients for the body functions. It should be noted that the digestive system is a long tube that runs from the mouth to the anus. The stomach, intestines, and esophagus are a few notable examples of this system. The urinary system maintains the fluid volume of the body, eliminates metabolic waste products, maintains water–salt balance, and helps regulate blood pressure. The kidneys, ureters, and urinary bladder are notable examples of this system. The nervous system (e.g., brain and spinal cord) regulates most of the body's actions with respect to internal and external stimuli. Our sense organs are also a major part of this system. The endocrine system essentially secretes hormones that initiate and control many bodily processes, such as growth, digestion, and reproduction. The thyroid and adrenals are examples of this system. The reproductive system produces eggs (female) or sperm (male) that allows for the continuation of life. Ovaries and testes are notable examples of this system. All these organ systems are equally important for life.

Glossary

Anatomy: The branch of science concerned with the structure of the body and the relationship of its organs.

Antibodies: Immunoglobin proteins secreted by B lymphocytes that have transformed into plasma cells.

Basement membrane: A thin sheet of extracellular substance to which the basal surfaces of membranous epithelial cells are attached; also called the basal lamina.
Blood: The fluid connective tissue that circulates through the cardiovascular system to transport substances throughout the body.
Blood vessel: A tube that carries blood through the body.
Bone: A solid, rigid, ossified connective tissue forming an organ of the skeletal system.
Brain: The enlarged superior portion of the central nervous system located in the cranial cavity of the skull.
Capillary: A microscopic blood vessel that connects an arteriole and a venule; the functional unit of the circulatory system.
Cartilage: A type of connective tissue with a solid elastic matrix.
Cell: The structural and functional unit of an organism; the smallest structure capable of performing all the functions necessary for life.
Central nervous system: Part of the nervous system consisting of the brain and the spinal cord.
Compact bone: The hard material that makes up the shaft of long bones and the outside surfaces of other bones.
Cytoplasm: In a cell, the protoplasm located outside of the nucleus.
Cytoskeleton: A latticework of structural proteins in the cytoplasm arranged in the form of microfilaments and microtubules.
Cytosol: A fluid matrix of water and dissolved substances such as proteins and nutrients.
Dermis: The second, or deep, layer of skin beneath the epidermis.
Effector: An organ, such as a gland or muscle, that responds to a motor stimulation.
Elastic fibers: Protein strands that are found in certain connective tissue that have contractile properties.
Enzyme: A protein catalyst that increases the rate of specific chemical reactions.
Epidermis: The outermost layer of the skin, composed of several stratified squamous epithelial layers.
Fibroblast: An elongated connective tissue cell with cytoplasmic extensions that is capable of forming collagenous fibers or elastic fibers.
Genetic transcription: The process by which RNA is produced with a sequence of nucleotide bases that is complementary to a region of DNA.
Genetic translation: The process by which proteins are produced with amino acid sequences specified by the sequence of codons in messenger RNA.
Gland: An organ that produces a specific substance or secretion.
Golgi apparatus: A network of stacked, flattened membranous sacs within the cytoplasm of cells. Its major function is to concentrate and package proteins for secretion from the cell.

Heart: A four-chambered, muscular, pumping organ positioned in the thoracic cavity, slightly to the left of midline.

Hormones: Chemical messengers produced by the endocrine system, such as pituitary glands and pancreas.

Integumentary system: The skin and its accessory organs, such as nail and hair.

Kidney: One of a pair of organs of the urinary system that contains nephrons and that filters waste from the blood in the formation of urine.

Lamella: A concentric ring of matrix surrounding the central canal in an osteon of mature bone tissue.

Lung: One of the two major organs of respiration positioned within the thoracic cavity on either side of the mediastinum.

Lymphocyte: A type of white blood cell characterized by agranular cytoplasm.

Lysosomes: Organelles containing digestive enzymes and responsible for intracellular digestion.

Mast cell: A type of connective tissue cell that produces and secretes histamine and heparin and promotes local inflammation.

Matrix: The intercellular substance of a tissue.

Metabolism: The breakdown of substances, the formation of new products, or the transferring of energy from one substance to another.

Microtubules: Protein fibers made of the protein tubulin and provide support and mobility for cellular activities found in the spindle apparatus.

Mitochondria: Cytoplasmic organelles that serve as sites for the production of most of the cellular energy; the so-called powerhouses of the cell.

Mitosis: The process of cell division that results in two identical daughter cells, containing the same number of chromosomes.

Molecules: Atoms chemically bound together.

Muscular system: Consists of skeletal muscles and their associated connective tissues.

Nerve: A bundle of nerve fibers outside the central nervous system.

Neuron: The structural and functional unit of the nervous system, composed of a cell body, dendrites, and an axon; also called a nerve cell.

Nucleolus: A dark-staining area within a cell nucleus; the site where ribosomal RNA is produced.

Nucleus: A spheroid body within a cell that contains the genetic factors of the cell.

Nutrients: Substances contained in the food consumed by the body from which the body absorbs energy for its functions.

Organ: A major part of the body consisting of a group of tissues (e.g., kidney and brain).

Organelle: A minute living structure of a cell with a specific function.

Osteoblast: A bone-forming cell.

Osteoclast: A cell that causes resorption of bone tissue.

Osteocyte: A mature bone cell.

Osteon: A group of osteocytes and concentric lamellae surrounding a central canal, constituting the basic unit of structure in osseous tissue; also called a Haversian system.

Pathogen: Any disease-producing microorganism or substance.

Physiology: The study of the function of body parts and the body as a whole.

Plasma: Liquid portion of the blood, which consists of water, proteins, waste products, nutrients, electrolytes, and respiratory gases.

Plasma membrane: A membrane that separates internal metabolic events from the external environment and controls the movement of materials into and out of the cell. It bounds the cell and encloses the nucleus and cytoplasm.

Proteins: A class of molecules that have varied functions. Eggs, muscles, antibodies, silk, fingernails, and many hormones are partially or entirely proteins.

Remodeling: A process of creating new bone and removing old bone.

Reproduction: Production of eggs and sperm and the processes leading to fertilization.

Respiration: The exchange of gases between the external environment and the cells of an organism.

Ribosome: A cytoplasmic organelle composed of protein and RNA in which protein synthesis occurs.

Skeletal system: Bones, cartilage, and the membranes that line the bones.

Spinal cord: The portion of the central nervous system that extends downward from the brain stem through the vertebral canal.

System: A group of organs that work together to perform a specific function.

Tissue: An aggregation of similar cells and their binding intercellular substance, joined to perform a specific function.

Trabeculae: A supporting framework of fibers crossing the substance of a structure, as in the lamellae of spongy bone.

Urinary system: A system that helps maintain homeostasis by regulating water balance and by removing harmful substances from the blood.

Zygote: The fusing of an egg and a sperm.

EXERCISES

2.1 What are the preliminary characterizations to be carried out for the study of *in vitro* and *in vivo* biological responses to biomaterials?

2.2 What are the different levels of structural organization of the human body?

2.3 What are the major elements associated with body weight?

2.4 What is meant by atomic number?

2.5 What is a cell and what are the various parts of the same?

2.6 What is the major role of cell membrane?

2.7 What is tissue and what are the major types of tissues in the human body?
2.8 Give some examples of soft tissue and hard tissue.
2.9 What is an organ? Provide some examples.
2.10 Classify various organ systems of the body.

References

http://www.blc.arizona.edu/Molecular%5FGraphics/DNA%5FStructure.
http://www.people.eku.edu/ritchisong/301notes1.htm.
http://biology-pages.info.
http://skincare.dermis.net.
Murugan, R. and S. Ramakrishna. 2005. Development of nanocomposites for bone grafting. *Comp. Sci. Tech.* 65:2385–2406.
______. 2006a. Nanoengineered biomimetic bone-building blocks. In *Handbook of molecular building blocks for nanotechnology*, ed. G. A. Mansoori, T. F. George, L. Assoufid, and G. Zhang, 301. Germany: Springer-Verlag.
______. 2006b. Nanophase biomaterials for tissue engineering. In *Tissue, cell, and organ engineering*. Vol. 9 of *Nanotechnologies for the life sciences*, ed. S. S. R. Challakumar, 216–56. Weinheim: Wiley-VCH.

Further Reading

Bruce, A. et al. 2003. *Essential cell biology*. New York: Garland Science/Taylor & Francis Group.
McKenzie, J. C. and R. M. Klein. 1999. *Basic concepts in cell biology and histology*. New York: McGraw-Hill.
Solomon, E. P. 2003. *Introduction to human anatomy and physiology*. Amsterdam: Elsevier.
Tortora, G. J. and S. R. Grabowski. 2001. *Introduction to the human body*. New York: John Wiley.

3

Degradation and Corrosion of Biomaterials

3.1 Introduction

All biomaterials when implanted in the human body induce a biomaterial–tissue response, which can be attributed to complex interactions from a vast array of material properties, including physicochemical, mechanical, morphology, and surface properties. Since the present biomaterials are neither truly inert nor totally integrated with tissues, the ultimate goal has been to minimize or control the host tissue response by modifying biomaterial properties. The surface properties of biomaterial have profound consequences on cellular and host responses. For this reason, we must understand the unique properties of surface and the methods to characterize surfaces in striving toward more "biocompatible materials," which either evokes a minimal inflammatory response or elicits a specific cellular response. Corrosion of biomaterials or implants is one of the important aspects of biocompatibility and greatly affects the service of medical devices. No metallic biomaterial is totally resistant to corrosion within the human body. All medical implants made of metals and alloys undergo chemical or electrochemical dissolution due to the complex and corrosive nature of the human body environment, which leads to failure of implants before fulfilling their intended function. Hence, it is highly desirable to fully discover corrosion-resistant biomaterials to minimize the failure rate of medical implants. In the following sections, we will discuss the degradation, corrosion, and biocompatibility aspects of biomaterials or implants.

3.2 Surface Properties

Some of the unique properties of the surface that are inevitably different from the bulk are its composition, structure, total mass, reactivity, and contaminants. Due to energy minimization, the surface composition is different from its bulk composition. This phenomenon is called surface segregation, which derives some of the elements of the bulk material to its surface, e.g., chromium in steels. The absence of periodic arrangement of atoms causes the organization of the outermost atomic layers of the surface to be different from the atomic structure of the bulk material. Relaxation of the atoms from their regular periodic position, rearrangement of atoms with different lattice spacing but with same periodicity, and reconstruction of a new periodic arrangement of atoms can occur at the surface. In view of the exposure to the atmospheres, the surfaces are readily covered with a few layers of the contamination of the vapor phase, such as hydrocarbons, adsorbed layers of oxygen, carbon, etc. So, for all practical purposes, the surface can be considered as an interface region with a different structure and composition than the bulk material and covered with a contaminant overlayer.

The surface zone usually scales with the size of the constituents of the material making up the surface and may extend from a few nanometers for atomic materials, such as metals, to 100 nm for molecular materials, such as polymers. A complete description of the surface zone therefore requires measurement of many parameters with the use of many techniques to compile all the needed information. As wettability, roughness, surface composition, etc., has been shown to play a major role in the biomaterial–tissue response, characterization of some these parameters are important.

The surface energy has been strongly correlated with biological interactions, such as adhesion of cells including bacteria. It can be quantitatively characterized through the contact angle of a liquid drop (θ) with the solid surface from Young's equation:

$$\gamma_s = \gamma_{sl} + \gamma_l \cdot \cos\theta,$$

where "s" and "l" stand for "solid" and "liquid," γ_s and γ_l describe the surface tension components of the two phases, and γ_{sl} represents the interfacial tension between the two phases. The contact angle is defined geometrically as the angle formed by the liquid at the phase boundary of the liquid, gas, and solid interacting phases, and it is determined by drawing a tangent at the contact where the liquid and solid phases intersect.

As surface tension can be thought of as the energy required to create a unit area of an interface, γ_s is the energy of the surface and the contact angle corresponds to the angle between vectors γ_l and γ_{sl}, as shown in Figure 3.1. The surface energy can be calculated from Young's equation by measuring the surface tension of the liquid and the contact angle, but the value of γ_{sl} must be known. So, to determine the surface energy of solids from contact angle measurements alone, a number of models have been developed. In the Zissman method (also called liquid homolog method), the contact angle of a series of homologous nonpolar liquids is measured on the solid surface of interest and the cosine of the angle is plotted vs. the liquid tension of the liquids. The surface tension at which the contact angle is zero, obtained by extrapolation,

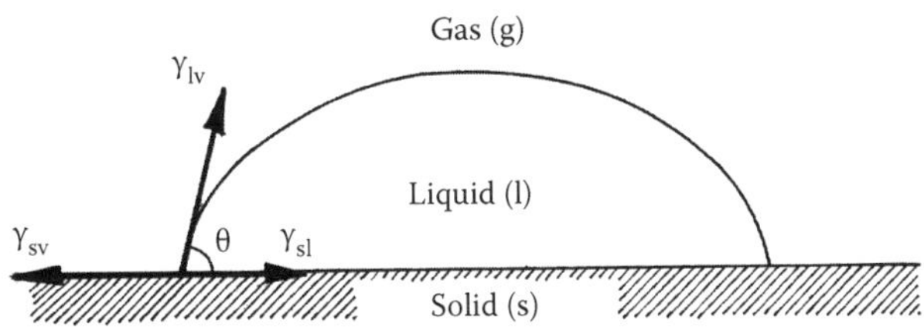

FIGURE 3.1
Contact angle formation on a solid surface.

is the critical surface tension of the solid. The surface tension (energy) of solids, which cannot be measured by similar methods as that of liquid because of the difficulty caused by the reversible formation of its surface, can thus be obtained. Based on the surface energy values, the solid surfaces can be divided into high-energy surfaces and low-energy surfaces. The high-energy surface materials are mainly comprised of metallic and inorganic materials and typically have a surface tension around 200–500 dynes/cm. Low-energy materials include organic compounds and polymeric materials with a critical surface tension less than 100 dynes/cm. Thus, low-energy materials, such as oils, contaminate high-energy solid surfaces due to a reduction in the free surface energy of the system and hence, it is essential to have a surface cleaning procedure or tailor the surfaces of implant materials. The goal of many treatments for adhesion of proteins or cells is to bring the surface to an intermediate state between water-repellent (hydrophobic) and completely wettable (hydrophilic). The contact angle measurement provides an easy and accurate way to determine the intermediate values (Sklodowska et al. 1999).

The contact angle represents the physical manifestation of more fundamental concepts of surface tension and surface energy, like the chemical bonding of the uppermost surface layers of a solid. The easy-to-measure indication of this bonding from contact angle values determines wettability, adhesion, surface cleanliness, effect of surface treatments, and properties of coatings. The wettability or wetting is the actual process of spreading of a liquid on a solid surface and is an important characteristic property of the surface for biomaterial applications. The contact angle, θ, is a quantitative measure of the wetting of a solid by a liquid, as schematically shown in Figure 3.2, i.e., when the contact angles are low, the liquid spreads, or wets well, meaning good wetting, and when the contact angles are high, this indicates poor wetting conditions. So, a zero θ represents complete wetting and if θ is less than 90° then the liquid is said to wet the solid, while if it is greater than 90° then it is said to be nonwetting. A spreading parameter S is also used to distinguish between total and partial wetting and it measures the difference between the surface energy of the sample under wet and dry conditions as

$$S = \gamma_s - (\gamma_l + \gamma_{sl}).$$

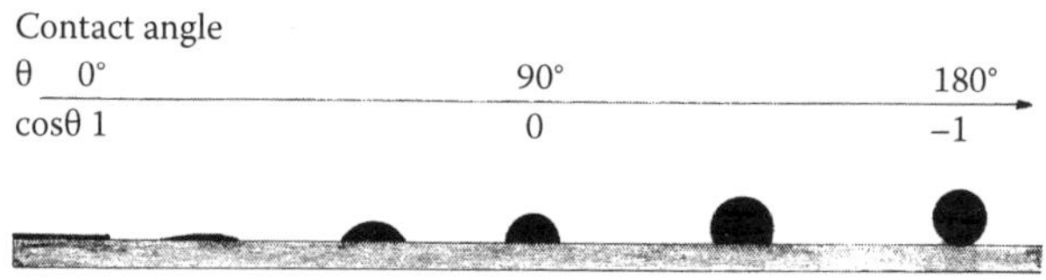

FIGURE 3.2
Schematic diagram on contact angle values and the corresponding wetting of a solid by a liquid.

For $S > 0$, the liquid spreads completely to lower its surface energy like ethanol, with a low value of γ_l spreading on a high value γ_s solid like glass. If $S < 0$, then the liquid does not spread, but forms a spherical drop resting on the surface of the solid. Thus, the contact angle is a direct measure of interactions taking place between a liquid, gas (or a second immiscible liquid), and solid phases.

Very often, the contact angle is one of the most sensitive, reliable, and inexpensive methods for the characterization of surface properties of solids—even powders. The various methods used to measure the contact angle are listed in Table 3.1, with a brief description of the technique. In all the methods, the solid is tested against a series of liquids and the angle θ of the liquid at the interface relative to the surface of the solid is measured. The sessile drop method is the most convenient and common technique to measure the contact angle. In this method, a drop of liquid of about 5 μL is placed on the surface and optics are used to measure the angle between the baseline of the drop and the tangent at the drop boundary. This static contact angle method is ideal for solids where one side has a different property from the other, or for curved surfaces, and can measure average θ as a function of time or temperature. In the dynamic contact angle technique, θ is measured while the volume of the drop is increasing until a plateau called "advancing contact angle" (θ_A) is reached. The "receding contact angle" (θ_R) is determined by immediately measuring the θ for successive removal of the equivalent volume of the fluid from the droplet just before the wetting is receding. Usually, θ for a liquid advancing across a surface is significantly higher than that for one receding from the surface (i.e., $\theta_A > \theta_R$) and the difference, $\theta_A - \theta_R$, is called contact angle hysteresis, as shown in Figure 3.3. On a tilted plane, a liquid drop can remain stuck despite gravity, due to contact angle hysteresis, i.e., if θ is larger at the front than at the rear of the drop. The capillary force, which exists due to the difference between the advancing angle and the receding angle, opposes the gravity force. In the "tilting plate method," θ_A and θ_R are measured as the surface is inclined until the drop starts rolling. Overall, contact angle measurement provides a simple way to index the surface properties, which allow comparison of various materials as well as preparing the surface of biomaterials for specific applications, such as cell spreading, etc.

TABLE 3.1
List of Methods for Contact Angle Measurements

Technique	Brief Description
Sessile drop	This method involves measurement of the contact angle optically and is used to estimate the wetting properties of a localized region on a solid surface. The angle between the baseline of the drop and the tangent of the drop boundary are determined. This technique is ideal for curved samples or when one side of the sample surface has different properties than the other side.
Dynamic Wilhelmy	This method requires uniform geometry for calculating average advancing and receding contact angles on solids. Both sides of the solid must have the same properties. Wetting force on the solid material is measured as the solid is submerged in, or withdrawn from, a liquid of given surface tension.
Single fiber Wilhelmy	This is a dynamic Wilhelmy method applied to single fibers to measure advancing and receding contact angles.
Powder contact angle	This procedure allows the measurement of average contact angle and adsorption speeds of powders and other porous species. The change in the weight as a function of time is measured.
Liquid homolog method (Zissman)	Called critical surface tension, it is based on measuring the contact angle of several liquids and plotting the cosine of the angle vs. surface tension of the liquids. The surface tension at which cosine of the contact angle is equal to one, obtained by extrapolation, is the critical surface tension of the solid.

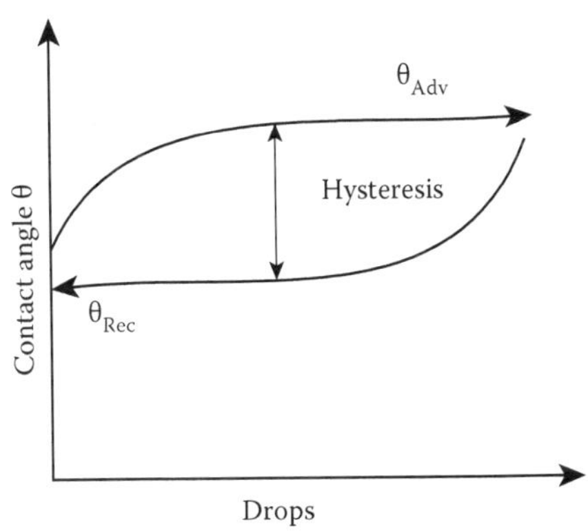

FIGURE 3.3
Contact angle plot showing the contact angle hysteresis. (Adapted with courtesy from Stein, J., University of Washington Engineered Biomaterials (UWEB), http://www.uweb.engr.washington.edu/research/tutorials/contact.html.)

3.3 Degradation of Biomaterials

The stability of biomaterials in the biological environment is a critical parameter for its biocompatibility. In fact, most biomaterials have been selected on the basis of their inertness, i.e., resistance to degradation. However, there are many active substances and components of the physiological environment that may have the potential to interact with and eventually degrade biomaterials. The degradation of biomaterials can have two broad consequences for biocompatibility (Williams 2003). Firstly, if the biomaterial is designed to be inert, then degradation can result in the loss of structural integrity, mostly with its eventual dissolution or removal, which is undesirable. But, if it is intentionally biodegradable, then it could be desirable. Secondly, the release of degradation products may affect the tissues, either locally or systemically when unintended, but the released products may have desirable and intended biological functions when intended. For example, degradation behavior can be exploited with the development of special materials to release active components, such as active molecules, enzymes, or growth factors during a specific degradation period. The degradation products from biomaterials may be of many different varieties. Metals may involve the release of soluble metal ions or particulate corrosion products and polymer may involve the release of small molecules resulting from depolymerization, fragments of polymer arising from heterogeneous degradation or release through leaching processes, additives used during polymerization and residual catalysts. Any of these degradation components can have an adverse effect on the surrounding tissue, which may take place over a prolonged period. Alternatively, the tissues that are often thought of as saline solutions as far as reactivity with synthetic materials is concerned may be more complex. For example, the inflammatory cells, which are the key feature of the tissue in response to a degrading material (Hunt et al. 1995), tend to produce a variety of active species, such as free radicals, peroxides, superoxides, and enzymes, all of which are able to influence or even initiate material degradation. Thus, there is a substantial implication that the degradation process and the tissue response to the degradation products are highly interdependent. Hence, understanding and assessments of the degradation process of biomaterials are necessary to prevent accidental degradation with improved biofunctionality and to develop new materials for the delivery of a variety of drugs, proteins, and genes (Black 1999). Degradation due to corrosion of biomaterials is one of the important parameters ensuring the quality of surgical implants and devices, which is discussed in the following section.

3.4 Corrosion of Biomaterials

In the absence of any reactions, the transfer of materials across the material–tissue interface is the basic response of the biomaterial–tissue interactions. This may cause swelling of the biomaterial if ions or fluid moves from the tissue into the biomaterial. The absorption of some component of the surrounding fluid may also cause the biomaterial to swell. The lipids present in the blood adsorbed by the silicone elastomer ball of the poppet-type aortic heart valves is an example of undesirable absorption that causes changes in color, volume, and mechanical properties like a reduction in wear resistance. If a component of the biomaterial dissolves in the surrounding biofluid or the fluid moves into the tissue, then the biomaterial is said to be leaching. Controlled leaching of biomaterials has been utilized in sustained drug delivery devices wherein the drug is diffused through a membrane from a drug reservoir of matrix through a barrier into the biological environment. However, released products from the unplanned leaching may effect undesirable local and systemic biological reactions. The coalescence of defects that are formed due to leaching into macroscopic voids may reduce the mechanical property, like the fracture strength of biomaterials. However, the effect due to leaching may be less pronounced than swelling.

Corrosion is the basic chemical reaction of the biomaterial with the hostile electrolytic environment in the human body resulting in its continued degradation to hydroxides, oxides, and other compounds. The clinical implication of the process of corrosion is that it can severely limit the fatigue life and ultimate strength of the material, leading to the mechanical failure of the implant. In the host, the released corrosion products may elicit an adverse biological reaction (e.g., discoloration, foreign body response), in some cases causing local pain and swelling in the region of the implant, in the absence of infection. Particularly for bone, the particulate corrosion and wear products may ultimately result in a cascade of events leading to periprosthetic bone loss. The slow release of excess metal species (especially chromium, cobalt, and nickel) is suspected to have a role in the induction of tumors, e.g., malignant fibrous histiocytoma. However, when toxicities (metabolic, bacteriological, immunological, or carcinogenic) of these elements are considered, they generally apply to soluble forms of the elements. The corrosion reaction of metallic biomaterials is briefly addressed in the following sections along with the dissolution of polymeric and ceramic biomaterials.

The human body presents a very aggressive environment in terms of corrosion with water, an abundant supply of dissolved oxygen, proteins, and a continuous flow of electrolytes of various ions, such as hydroxide and chloride. The two fundamental characteristics that decide why implant material corrodes involves the thermodynamic driving forces that cause corrosion (oxidation and reduction) reactions and the kinetic barriers to corrosion that limit the rate of these reactions. For metallic biomaterials, oxidation with the loss of electrons of the metal atom to form an ion, as expressed by Equation 3.1, is the basic reaction that occurs during corrosion:

$$M \rightarrow M^{n+} + ne^{-}. \tag{3.1}$$

The resulting free ions in the solution can migrate away from the metal surface or can form chemical species, such as metal oxides, chlorides, phosphates, etc. The species may form adherent compact oxide films or can precipitate away from the metal surface as nonadherent oxide, chloride, phosphate, or other particles. The thermodynamic driving force for all of these possible reactions is the free energy resulting from the oxidation of metal atoms to their ionic form, e.g., in the alloys used for orthopedic implants to their ionic form. Apart from the chemical driving force, the second source of energy occurs from the separation of the positive metal ions and the negative electrons, which contributes as the electrical double layer and creates an electrical potential across the metal–solution interface. This potential is the driving force for the oxidation of metals and at equilibrium, the electrical energy balances with chemical energy. This is the basis of the Nernst equation, which states that when metals are immersed in a solution, there is an electrical potential across the interface between the metal and the solution. This equilibrium potential is called the Nernst potential, which can be used to express a scale of tendency of metals to corrode, known as the electrochemical series, as shown in Table 3.2. The Nernst potentials are measured using an electrochemical cell with reference to a standard hydrogen electrode and the potential of this reference electrode is defined as zero. From their equilibrium potentials, the metals are ranked from most noble or least reactive (having positive potential) to most reactive or most base (having most negative potential). Metals like gold and platinum, etc., have corrosion resistance because their equilibrium potentials are very positive, indicating that they have little or no driving force for oxidation in aqueous solutions. Hence, in the human body, they tend to remain in metallic form indefinitely. But many metals that are used as orthopedic implants have more negative potentials and are therefore much more susceptible to corrosion. However, it should be noted that the potentials are across the metal–solution interface and are based only on thermodynamic considerations with the assumption that there is no barrier to the oxidation of the metals.

The corrosion of metallic biomaterials is also governed by the kinetic barriers to corrosion that prevent or impede corrosion by physical limitation of the rate at which oxidation or reduction processes can take place and not by energetic mechanisms. The formation of a compact oxide film on a metal surface, called passivation, is a well-known example of a kinetic limitation to

TABLE 3.2

Electrochemical Series for Selected Metals

Reaction			Potential (V)
Noble			
$Au^{3+} + 3e^-$	⇔	Au	1.42
$Pt^{2+} + 2e^-$	⇔	Pt	1.20
$Ag^+ + e^-$	⇔	Ag	0.80
$O_2 + 2H_2O + 4e^-$	⇔	OH^-	0.40
$Ti(OH)^{3+} + H^+ + e^-$	⇔	$Ti^{3+} + H_2O$	0.06
$H^+ + e^-$	⇔	$1/2\ H_2$	0.00
$Fe^{3+} + 3e^-$	⇔	Fe	−0.04
$Co^{2+} + 2e^-$	⇔	Co	−0.28
$Fe^{2+} + 2e^-$	⇔	Fe	−0.41
$Cr^{2+} + 2e^-$	⇔	Cr	−0.56
$Cr^{3+} + 3e^-$	⇔	Cr	−0.74
$2H_2O + 2e^-$	⇔	$2OH^-$	−0.83
$TiO_2 + 4H^+ + 4e^-$	⇔	$Ti + 2H_2O$	−0.86
$Ti^{2+} + 2e^-$	⇔	Ti	−1.60
$Mg^+ + e^-$	⇔	Mg	−2.37
Active			
$Na^+ + e^-$	⇔	Na	−2.71

Source: Compiled from Jacobs, J. J. et al., *J. Bone Joint Surg. Am.*, 80, 268, 1998. With permission.

corrosion. Passive oxide films are the best kinetic barriers to corrosion to prevent the migration of metal ions from the metal to the solution, the migration of anions from the solution to the metal, and the migration of electrons across the metal–solution interface. So, only those metals that have the capacity to spontaneously form a protective passive film on the metal surface to prevent transport of metal ions and electrons across the film are used as biomaterials. The passive films must be nonporous, fully cover the metal surface, and must have an atomic structure to prevent migration of ionic species across the metal oxide–solution interface to limit corrosion. As titanium dioxide is very close to stoichiometry, it has an increased resistance to ionic transport. For orthopedic applications, the oxide layer must also be able to remain on the material surface even with mechanical stressing or abrasion, such as fretting, micromotion, or applied stresses, which may cause the film to abrade or fracture. Rupturing of the oxide film exposes the unoxidized metal to solution. But such films tend to repassivate with large driving forces that are present for the oxidation process due to the removal of the kinetic barrier. So, for orthopedic applications, the mechanical stability of the passive oxide film and its ability to repassivate are essential for corrosion protection.

Although passivation inhibits corrosion and keeps the release of corrosion products at a very low level, due to the complex corrosive environment of the body, all implant materials undergo corrosion at some finite rate. The various types of corrosion that are pertinent to the biomaterials will be briefly explained below with examples: Uniform attack or overall general corrosion refers to the inevitable corrosion occurring to all the materials immersed in electrolytic solutions with the removal of the metal from the implants. However, its effect may not be noticed unless there is a significant loss of metal, but it reiterates that all materials have a finite corrosion rate *in vivo*. Generally, titanium and its alloys have lower overall corrosion rates when compared with stainless steel and cobalt-chromium alloys.

3.4.1 Galvanic Corrosion

Galvanic corrosion or couple corrosion occurs when two different metals are in physical contact in an ionic-conducting fluid medium, such as interstitial fluid or serum, because of the differences in their electrochemical potentials. In this two-metal corrosion, the metal that is less noble than the other becomes anodic and undergoes uniform attack. Hence, it is safe to assume that galvanic corrosion will occur in any dissimilar metal pair in acidic pH and the inappropriate use of the contact of dissimilar materials in many implant applications, such as a titanium-alloy screw in contact with a stainless-steel plate, a cobalt-alloy femoral head in contact with a titanium-alloy femoral stem, etc., should be avoided.

3.4.2 Crevice Corrosion

Crevice corrosion is a form of local corrosion due to oxygen depletion in a confined space, such as between a plate and screw head, incomplete fatigue crack, etc. The static nonflowing condition of the electrolyte at the crevice (a deep and narrow crack) leading to a concentration gradient of the metallic ions from the open end of the crevice seems to favor crevice corrosion; this is frequently observed in retrieved multipart internal fixation devices. So, appropriate design of the interface between the parts of an implant can often eliminate crevice corrosion.

3.4.3 Pitting Corrosion

Pitting corrosion is a special case of localized corrosion initiated by scratches, inclusions, or damages due to handling of the implant surface. Pitting refers to the formation of small cavities/holes at the surface of a material, which is attributed to the interaction of certain aggressive ions with the passive film at locations where it is defective or weak in nature. Thus, autocatalysis seems to play a major role in pitting rather than reduced oxygen content and static conditions as in crevice corrosion. The mechanism of pitting attack is shown in Figure 3.4, along with the formation and breakdown of passive oxide film (Mudali 2003). Pits constitute points of stress concentration

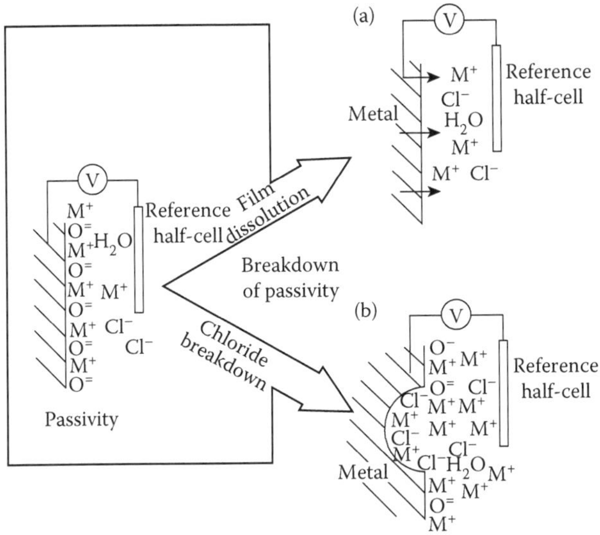

FIGURE 3.4
Schematic diagram on the breakdown of passivity: (a) metal undergoes general corrosion with film dissolution and (b) metal undergoes pitting corrosion.

and are dangerous to the extent that they can allow the formation of stress corrosion cracking (SCC) or fatigue cracks, leading to the failure of highly stressed implants. Cleanliness and careful of handling of multipart implants has declined the prevalence of these corrosion.

3.4.4 Intergranular Corrosion

Intergranular corrosion is a form of galvanic corrosion due to impurities and inclusions in an alloy, which are preferentially deposited between the grains during solidification. So, the grain and its boundary probably have different electrochemical potential resulting in an intergranular attack in a corrosive environment resembling crevice corrosion. Stainless steels are prone to intergranular corrosion if not properly heat treated due to sensitization. Welding of alloys often results in a compositional gradient because of local melting and resolidification, which can also lead to a variant of this process, called knife-edge attack. Proper heat treatment can prevent or reduce such corrosion.

3.4.5 Stress Corrosion

Stress corrosion occurs due to an increase in the chemical activity of metals under tensile stress. An electrochemical potential is created between stressed and unstressed regions of the same material, which accelerates the corrosion two to threefold over the uniform corrosion rate. Since the formation of a small crack will concentrate stress in a loaded structure, the stress corrosion tends to initiate cracks that grow rapidly, leading to implant fracture. The stress corrosion cracks extend between grains and have a branched structure compared to intergranular cracking. For example, the screw holes in fracture fixation plates will act as stress risers under load and will corrode at the expense of the surrounding less stressed material.

3.4.6 Fretting Corrosion

Fretting corrosion occurs at the contact area between materials under load when subjected to repeated, small relative surface motion in the body environment. In the presence of the relative motion (fretting) as induced for example by vibration, the passivating oxide layer may be removed by the rubbing action exposing the fresh, active metal to the corrosive environment. So, accelerated corrosion may occur with any combination of metals, depending on the nature of the fretting motion, the local solution chemistry, and the microstructure of the metals. The clinical consequence of the fretting corrosion lies not only as a major factor in crack initiation leading to implant failure, but with the large amount of corrosion products in adjacent tissues.

Overall, metallic biomaterials release cations by these corrosive reactions, which form a wide variety of organometallic complexes. Some of these complexes are soluble, while some have biological roles as trace elements. Others, even when they are in higher concentrations than the normal value or even small particles are released in the body. The rate of failure of the implant or its function due to corrosive attack is quite small. For nonmetallic materials such as ceramics and polymers, dissolution due to corrosion tends to dominate compared to the corrosive reactions of metallic biomaterials. But these soluble and particulate materials are also released. Interestingly, for some biomaterial applications, the release of the corrosion products is necessary for the successful functioning of the implant. For example, the contraceptive property of the copper intrauterine device (IUD) depends on the release of the copper ions due to corrosion in body fluids.

3.5 Methods of Corrosion Testing

Corrosion is the process of oxidation when moisture is present. In order for corrosion to occur, there needs to be a corrosive metal, water, and oxygen. The rate of corrosion differs from material to material. For example, Al is prone to corrode more than Fe. Au and Ag are less prone to corroding. Most corrosion occurs via electrochemical reactions at the interface between the metallic biomaterials and an electrolyte solution. A thin film of moisture present on a metal surface forms the electrolyte for corrosion. Electrochemical corrosion tests rely on electrochemical theory and electrochemical corrosion measurements to characterize corrosion damage and, where possible, estimate corrosion rates. Corrosion normally occurs at a rate determined by equilibrium between opposing electrochemical reactions. The first is the anodic reaction, in which a metal is oxidized, releasing electrons into the metal. The second is the cathodic reaction, in which a solution species is reduced, removing electrons from the metal. When these two reactions are in equilibrium, the flow of electrons from each reaction is balanced, and no net electron flow (i.e., electrical current) occurs. The potential of the metal is the means by which the anodic and cathodic reactions are kept in balance. Because corrosion occurs via electrochemical reactions, electrochemical techniques are ideal for the study of the corrosion processes.

Because corrosion of metallic biomaterials is an electrochemical process, the following are some of the accepted and standard electrochemical testing techniques employed for evaluating the corrosion performance of metallic biomaterials. These include American Society for Testing and Materials (ASTM) G5, G31, G61, F746, and F2129.

ASTM G5 is a standard reference test method for making potentiostaic and potentiodynamic anodic polarization measurements. The ASTM G5 standard is based on the testing of 430 stainless steel in 0.1 N sulfuric acid under a nitrogen purge condition at room temperature. The implant alloys are subject to very controlled surface preparation and passivation processes and do not exhibit the active–passive transition exhibited by the 430 stainless steel. While ASTM G5 is still the governing standard for corrosion testing of materials, it is imperative that the environment in which the tests are conducted and examples of data used to explain the analytical process be representative of the end application.

ASTM G31 is an immersion test procedure that typically requires extended exposure periods to evaluate the resistance of biomedical materials to corrosion. This test involves alternate immersions/drying in the form of cyclical tests. The acceleration of corrosion damage can be achieved from the length of immersion in the corrosive medium and other accelerating factors, such as temperature, humidity, and the chemical environment.

ASTM G61 is a modified test method of ASTM G5 standard. This standard test method is used for conducting cyclic potentiodynamic polarization measurements to examine susceptibility to localized pitting and crevice corrosion. Stainless steel and Ni-Ti alloy stents for cardiac, biliary, and prostatic medical applications are often tested by this method.

ASTM F746 is a standard test method for the determination of resistance to either pitting or crevice corrosion, or both, of metal and alloy-based surgical implants under specific conditions. It is generally used as a screening test to rank surgical implant alloys in order of their resistance to localized corrosion. The test conditions were intentionally designed to cause breakdown of Type 316L stainless steel, then considered acceptable for surgical implant use. The test results realized that those alloys that suffered localized attack during the test do not necessarily undergo localized corrosion when placed in the human body as an implant. This test method applies only to passive metallic biomaterials. Note that nonpassive metallic materials (other than noble alloys) are susceptible to general corrosion and are not normally suitable for medical use. The test consisted of placing a nonmetallic collar around a test specimen that was immersed in a 0.9% NaCl solution for 1 h while measuring the potential (E1) with respect to a saturated calomel electrode (SCE). After 1 h, the potential of the specimen was shifted to + 0.8 V (SCE) and held there for a specific period of time. Depending on the resulting current change over the course of time, the resistance to localized attack could be assessed.

ASTM F2129 is a standard test method for the determination of corrosion resistance of small metallic devices or components specific to implants. The devices that are anticipated to be evaluated by this test method include vascular stents, filters, support segments of endovascular grafts, cardiac occluders, aneurysm or ligation clips and staples. In this test method, the metallic device is exposed to simulated physiological solution and the open circuit (rest) potential (Er) is measured for 1 h. Then, a potentiodynamic polarization scan is made from an initial potential of negative 100 mV from the 1-h potential. The scan is in the positive, active to noble, direction at a rate of 0.16 mV per second. The scan is reversed when the current has reached two decades greater than that of the breakdown potential (Eb), which is defined as a rapid increase of current per increment of applied potential. The reverse scan is stopped when the current becomes less than the current in the forward scan (defined as the protection potential, Ep) or the potential reaches the initial potential. The data is plotted on an x-y semilogarithmic diagram with the current density on the x-axis and the potential vs. a SCE on the y-axis, allowing the resulting curve to be analyzed for key-point voltages and currents.

3.6 Biocompatibility of Implants

Biocompatibility is the primary requirement for any biomaterials or implants. The success of implants in the body depends on the biocompatibility, design, and properties of the material used. Biocompatibility has been defined as "the ability of a material to perform with an appropriate host response in a specific application" (Williams 1992). Fundamentally, it means the acceptance of the material by the surrounding tissues and by the body as a whole. It also clearly indicates that there is no absolute "biocompatibility" and it is not a property of the material, i.e., materials such as bioactive ceramics used for bone would not be safe in contact with flowing blood. The definition also calls for "appropriate host response," which in addition to the response of the host organism (local and systemic) to the implanted material or device, also incorporates lack of blood clotting, resistance to bacterial colonization and normal healing. As only few materials provoke no response from the body, a thin fibrous encapsulation with little or no chronic inflammation will then be biocompatible in such cases. Also, to achieve acceptance, the biocompatible materials should not irritate, cause abnormal inflammatory response, or provoke allergic or immunologic reactions and cancer. Additionally, the biomaterial must have adequate mechanical properties, such as strength, stiffness, and fatigue, and appropriate properties for its intended use, e.g., optical properties if the material is to be used in the eye. The design aspects, manufacturability, sterilizability, and long-term storage stability also play a role in compatibility.

International organizations give recommendations and standards for the manufacturing and testing of biomaterials, such as ISO 10993 (International Standards Organization), ASTM 1999 (American Society for Testing and Materials), etc. Government organizations also supervise biomaterial applications for human use, like the Food and Drug Administration of the USA (FDA) and US Pharmacopeia (USP) (ISO 10993, ASTM 1999, MDDI 1998). It should be noted that the FDA does not regulate the materials used in medical devices, but rather the devices themselves (FDA G95-1).

The biocompatibility of the material is a central factor in devices intended for use inside the body. There are two main factors that determine the biocompatibility of a material: the host reactions induced by the material and the degradation of the material in the body environment. The evaluation of biomaterials to determine that they will function in a biologically appropriate manner can be divided as *in vitro* (laboratory based) and *in vivo* (animal and clinical trials) test methods. The single most important function of biocompatibility tests is that it excludes materials that exert toxic or injurious effects on biological systems, i.e., materials that release anything in sufficient quantities that affect normal cellular biochemical functions, from killing the cells directly or indirectly through inhibition of metabolic pathways (Kirkpatrick 1990).

3.6.1 *In Vitro* Test Methods

The *in vitro* ("in glass" conditions; i.e., in laboratory glassware) tests are conducted outside the living system where certain environmental conditions, such as pH, temperature, cells, are maintained as necessary, while *in vivo* ("in live" conditions; i.e., in a live animal or human) tests are conducted within the normal physiological environments. The *in vitro* tests are quick and inexpensive initial screening methods. They involve the evaluation of mechanical, physical, chemical, and biological properties of materials. Emphasis is placed on studying environmental effects and manipulative procedures on materials. The principle component of the human body is water. Hence, the solubility characteristics of the biomaterial are evaluated in buffered solutions under physiological conditions of pH 7.4 and body temperature of 37°C. Most of the biomaterials in the medical devices are water-insoluble materials (polymers, metals, and ceramics), meaning that less than one part of the material is soluble in 10,000 parts of water. Often, the bone-bonding ability of a material is evaluated *in vitro* by the ability of hydroxyapatite (mineral component of bone) to form on its surface in a simulated body fluid (SBF) with ion concentrations nearly equal to human blood plasma (Kokubo 2006). This method is called a bioactivity test and is useful for predicting not only qualitatively, but also quantitatively, the *in vivo* bone bioactivity of the material. The bone bioactive materials can thus be effectively screened by the *in vitro* tests before animal testing, with a reduction in the number of animals used and the duration of animal experiments.

Basically, *in vitro* tests minimize the use of animals and evaluate the response (cytotoxicity) of the material to cells. The cell culture methods have been used for more than two decades to evaluate the biological compatibility of materials (Northup 1986). The term "cytotoxicity" means to cause toxic effects like death, alterations in cellular membrane permeability, enzymatic inhibition, etc., at the cellular level. Many of these cytotoxicity test methods are extensively accepted in biomaterial screening and quality control. A variety of cell types are used for the *in vitro* techniques, which differ in relative sensitivity and the time required to conduct the assay. Three primary cell culture assays/methods are used for evaluating cytotoxicity: direct contact, agar diffusion, and elution (also known as dilution) tests. Positive and negative controls are often included in the assays to ensure the operation and suitability of the test system. In the direct contact test method, the required amount of cell type is grown in cell culture flasks. The sample materials along with positive and negative controls are placed in direct contact with the cells and incubated for 24 h at 37°C. The sample is then removed and the cells are fixed and stained. The dead cells lose their adherence and the live cells adhere to the culture plate and to the sample. The toxicity is evaluated by examining microscopically for the presence of morphological changes, reduction in cell density, or lysis induced by the test material. The required amount of cells is grown in a culture medium initially in the agar diffusion test method. The cells are then spread on a culture medium containing 2% agar and the material is placed on the surface of the agar plate along with the controls. Following incubation for 1 day, the toxicity is evaluated by the cell loss under and around the periphery of the sample. In the elution test, an extract of the material is initially prepared by using 0.9% sodium chloride or serum-free culture medium. The extract in then added to the culture medium containing the cells. The viability of the cells is evaluated after incubation for two days.

The *in vitro* assessment tests are the primary screening tests for a wide variety of biomaterials used as implants or in medical devices. Once the cytotoxicity of the materials has been evaluated, more application-specific tests of the biomaterials are then performed. For example, a new material to be used as a scaffold in tissue-engineering applications would be initially tested for cytotoxicity, followed by specific assays to compare the growth rates of cells on the new material with other currently used materials. In general, *in vitro* cell culture test methods are more sensitive to toxic materials and have shown good correlations with animal assays. The major drawback is that it only evaluates intrinsic toxicity of the biomaterial and does not test the metabolic products that may have different toxic potential. But, in reality, the leachable chemicals are transported to the distant tissues that are metabolically active and the biological effect is that these chemicals are more clinically relevant (Northup 2004). Some of the other drawbacks of the *in vitro* test are that there is no local circulation; the cells are never more than ~100 microns from a capillary, the cell types tend to differentiate, and use antibiotics, fungicides. Overall, it can only test early and acute responses of biomaterial, minimizing the use of animals for tests as required by regulatory agencies.

3.6.2 *In Vivo* Test Methods

The *in vivo* test is a critical element in the development and implementation of implants for human use after satisfactory *in vitro* screening. The goal of the test is to expose the biomaterial to systemic physiological processes and the assessment of tissue compatibility of the biomaterials in animal models, to determine that the material performs as intended and presents no harm to the user. There is great range in animal anatomy, physiology, and biochemistry. So, the animal model that offers a reasonably parallel anatomical, physiological, or biochemical situation in humans is selected. The test is categorized by the nature of tissue contact of the biomaterial as surface (skin, mucosal membrane), external communicating (blood path), or implant (bone, blood) type, and duration of contact as limited ($\leq$ 24 h), prolonged (1–30 days), or permanent ($\geq$ 30 days). There are two types of *in vivo* tests: nonfunctional and functional. The implant in a specific shape floats passively in the tissue site in nonfunctional tests, while the interaction between the implant material and the biochemical implant environment are focused in functional tests.

Usually, the initial nonfunctional testing is carried out in soft tissue because soft tissue sites can be approached in animals with relatively minor surgery and the cytotoxic effects have a generality of action. The subcutaneous, intramuscular, intraperitoneal, transcortical (e.g., femur, cranium), and intramedullary (e.g., femur, tibia) are the most popular sites for the tests. The functional tests require that the implanted material be placed in the functional mode so that it experiences the real effects as a human implant. The biomaterial component of certain devices may fall into more than one category. So, a structured program that indicates required tests according to specific types of tissue contact and contact duration are provided by the regulatory bodies, such as ISO, ASTM, and USP (ISO 10993, ASTM 1999, MDDI 1998).

In the implantation test, the biological responses of the tissue induced by the biomaterial are determined by histological (microscopic) evaluation. The usual animals for short-term implantation tests up to 12 weeks are mice, rats, guinea pigs, or rabbits. Animals such as rats, guinea pigs, rabbits, dogs, sheep, and goats are used for long-term tests in subcutaneous tissue, muscle, or bone. The actual medical devices are evaluated in larger species, e.g., artificial hearts are tested in calves. Compared to nonfunctional tests, the functional tests are more complex and test animals have shorter life spans and higher metabolic rates than humans, which introduces additional uncertainty into the results. So, clinical testing seems to be the appropriate technique for the determination of the true biological performance of any implantable biomaterials (Black 1999).

3.7 Case Study

Copper metal, either as ions or as in copper complexes, have been used for centuries to disinfect liquids, solids, and human tissue. The ancient Greeks (400 BC) were the first to discover the sanitizing power of copper and prescribed copper for pulmonary diseases and for purifying drinking water. Whisky was produced in copper vessels in Scotland around 800 AD and this practice has continued to the present day. The sacred water of the river Ganga is stored in copper utensils in every Hindu household due to the antifouling and bacteriostatic properties of copper. By the eighteenth century, copper had come into wide clinical use for the treatment of mental disorders and afflictions of the lungs. Today, copper is considered safe to humans, as demonstrated by the widespread and prolonged use of copper IUDs by women from 1969 [Population Council]. The IUD is a small, flexible, plastic frame inserted into the uterine cavity to avoid pregnancy, as shown in Figure 3.5. The IUD mainly works by changing the intrauterine environment, making it spermicidal. In copper-containing intrauterine devices (Cu-IUD), copper wire or copper sleeves are put on the plastic frame (polyethylene frame). A monofilament polyethylene thread is tied at the tip of the T, to aid in detection and removal of the device as shown in Figure 3.6. The contraceptive action of Cu-IUD is based on the dissolution of copper in uterine secretions and the formation of cupric ions leads to the inactivation of sperm and the suppression of myometrial contractions. A sterile inflammation that is enhanced by copper is also considered (Moraa et al. 2002). As the IUD's contraceptive action is local, within the uterine cavity, it is popular with users as there is no associated weight gain or other hormonal side effects.

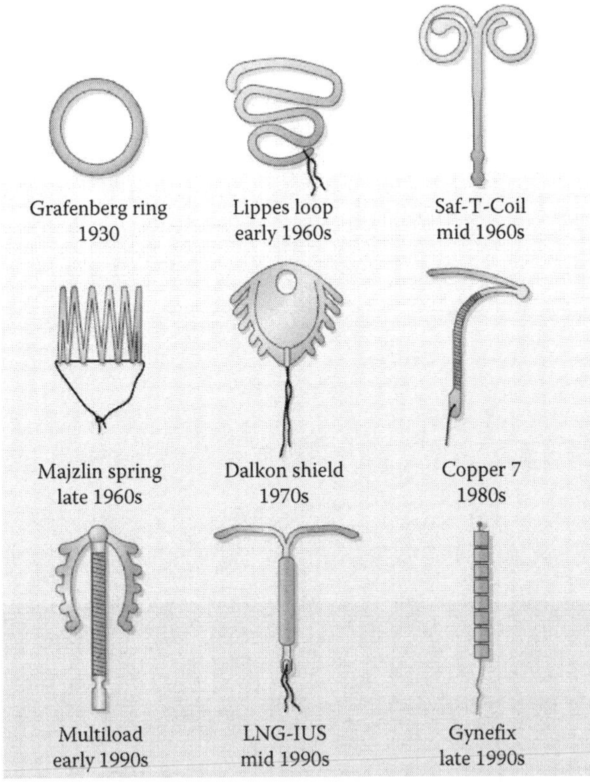

FIGURE 3.5
Developments of intrauterine devices through the twentieth century. Dates represent roughly the time of first availability in the U.K. or USA. (Adapted with courtesy from Glasier, A., www.nature.com/fertility.)

The various types of Cu-IUDs differ from each other by the amount of copper. The initial Cu-IUDs were wound with 200–250 mm^2 wire (Copper T 200). The Copper T 200 is the first of the Cu-IUDs that combined a plastic IUD in the shape of a "T" and the contraceptive action of intrauterine copper (Population Council). Modern Cu-IUDs are much smaller with most having a central frame made of polyethylene and containing more copper in the form of solid tubal sleeves rather than wire. These come in varying shapes and sizes, including a frameless device. Most devices now have a surface area of 300 mm^2 copper, making them a highly effective, reversible, inexpensive contraceptive option for women. This increases the efficacy and lifespan, as in Copper T 380A, which is a flexible polyethylene T-shaped frame holding 380 mm^2 of exposed surface area of copper (approximately 66.5 mg of copper on each of its transverse arms and 176 mg of copper wire coiled around its vertical shaft). The Copper T 380 slimline has copper sleeves flushed at the ends of horizontal arms to facilitate easier

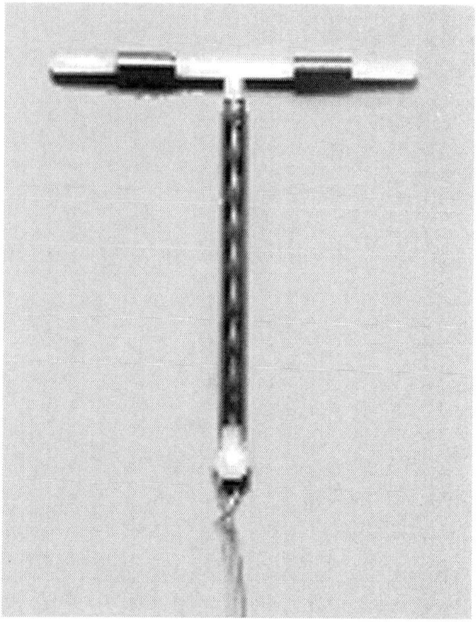

FIGURE 3.6
Copper T intrauterine device. (The Population Council, Inc., USA. *Momentum*, New York, 5, 2002. With permission.)

loading and insertion. The IUD frame also contains barium sulphate, thus making it radio-opaque. The Copper T 380Ag is identical to 380A except that the copper wire on the stem has a silver core to prevent fragmentation and extend the life span of the copper. Multiload 375 has 375 mm^2 of copper wire wound around its stem. The flexible arms are designed to minimize expulsions.

The Copper T 380A IUD is seen as the gold standard and the preferred choice for most women. Copper wire is wound around the vertical polyethylene arm and an additional copper collar is placed on each of the two transverse arms. The more surface area of exposed copper results in immediate contraception with very low failures and this efficacy lasts for at least 10 years. The pregnancy rate associated with the use of IUDs containing 380 mm^2 copper is very low (less than one pregnancy per 100 women during the first year and during each subsequent year) and there is no evidence of a delay in the return of fertility following removal or expulsion of IUDs. Thus, Cu-IUDs are an ideal choice for family spacing and as a contraceptive method once a family is complete. The copper IUDs also seem to have additional noncontraceptive benefits, such as a 50–60% reduction in the risk of endometrial adenocarcinoma regardless of the duration of use and age at first and last use. Continuous Cu-IUD use is known to cause a significant reduction in endometrial mitotic activity and endometrial estrogen receptor concentration. Also, IUD use causes an intense local inflammatory reaction along with complete endometrial shedding every menses. One or more of these factors seems to play a role for the noncontraceptive benefits of Cu-IUDs (Mansour 2007).

3.8 Summary

Corrosion of biomaterials is a pertinent clinical issue because success of the surgery depends on the performance of the implants. Localized corrosion through galvanic corrosion, crevice formation, pitting, intergranular corrosion, corrosion cracking, corrosion fatigue, and fretting and wear corrosion are the most prevalent corrosion types that cause the medical implants to fail from their indented function. Improving the surface properties of the implants by surface modification is one of the ways to reduce the corrosion and to increase their bioactive performance in the living environment. In spite of a few complex and complicated clinical results, owing to the corrosion of implants and the biocompatibility of their by-products, innovative technological developments have been taking place to better provide suitable corrosion resistance biomaterials with minimal reaction and rejection by the host tissues.

Glossary

Biocompatibility: The ability of a material to perform with an appropriate host response in a specific application.

Biodegradation: A process by which substances are broken down by living organisms.

Contact angle: An angle at which a liquid interface meets the solid surface.

Corrosion: A process that leads to the breaking down of essential properties in a material due to chemical or biochemical reaction with its surroundings.

Cytotoxicity: The degree to which something is toxic to living cells.

Enzymes: Enzymes are biomolecules (e.g., proteins) that function as biochemical catalysts.

Histology: The study dealing with the microscopic anatomy of cells and tissues.

Hydrophilic: An important property of biomaterials; means "water loving." Hydrophilic substances are attracted to and dissolve well in water.

Hydrophobic: An important property of biomaterials; means "water hating." Hydrophilic substances are repelled by water.

Inflammation: A biological process in which the body reacts to infection due to harmful stimuli.

Intrauterine device: A birth control device placed in the uterus, often called an IUD.

***In vitro*:** A biological study performed in the laboratory. In other words, outside the living body.

***In vivo*:** A biological study performed inside the living body.

Metabolism: A series of biochemical reactions that occur in living organisms in order to maintain life.

Toxicity: The measure to which a substance is able to damage an exposed organism.

Wettability: The contact angle between a droplet of the liquid in thermal equilibrium on a horizontal surface.

EXERCISES

3.1 Why does the surface of a material have more unique properties than its bulk?

3.2 How are contact angle measurements used to determine the surface energy of a solid?

3.3 How is the wettability of a solid characterized?

3.4 What are the consequences of the degradation of a biomaterial?

3.5 What are the driving forces for the corrosion of implant materials?

3.6 What are the different types of localized corrosion observed in surgical implants?

3.7 How is the corrosion of biomaterials avoided?

3.8 What is the difference between *in vitro* and *in vivo* studies?

3.9 What tests are performed to evaluate the cytotoxicity of a material?

3.10 What design aspects are used in a Cu-IUD device?

References

ASTM. 1999. http://www.astm.org/cgibin/SoftCart.exe/DATABASE.CART/MARKETINGCODES/HC2.htm?U+mystore+kkjr2104.

http://www.blc.arizona.edu/Molecular%5FGraphics/DNA%5FStructure.

http://www.people.eku.edu/ritchisong/301notes1.htm.

http://biology-pages.info.

http://skincare.dermis.net.

ASTM. 1999. *Corrosion testing and evaluation, STP 1000*, ed. R. Baboian and S. W. Dean. Philadelphia, PA: American Society for Testing and Materials.

Black, J. 1999. *Biological performance of materials: Fundamentals of biocompatibility*. 3rd ed. New York: Marcel Dekker.

ISO. 10993. http://www.iso.ch/iso/en/CatalogueDetailPage.CatalogueDetail?CSNUMBER=37875.

Jacobs, J. J. et al. 1998. Corrosion of metal orthopaedic implants. *J. Bone Joint Surg. Am.* 80:268.
Kokubo, T. and H. Takadama. 2006. How useful is SBF in predicting in vivo bone bioactivity? *Biomaterials* 27:2907.
Kirkpatrick, C. J. and C. Mittermayer. 1990. Theoretical and practical aspects of testing potential biomaterials in vitro. *J. Mat. Sci.: Mat. Med.* 1:9.
Mansour, D. 2007. Copper IUD and LNG IUS compared with tubal occlusion. *Contraception* 75:S144.
MDDI. 1998. http://www.devicelink.com/mddi/archive/98/01/023.html.
Mora, N., Cano, E., Mora, E. M. et al. 2002. Influence of pH and oxygen on copper corrosion in simulated uterine fluid. *Biomaterials*, 23:667–71.
Mudali, U. K. et al. 2003. Corrosion of bioimplants. *Sadhana* 28:601.
Murugan, R. and S. Ramakrishna. 2005. Development of nanocomposites for bone grafting. *Comp. Sci. Tech.* 65:2385–2406.
———. 2006a. Nanoengineered biomimetic bone-building blocks. In *Handbook of molecular building blocks for nanotechnology*, ed. G. A. Mansoori, T. F. George, L. Assoufid, and G. Zhang, 301. Germany: Springer-Verlag.
———. Nanophase biomaterials for tissue engineering. In *Tissue, cell, and organ engineering*. Vol. 9 of *Nanotechnologies for the life sciences*, ed. S. S. R. Challakumar, 216–56. Weinheim: Wiley-VCH.
Northup, S. J. 1986. Mammalian cell culture models. In *Handbook of biomaterials evaluation*, ed. A. F. von Recum, 209–25. New York: Macmillan.
———. 2004. In vitro assessments of tissue compatibility. In *Biomaterials science: An introduction to materials in medicine*, ed. B. D. Ratner, A. S. Hoffman, F. J. Schoen, and J. E. Lemons, 357–67. San Diego, CA: Elsevier Academic Press.
Population Council, Inc., USA. 1995–2010. http://www.popcouncil.org/biomed/cut380.html.
Sharan, D. 1999. The problem of corrosion in orthopaedic implants. *Ortho. Update (India)* 9:1.
Sklodowska, A. et al. 1999. The method of contact angle measurement and estimation of work adhesion in bioleaching of metals. *Biol. Proc. Online* 1:114.
Stein, J. 1995–2010. http://www.uweb.engr.washington.edu/research/tutorials/contact.html.
The Population Council, Inc., USA. 2002. *Momentum*, 5. New York.
Williams D. F., ed. 1992. *Materials science and technology. A comprehensive treatment. Medical and dental materials*, Vol. 14. New York: VCH.
Williams, D. F. 2003. Biomaterials and tissue engineering in reconstructive surgery. *Sadhana* 28:563.

Further Reading

Fontana, M. G. and N. D. Greene. 1987. *Corrosion engineering*. New York: McGraw-Hill.
Glasier, A. www.nature.com/fertility.
Hench, L. L. and E. C. Ethridge. 1982. *Biomaterials: An interfacial approach*. New York: Academic Press.

Kruger, J. 1979. Fundamental aspects of corrosion of metallic implants. In *Corrosion and degradation of implant materials*, ASTM STP 684, ed. B. C. Syrett, and A. Acharya, 107–113. Baltimore, MD: American Society for Testing and Materials.

Park, J. P. and R. S. Lakes. 1992. *Biomaterials: An introduction*, 2nd ed. New York: Plenum Press.

Population Council USA., http://www.popcouncil.org/biomed/cut380.html.

Shreir, L. L. R. A. Jarman, and G. T. Brustein. 1994. *Corrosion*. Vol. 1, *Metal/environment reactions*. Vol. 2, *Corrosion control*. 3rd ed. London: Butterworth Heinemann.

Silver, F. H. 1994. *Biomaterials medical devices and tissue engineering: An integrated approach*. London: Chapman & Hall.

4

Failure and Tribology of Biomaterials

4.1 Introduction

As discussed in the previous chapters, materials that are used in the fabrication of medical implants or devices must not only be biologically compatible, but also mechanically strong enough to endure *in vivo* mechanical stimulus upon implantation, particularly to suit them in load-bearing orthopedic and dental applications. An understanding of the basic mechanics of biomaterials is therefore important to both the development of new biomaterials and the selection of appropriate materials for a specific structural application. Mechanical behaviors, in particular deformation, fracture, fatigue, and tribological aspects, of structural biomaterials are considered the most important characteristics responsible for the success of long-term biomedical implants or devices. The implants or devices may be of metal, ceramic, polymer, or their composites. Among them, metals are often used in load-bearing applications, either in monolithic or in composite form, primarily due to their superior strength. For instance, titanium (Ti) and Ti-based alloys are extensively used in the manufacture of prosthetic devices for use in humans, owing to their tissue compatibility and mechanical reliability. The mechanical properties of pure Ti and its alloys are given in Table 4.1 (Niinomi 1998). Although several Ti-based alloys have been developed in recent years, Ti-6Al-4V is one of the well-established alloys widely used in orthopedic applications, particularly hip replacement surgery, owing to its high strength, high resistance to fatigue and wear, low specific weight, excellent corrosion resistance, exceptional biocompatibility, and it also develops a good interfacial strength with host tissues. Some of the prosthetic devices, such as hip joints, bone plates, screws, and dental post, made from Ti-based biomaterials are shown in Figure 4.1. However, the biomedical community often experiences failure of biomaterials to a variety of loading conditions upon implantation, which will be discussed in Section 4.13 with clinical examples. This is because biomaterials are subject to forces (loads) when they were implanted at the load-bearing sites. For instance, mechanical mismatch between the metallic implant and bone tissue could result in uneven stress distribution at the bone–metal interface. This is called stress-shielding effect.

TABLE 4.1

Mechanical Properties of Pure Titanium (Ti) and Its Alloys

Alloy	Young's Modulus (GPa)	Yield Strength (MPa)	Ultimate Strength (MPa)	Ultimate Strain (%)
Ti pure – Grade 1	102.7	170	240	24
Ti pure – Grade 2	102.7	275	345	20
Ti pure – Grade 3	103.4	380	450	18
Ti pure – Grade 4	104.1	485	550	15
Ti-6Al-4V (annealed)	110–114	825–869	895–930	6–10
Ti-6Al-7Nb	114	880–950	900–1050	8–15
Ti-5Al-2.5Fe	112	895	1020	15
Ti-5Al-1.5B	110	820–930	925–1080	15–17
Ti-15Zr-4Nb-4Ta-0.2Pd (annealed)	99	693	715	28
Ti-15Zr-4Nb-4Ta-0.2Pd (aged)	94	806	919	18
Ti-13Nb-13Zr (aged)	79–84	836–908	973–1037	10–16
Ti-12Mo-6Zr-2Fe (annealed)	74–85	1000–1060	1060–1100	18–22
Ti-15Mo (annealed)	78	544	874	21
Ti-15Mo-5Zr-3Al (solubilized)	80	838	852	25
Ti-15Mo-5Zr-3Al (aged)	80	1000–1060	1060–1100	18–22
Ti-15Mo-2.8Nb-0.2Si (annealed)	83	945–987	979–999	16–18
Ti-35.3Nb-5.1Ta-7.1Zr	55	547	597	19
Ti-29Nb-13Ta-4.6Zr (aged)	80	864	911	13.2

Source: Reprinted from Niinomi, M., *Mater. Sci. Eng.*, A243, 231, 1998. With permission from Elsevier.

The part of the bone not stressed is subject to necrosis that eventually causes implant loosening and more susceptibility to fracture. In this regard, one has to be well versed in the fundamental aspects of biomechanics while designing the structural biomaterials for a given application, as it is an important tool in improving the mechanical performance and durability of biomedical implants. The following sections describe the fundamental aspects of deformation, fracture, fatigue, and tribological behaviors from the biomaterials point of view.

4.2 Deformation Mechanics

The mechanical behavior of materials may be best described by integrating basis phenomena of deformation and fracture produced by an applied force. The deformation or strain can be produced by an applied stress. Such behavior can be plotted on a stress–strain diagram. A schematic of stress–strain relationship is illustrated in Figure 4.2, which represents how

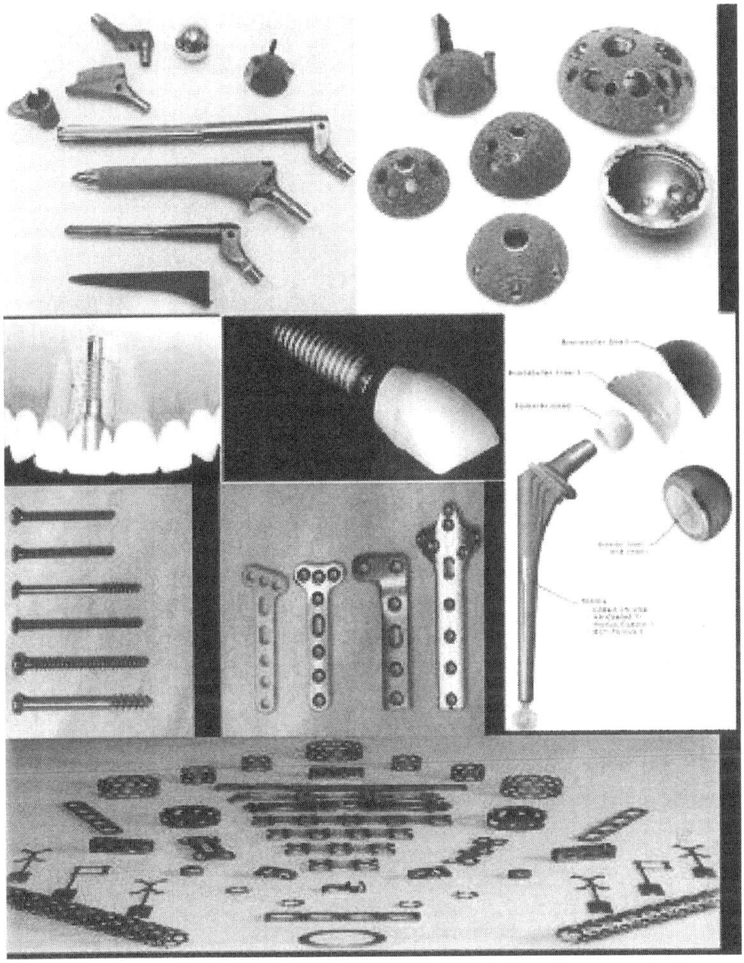

FIGURE 4.1
Biomedical implants made of titanium (Ti)-based biomaterials. (Adapted with courtesy from http://images.google.com/images?um=1&hl=en&q=implants+titanium.)

a typical ductile material undergoes different stages of deformation phenotypes. It should be noted that all solid materials could be deformed when subjected to external force. The force on materials can be externally applied in three different ways, namely, tension, compression, and shear. As a result, solid materials tend to either deform or to fracture, depending upon the strength of the force applied. Deformation is therefore defined as changes in the shape and size of a material due to an external mechanical force. Deformation of material can be broadly classified into two types, namely elastic and plastic, depending on the size and geometry of the solid material, and the external mechanical forces applied. The deformation is called elastic if the material is capable of returning to its original shape and size

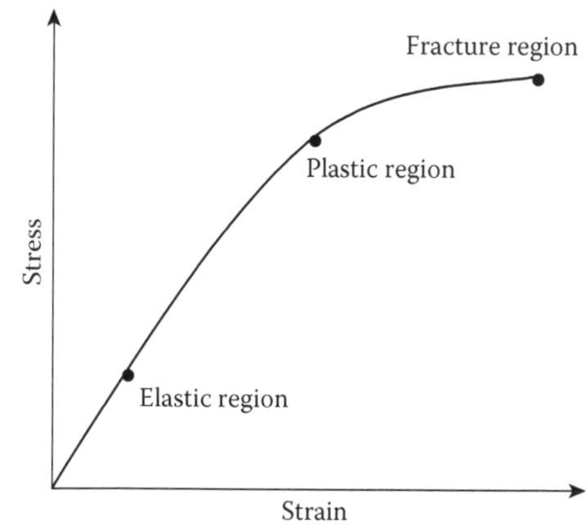

FIGURE 4.2
Schematic representation of deformation changes under external force.

upon removal of the external mechanical force. The deformation is called plastic (also called inelastic) if the material is unable to return to its original shape and size even if the external force is completely removed. The following subsections describe these two types of deformation with illustrated examples.

4.2.1 Elastic Deformation

A temporary change in the shape and size of a material, due to an external force, that is capable of gradually restoring its equilibrium position is called elastic deformation of the particular material. This type of deformation involves stretching of atomic bonds within the solid material but the bonds are not broken, so that the material is capable of snapping back to its original shape and size. A rubber band is a typical example of an elastic deformation because it changes in shape and size upon applying force and is also capable of rapidly returning to its original shape and size when the force is removed. There are several materials that undergo elastic deformation, including certain thermoplastic polymers (e.g., polyurethane) and metals (e.g., aluminium).

The elastic deformation is governed by Hooke's law, which states that strain is proportional to applied stress in an elastic material. For example, if you consider a bar that is subjected to external mechanical force, then the elongation of the bar can be said to be directly proportional to the tensile force and the length of the bar, and inversely proportional to the cross-sectional area and the elastic modulus (also called Young's modulus) of the bar. Therefore, stress can be written as

$$\delta = P\iota/AE. \tag{4.1}$$

Here, P is the tensile force responsible for the extension of the bar, ι is the length of the bar, A is the cross-sectional area of the bar, and E is the Young's modulus of the bar.

The stress can be considered to be the force per unit area, and thus it can be written as

$$\sigma = P/A.$$

If this stress equation is substituted into Equation 4.1, then it becomes

$$\delta = \sigma\iota/E.$$

By rearranging the stress equation, we get

$$\sigma = \delta E/\iota.$$

The strain or the elongation of the bar per unit length can be written as

$$\varepsilon = \delta/\iota.$$

According to Hooke's law, the stress can also be written as

$$\sigma = E\varepsilon,$$

$$E = \sigma/\varepsilon.$$

Here, σ is the applied stress, E is the Young's modulus, and ε is the resulting strain. If the modulus relationship is not linear, then E can be defined alternatively as the local slope.

That is,

$$E = d\sigma/d\varepsilon.$$

Note that this stress–strain relationship only applies to elastic materials, not all materials.

4.2.2 Plastic Deformation

The deformation is called plastic if the material is unable to return to its original shape and size even if the applied force is completely released. Therefore, unlike elastic deformation, plastic deformation is not a reversible process, which means the change that occurred due to the deformation is permanent. However, any material that reaches plastic deformation must have undergone elastic deformation. In certain types of materials, the elastic behavior ends when the material reaches its yield strength (YS). Notice that stress at the yield point is called yield stress. At this point, plastic deformation begins. So, the yield stress measures the resistance to plastic deformation of a material. Here, Hooke's law does not apply at the yield stress because shear stress exceeds shear YS. That is why in Section 4.2.1 we mentioned that Hooke's law only applies to elastic materials, not all materials. Some polymers (e.g., polystyrene), ceramics (e.g., strontium titanate), and metals (e.g., Cu, Ag, and Au) are notable plastic deformation materials.

Unlike elastic deformation, the primary reason for the cause of plastic deformation is the motion of dislocations, which involves breaking of atomic bonds within the solid material. Plastic deformation in metals and other crystalline materials is closely associated with their strain hardening. The larger the deformation, the higher the metal strength and the lower the reverse of the metal's plasticity. The plasticity of a metal permits it to be shaped into various useful forms that are retained even after the applied forces have been removed. Plastic deformation of metals requires an understanding of (i) the mechanism by which plastic deformation occurs in metals, (ii) the way in which different metals respond to a variety of applied loads, and (iii) the relation between the internal structure of a metal and its ability to plastically deform under a given set of conditions. Most metals and alloys that can undergo significant amounts of plastic deformation have their atoms orderly packed in a crystal structure (crystalline materials). The primary step in the plastic deformation of crystalline metals is the translation or slip of one part of the crystal with respect to the other across one of a set of crystallographically equivalent planes (called slip plane), and in one of several possible crystallographically equivalent directions (called slip direction). The particular direction and plane orientation differ from one metal to another, depending on the crystalline structure, the atom packing, and the temperature. Metals with equivalent crystal structures have the tendency to exhibit a similar kind of plastic response to the applied stresses, even though the actual strength and temperature response will differ from one metal to another. When a metal consists of a single crystal, it deforms anisotropically when subjected to stress, depending on the orientation of the operative slip system. Grain size and shape of a material also greatly influences the deformation behavior in metals.

4.3 Deformation Analysis of Biomaterials

The quantitative understanding of deformation behaviors, such as elastic and plastic, helps biomaterialists predict the mechanical stability of metallic implants used for biomedical applications, and thus one can easily choose the right implants with the required durability and longevity. The elastic and plastic deformation behaviors of several biomaterials have long been investigated. In a notable study, Zhang et al. (2001) determined both the elastic and plastic deformation of Ti-6Al-4V substrates, either as such or surface modified ones, quantitatively from the data of tensile and compression measurements. Hydroxyapatite (HA) was chosen as a coating material for surface modification. The authors have introduced a novel approach that combines the indentation tests (Hertzian indentation) with nonlinear finite element modeling (FEM) in order to estimate the elastic/plastic constitutive equation (i.e., stress/strain relation) of HA-coated Ti-6Al-4V substrates. Hertzian indentation tests were performed on both Ti-6Al-4V (as a control) and HA-coated Ti-6Al-4V substrates under the load-control mode using a universal testing machine. The indentation stress as a function of the indentation strain was obtained from the measurements, and simulations for the Hertzian indentation measurements were performed by FEM.

The FEM simulations of the indentation stress and indentation strain curves of test substrates are shown in Figure 4.3 (Zhang 2001). The results indicate that the Ti alloy exhibits higher resistance to elastic and plastic deformation than the free-standing HA coatings. The poor resistance to plastic deformation in the HA coatings is partially attributed to their microscopic pores and micro cracks, which were formed from the coating process. At low strain levels, the curves of HA-coated Ti-6Al-4V substrates initially coincide with that of the corresponding free-standing HA coating, and then with increasing load, gradually deviate from it and approach that of Ti alloy. This tendency is more obvious among the 90-μm thick coating

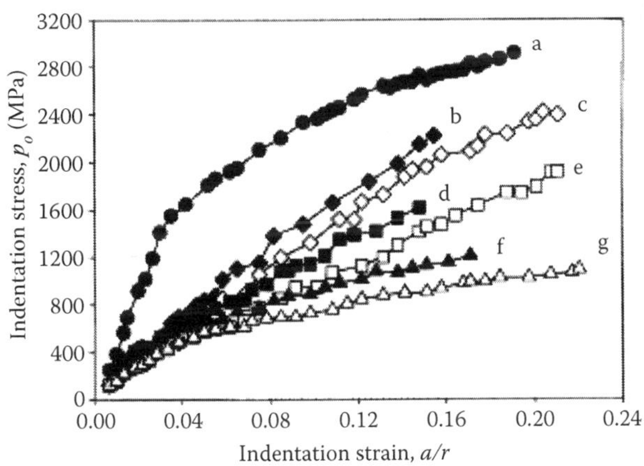

FIGURE 4.3
Comparison of FEM simulation: (a) Ti-6Al-4V, (b) posttreated 90-μm thick HA/Ti-6Al-4V, (c) as-sprayed 90-μm thick HA/Ti-6Al-4V, (d) posttreated 200-μm thick HA/Ti-6Al-4V, (e) as-sprayed 200-μm thick HA/Ti-6Al-4V, (f) free-standing posttreated HA coating, and (g) free-standing as-sprayed HA coating. (Reprinted from Zhang, C., Leng, Y., and Chen, J., *Biomaterials*, 22, 1357, 2001. With permission from Elsevier.)

TABLE 4.2

RO Equation Parameters of Plasma-Sprayed HA Coatings

Coating Crystallinity (%)	E (GPa)	σ_0 (MPa)	α	n
10	70.8	120	0.45	3
80	95.0	140	0.45	3

Source: Reprinted from Zhang, C., Leng, Y., and Chen, J., *Biomaterials*, 22, 1357, 2001. With permission from Elsevier.

substrates than the 200-μm thick ones. This phenomenon is rational and predictable because the effect of substrates on the mechanical behavior of coating systems should be more evident with increasing indentation load and reduced coating thickness. The elastic/plastic deformation of HA coatings on Ti-6Al-4V substrates can be quantitatively described by the Ramberg–Osgood (RO) equations. The RO equation of plasma-sprayed HA coatings on a Ti-6Al-4V substrate, estimated by combining indentation tests and FEM, can be written as:

$$\varepsilon = \sigma/E + A\sigma^3/E,$$

where $A = 2.296 \times 10^{-17}$ or 3.125×10^{-17} Pa^{-2} and $E = 95.0 \times 10^9$ or 70.8×10^9 Pa for coatings with crystallinity of 80 or 10 wt.%, respectively (see Table 4.2) (Zhang 2001). Notice that this equation is independent of coating thickness. The posttreated coating with higher crystallinity exhibits higher resistance to elastic and plastic deformation, as indicated by the RO equation. The quantitative analysis investigated in this study provides insights into coating deformation behavior, which could help to predict the mechanical behaviors of coated metallic systems as well as to identify their failure mechanism. Note that surface-coated metallic biomaterials are the most used hip joint system in load-bearing orthopedics.

4.4 Fracture Mechanics

Fracture (also called rupture) is a phenomenon wherein a structural material tends to break into two or more pieces with respect to an external mechanical force applied. Fracture behavior of structural biomaterials is one of the important characteristics for use in load-bearing applications. An understanding of the basic concept and methods of fracture behavior could help in designing mechanically enhanced biomedical implants or devices. Fracture is generally considered a complex process that includes several steps, such as crack initiation, crack nucleation, crack propagation, and finally fracture formation. To better understand the complex nature of fracture, one must know the stress needed to initiate the crack and the distribution of internal stress

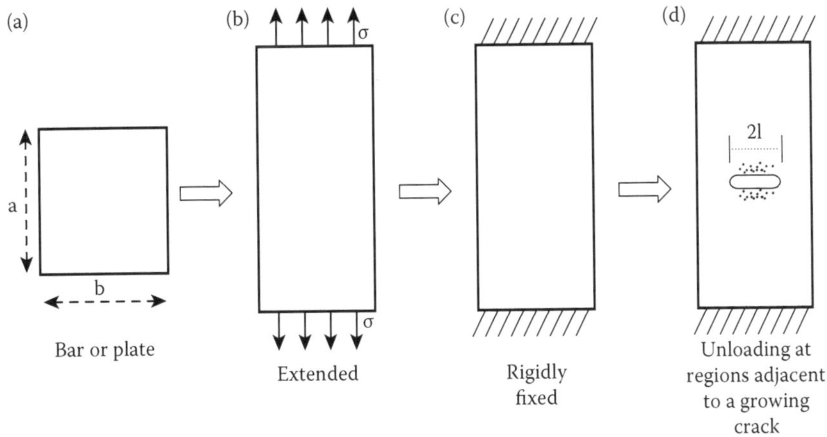

FIGURE 4.4
A plate with a crack growing with an applied stress. (Modified from Parton, V. Z., *Fracture mechanics: From theory to practice*, Gordon and Breach Science, Philadelphia, PA, 1992.)

within the solids, as shown in Figure 4.4 (Parton 1992). Each of these stages occurs progressively over time, depending on the strength of the applied mechanical force.

Fracture mechanics is the subfield of materials science and engineering that deals with how the structural materials break under the action of stress and strain. Fracture mechanics was introduced in the 1920s by A. A. Griffith, who wanted to explain why structures fail when containing a crack, and he extensively discussed the notion of critical crack length. Griffith postulated that the fracture occurs when the energy release rate exceeds the rate that energy is required during crack propagation. That is, if the change in elastic strain energy due to crack extension is larger than the energy required creating new crack surfaces, crack propagation will take place. Griffith's theory of failure is based on the assumption that the low order of tensile strength in common materials is due to the presence of small cracks or flaws. Actual stresses may occur around these cracks, which are of the order of magnitude of molecular cohesion values, while the average tensile strength may be quite low. Griffith's theory should not be confused with Mohr's theory. Notice that Mohr's theory (also known as the Coulomb–Mohr theory) predicts that failure of materials is due to failure in shear, whereas Griffith's theory postulates that it is due to failure at crack tips.

In the 1940s, Irwin extended Griffith's theory and postulated that, in ductile materials, the energy due to plastic deformation must be added to the surface energy associated with the creation of new crack surfaces. He recognized that the surface energy is often negligible compared to the energy associated with plastic deformation. In the 1950s, Irwin made another significant contribution when he introduced two new terms, by modifying Griffith's solids theory, namely "stress intensity," which replaced strain energy release rate and "fracture toughness," which replaced surface weakness energy. Note that the term stress intensity is not to be confused with stress concentration of Griffith's theory. The stress concentration is how the stress is amplified at a crack tip, whereas the stress intensity is used to describe the distribution of stress around a particular flaw. This term is used when investigating modes of fracture (K_{Ic}), in particular, mode I fracture. Details of fracture toughness of biomaterials are discussed in Sections 4.7 and 4.8.

According to the modified Griffith's theory, the strain energy release rate of a rectangular plate with a crack perpendicular to the load can be written as

$$G = \pi\sigma^2 a/E.$$

Here, G is the strain energy release rate, σ is the applied stress, a is half the crack length, and E is the Young's modulus.

The above equation can be rearranged as

$$\sigma^2 = EG/\pi a,$$

$$\sigma = \sqrt{EG/\pi a}.$$

At fracture $G=G_c$, the critical stress required for the crack to propagate in the plane-stress situation can be written as

$$\sigma_c = \sqrt{EG_c/\pi a}.$$

Here, σ_c is the critical stress at fracture, G_c is the critical strain energy rate, a is half the crack length, and E is the Young's modulus.

In the case of plane-strain situation, we need to introduce the factor $(1-\nu^2)$ because of the confinement in the direction of thickness of the plate.

Therefore,

$$\sigma_c = \sqrt{EG_c/\pi a(1-\nu^2)}.$$

From the plane-stress and plane-strain equations, we get

$$G_c = 2(\nu_s + \nu_p).$$

If $G \geq G_c$, the crack propagation will take place. Griffith postulated that the condition for the crack to propagate is that the energy released must be sufficient for the destruction of a material when G is equal or greater than a critical value G_c. Note that this condition applies only to elastic and brittle materials, in which there won't be any noticeable sign of plastic deformation.

4.5 Classification of Fracture

Depending on the ability of a material to undergo plastic deformation before fracture, the fracture can be classified into two types: (i) ductile fracture and (ii) brittle fracture. These two fractures are the best-known failure modes of load-bearing structural biomaterials. The basic difference is, however, that in ductile materials, an extensive plastic deformation and energy absorption (i.e., toughness) takes place before fracture occurs. On the other hand, in brittle materials, a little plastic deformation and low energy absorption takes place before fracture. Figure 4.5 schematically describes basic fracture morphologies and how they occur in different types of materials (Mayers 1999). It can be seen from Figure 4.5 that two modes of crack propagation

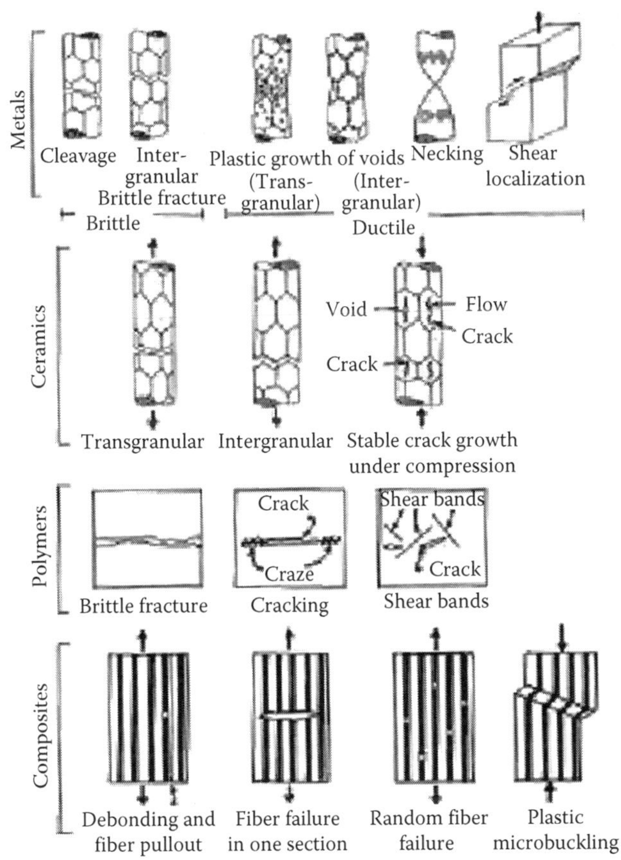

FIGURE 4.5
Schematic representation of fracture morphologies and how they occur in different materials. (Adapted from Meyers, M. A. and Chawla, K. K., *Mechanical behavior of materials*, 2nd Edition. Cambridge University Press, Cambridge, England, 2009. With permission.)

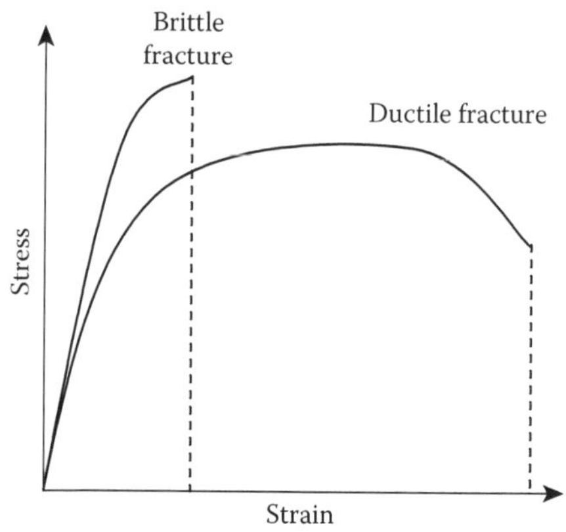

FIGURE 4.6
Stress–strain curve represents ductile and brittle fracture.

occur for metallic and ceramic materials, namely transgranular (also called cleavage) and intergranular modes. Polymeric materials undergo a mode of fracture called crazing, in which the polymer chains ahead of a crack align themselves along the tensile axis, so that the stress concentration is released. Also shear-banding mode (also called localization) of deformation takes place in polymers prior to fracture. On the other hand, composite materials undergo a series of failure modes, as shown in Figure 4.5, depending on the key components used to make the composites. If the atomic bonding between the components is weak, then the composite undergoes atomic debonding that greatly causes fiber breaking and microbucking, resulting in structural collapse and finally composite failure in many cases. Note that ductile fracture is better than brittle fracture, because ductile fracture occurs over a period of time, whereas brittle fracture is fast, and can occur at lower stress levels (see Figure 4.6).

4.5.1 Brittle Fracture

Brittle fracture is a sudden separation of a stressed body into two or more pieces without any measurable plastic deformation. Brittle fracture generally initiates as a result of cleavage by breaking of the atomic bonds. According to Griffith's theory, it occurs due to minute crack-like defects. When brittle cracks become unstable and acceptable toward eventual fracture, they gather velocities that reach an appreciable fraction of the velocity of sound in the medium. Under certain conditions, especially at high stress levels, the crack front can split into a number of diverging fronts. Brittle fracture looks generally flat in nature with very little or no noticeable evidence of localized necking, as observed in the case of ductile fracture (see Figure 4.5) (Mayers 1999). So, the brittle fracture is characterized by rapid crack propagation with low energy release and without significant plastic deformation.

The fracture can also be explained in terms of crystallinity. For instance, in brittle crystalline materials, fracture can occur by cleavage as the result of tensile stress acting normal to crystallographic planes with low bonding (cleavage planes). Whereas, in amorphous materials, by contrast, the lack of a crystalline structure results in a conchoidal fracture, with cracks proceeding normal to the applied tension. The theoretical strength of a crystalline material can be written as:

$$\sigma_{\text{theoretical}} = \sqrt{E\gamma/r_o}. \tag{4.2}$$

Here, E is the Young's modulus of the material, γ is the surface energy, and r_o is the equilibrium distance between atomic centers.

On the other hand, a crack introduces a stress concentration modeled by

$$\begin{aligned}\sigma_{\text{elliptical crack}} &= \sigma_{\text{applied}}(1+2\sqrt{a/\rho})\\ &= \sigma_{\text{applied}} + 2\sigma_{\text{applied}}\sqrt{a/\rho}.\end{aligned}$$

Here, σ_{applied} is the loading stress, a is half the length of the crack, and ρ is the radius of curvature at the crack tip. For sharp cracks, the above equation becomes:

$$\sigma_{\text{elliptical crack}} = 2\sigma_{\text{applied}}\sqrt{a/\rho}. \tag{4.3}$$

By combining Equations 4.2 and 4.3, we get:

$$\sigma_{\text{fracture}} = \sqrt{E\gamma\rho/4ar_o}.$$

This equation implies that sharp cracks (small ρ) and large defects (large a) both lower the fracture strength of the material.

4.5.2 Ductile Fracture

Ductile fracture is a rapid propagation of cracks through a stressed material. Ductile fracture results from an excessive mechanical force applied to a material, which has the ability to deform permanently prior to fracture. In ductile fracture, extensive plastic deformation takes place before fracture. The property of ductility is therefore the ability of the material to deform depending on the magnitude of the applied force. In metals, the ductile fracture is characterized by tearing of metal accompanied by appreciable gross plastic deformation and outflow of considerable energy, which is in contrast to brittle fracture. Many ductile metals, especially materials with high purity, can sustain very large deformation (more than 50%) or more strain before fracture under favorable loading condition.

Since ductile fracture involves a high degree of plastic deformation, the fracture behavior of a propagating crack, as modeled above, changes fundamentally. Some of the energy from stress concentrations at the crack tips is dissipated by plastic deformation before the crack actually propagates. A schematic representation of the basic steps involved in ductile fracture is shown in Figure 4.5 (Mayers 1999). The basic steps of ductile fracture include necking or distortion, which results in stress localization at the point on the sample of smallest cross-sectional area followed by void formation. Ductile fracture generally occurs by a series process of microvoid initiation, nucleation, growth, and coalescence mechanism (also called crack formation). The crack is further propagated along the direction of the stress until the remaining area becomes too small to support the applied load, leading to fracture failure.

4.6 Brittle to Ductile Transition of Biomaterials

Many factors determine the nature of fracture that occurs in a material. Among them, temperature, dislocation density, crack propagation, and grain size primarily influence the nature of fracture that pertains to whether it is brittle or ductile. From a temperature point of view, the YS is lowered at higher temperatures and thus fracture is more ductile in nature. At lower temperatures, on the other hand, the YS is greater and thus fracture is more brittle in nature. From a dislocation point of view, the higher the dislocation density, the greater the chance of brittle fracture occurring, and, on the other hand, the lower the dislocation density, the greater the chance of ductile fracture occurring. From a crystal grains point of view, the smaller the grain size, the greater the brittle fracture, and, on the other hand, the larger the grain size, the greater the ductile fracture. So, transition from ductile to brittle fracture mode occurs when a transitional change occurs either in temperature or other factors that influence dislocation density or grain size of a material.

In a recent study, Peterlik et al. (2006) experimentally described the transitional changes from brittle to ductile fracture behavior of bone materials. They employed a controlled crack-extension in three-point bending experiments to determine the energy required to propagate a crack in different directions. The results were then correlated to the main origin of anisotropy, the so-called collagen angle (γ). This method allows for the determination of the energy per area with a local resolution of 20–500 μm, depending on the amount of local crack extension (see Figure 4.7) (Peterlik et al. 2006). The crack-extension energy per area was found to be strongly dependent on the collagen angle with respect to the loading axis, as defined in Figure 4.8a (Peterlik et al. 2006). To extend the crack along the direction of the collagen fibrils with a misalignment between 0° and 5°, only 375 J m^{-2} are required

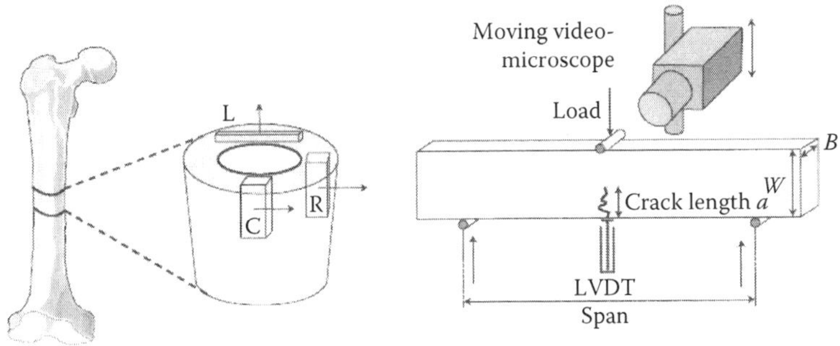

FIGURE 4.7
The experimental setup of the controlled crack-extension experiment. Longitudinal (L), radial (R), and circumferential (C) denote the respective directions of crack propagation. Rectangular slabs were prepared from fragments of cortical bone from femoral and tibial diaphysis of a 52-year-old woman, which were wet-machined in different directions to give final dimensions of approximately $15 \times 1.5 \times 2$ mm^3; they were then loaded under three-point bending. With a closed-loop control, a linear variable differential transducer (LVDT) ensured a constant displacement rate of 3 μm s^{-1} corresponding to a peak strain rate of approximately 200 microstrain s^{-1}. In several cycles, the specimens were increasingly loaded to propagate the crack and then immediately unloaded. A distinction from other experimental methods is that no artificial starting notch was used, but the crack was initiated by the load of the as-machined specimens. Furthermore, the crack was filled with a wetting fluid containing the dyestuff rhodamine B after each cycle for a better visualization of the crack tip. (Reprinted from Peterlik, H. et al., *Nat. Mater.*, 5, 52, 2006. With permission from Macmillan Publishers Ltd.)

(with a lowest value of 110 J m^{-2} for the lowest misalignment angle of 1.5°), whereas 9920 J m^{-2} are needed for a propagation perpendicular to the fibrils (see Figure 4.8a), which is nearly an increase of two orders of magnitude. Whereas, only a slight increase of the crack-extension energy was observed with increasing the collagen angle up to a level of about 50°. At this point, a considerable jump in the crack-extension energy per area is visible, followed by an increase up to an angle where the collagen fibrils are oriented perpendicular to the direction of crack extension. Accordingly, the crack path angle (α) changes its appearance from straight to zig-zag (see Figure 4.8b). Its standard deviation, calculated from the distribution observed in the scanning electron microscopy (SEM) within the respective ranges of constant collagen angles, shows low values (that is, a straight and smooth crack path) for the case of collagen angles lower than about 50° and high values otherwise (that is, a deflected and zig-zag crack path). The sudden increase in the crack-extension energy per area and the appearance of the cracks cannot be related to just one of the various toughening mechanisms proposed for bone tissue; it's complex! However, the sudden increase in energy values suggests a transition from a brittle to a quasi-ductile fracture mode. The authors found that the fracture energy changes by two orders of magnitude depending on the collagen orientation, and the angle between collagen and crack propagation direction is decisive in switching between different toughening mechanisms.

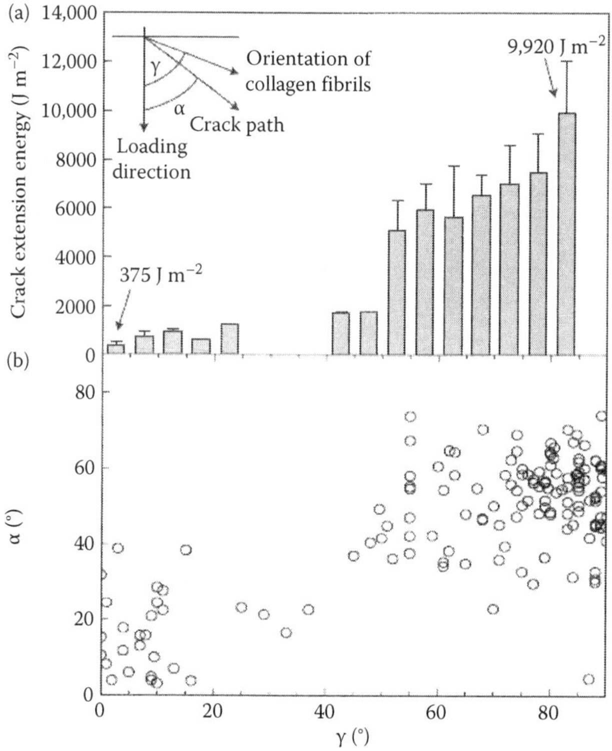

FIGURE 4.8
Crack extension as a function of the collagen angle (γ). (a) The energy required for crack extension and (b) the standard deviation of the crack path angle α. The total number of values is 76 for (a), showing the mean and standard error, and 169 for (b). A significant jump for both parameters is observed at approximately 50°. The standard deviation was calculated from the distribution of the crack path angles (obtained from digitized SEM images with a resolution of about 1 μm), which were overlaid with the digitized images from polarization light microscopy, on which the ranges of constant collagen angles were identified (which are typically in the range of about 10 μm, but significantly larger, up to 100 μm, for specimens cut out in the longitudinal direction). Thus, a distribution of crack path angles was obtained within each interval of approximately constant collagen angle, from which mean values and a standard deviation could be calculated. (Reprinted from Peterlik, H. et al., *Nat. Mater.*, 5, 52, 2006. With permission from Macmillan Publishers Ltd.)

4.7 Fracture Toughness

Fracture toughness is a quantitative way of expressing a material's resistance to brittle fracture when a crack exists. Therefore, the resistance of a material to fracture is known as its fracture toughness. The unit of fracture toughness is $MPa.m^{1/2}$. It is one of the most important properties of any structural material for virtually all load-bearing orthopedic applications. If a material has a large value of fracture toughness, it will probably undergo ductile fracture, whereas a material with a low value of fracture toughness undergoes brittle fracture. Fracture toughness generally depends on temperature, environment, applied force, composition of the material and its microstructural features. A parameter, called the stress intensity factor (K), is used to determine the fracture toughness of most materials. It is a function of loading, crack size, and structural geometry.

The fracture toughness can be commonly categorized into three types, namely, K_{IC}, K_{IIC}, and K_{IIIC}. These types are based on the different loading modes. Here, K_C is the critical stress intensity factor. The value of the stress intensity factor in which the crack propagates to fracture failure is called critical stress intensity factor. K_C is used to measure the fracture toughness of a material that has a thickness less than that of some critical value. The critical value is denoted as B. If the thickness of a material is less than B, and stress is applied, the material is in a state called plane stress. Note that plane stress is different from plane strain. Plane stress is a condition of a body in which the state of stress is such that two of the principal stresses are always parallel to a given plane and are constant in the normal direction. Whereas, plane strain is a condition of a body in which the displacements of all points in the body are parallel to a given plane, and the values of these displacements do not depend on the distance perpendicular to the plane. The critical value of B can be written as

$$B \geq 2.5(K_{IC}/\sigma_y)^2.$$

Here, B is the minimum thickness to distinguish between K_C and K_{IC} (in mode I loading), K_C is the fracture toughness if the thickness of the material is less than B, and σ_y is the yield stress of the material.

The thickness of the material is related to its fracture toughness, which is graphically depicted in Figure 4.9. The fracture toughness of a material in relation to the material's thickness can be written as

$$K_C = Y\sigma\sqrt{\pi a}.$$

Here, K_C is the fracture toughness if the thickness of the material is less than B, Y is the constant factor related to the geometry of the test material, a is the characteristic dimension of the crack (i.e., crack length), and σ is the stress applied to the material.

On the other hand, K_{IC}, K_{IIC}, and K_{IIIC} all represent fracture toughness of a material if the material thickness is greater than B. If a stress is applied to the material with a thickness greater than B, it is in a state called plane strain. The differences between K_{IC}, K_{IIC}, and K_{IIIC}, however, do not depend on the thickness of the material. Instead, K_{IC}, K_{IIC}, and K_{IIIC} are the fracture toughness of a material under the three different modes of loading, mode I, mode II, and mode III, respectively. These three modes enable a crack to

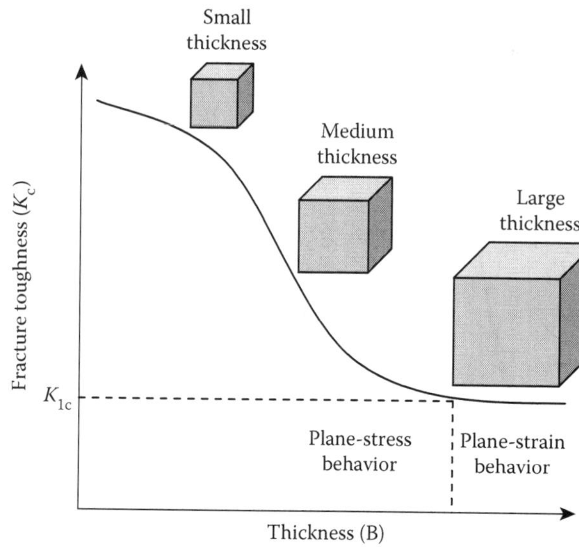

FIGURE 4.9
Fracture toughness as a function of material thickness.

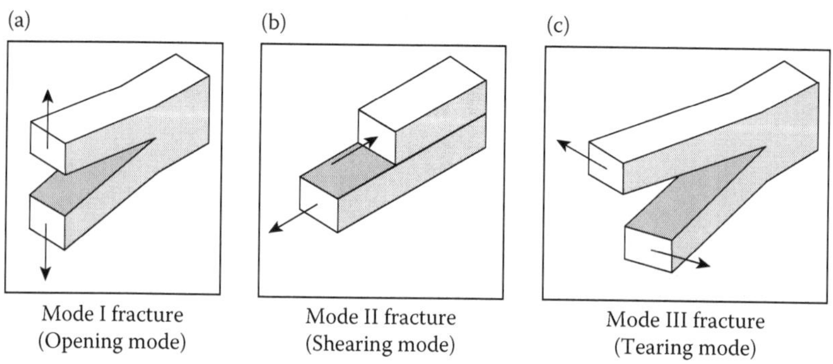

FIGURE 4.10
Fracture mechanism under three modes of loading.

propagate in structural materials. The three different modes of loading are schematically illustrated in Figure 4.10. Mode I (see Figure 4.10a) is called opening or tensile mode, where the crack surfaces move directly apart. Mode II (see Figure 4.10b) is called sliding or in-plane shear mode, where the crack surfaces slide over one another in a perpendicular direction to the crack front. Mode III (see Figure 4.10c) is called tearing or antiplane shear mode, where the crack surfaces move parallel to the plane of the crack front.

The fracture toughness of a material with a thickness equal to or greater than B can be written as

$$K_{IC} = Y\sigma\sqrt{\pi a}.$$

Here, K_{IC} is the fracture toughness in mode I loading, Y is the constant factor related to the geometry of the test material, a is the characteristic dimension of the crack, and σ is the stress applied to the material.

K_{IC} values can be used to determine critical lengths given an applied stress, or critical stress values can be calculated given a crack length already in the material. The critical applied stress required to cause failure in a material can be written as

$$\sigma_c \leq K_{IC}/Y\sqrt{\pi a}.$$

Here, σ_c is the critical applied stress required for failure in a material, K_{IC} is the fracture toughness in mode I loading (with a thickness less than B), Y is the constant factor related to the geometry of the material, and a is the crack length.

The critical crack length that causes the material to fail can be calculated from the following equation:

$$a_c = 1/\pi(K_{IC}/\sigma Y)^2.$$

Here, a_c is the critical crack length, K_{IC} is the fracture toughness in mode I loading (with a thickness less than B), σ is the stress applied to the material, and Y is the constant factor related to the geometry of the material.

Fracture toughness (K_{IC} values) of some of the structural materials is given in Table 4.3 (Callister 1994). Notice that the ceramic and polymeric materials have much lower fracture toughness than the metals. The fracture toughness

TABLE 4.3

Fracture Toughness (K_{IC}) of Structural Materials

	Fracture Toughness (K_{IC})	
Materials	**MPa m**	**Psi in**
Metals		
2024-T351 Aluminum	36	33,000
4340 Steel (tempered at 260°C)	50.0	45,800
Titanium Alloy (Ti-6Al-4V)	44–66	40,000–60,000
Ceramics		
Aluminum oxide	3.0–5.3	2700–4800
Soda-lime glass	0.7–0.8	640–730
Concrete	0.2–1.4	180–1270
Polymers		
Polymethylmethacrylate (PMMA)	1.0	900
Polystyrene (PS)	0.8–1.1	730–1000

Source: Adapted from Callister, W. D., *Materials science and engineering: An introduction*, John Wiley, New York, 1994. Reprinted by permission of John Wiley & Sons, Inc.

values imply the fact that ceramic materials are more susceptible to cracks followed by brittle fracture, whereas the metals undergo ductile fracture due to their high fracture toughness values. In this regard, composites made of metals, ceramics, and/or polymers might be better than their monolithic components due to their moderate fracture toughness values. In this way, biomaterials could be extended to many biomedical applications where monolithic materials do not possess the required fracture toughness for a given structural application. This concept introduces the toughening mechanisms in biomaterials.

4.8 Toughness Analysis of Biomaterials

The most critical property of biomaterials, in particular ceramics, is their brittleness, as characterized by their poor tensile strength, low tensile strain to failure, and corresponding fracture toughness. For example, HA has a low fracture toughness value that restricts its usage in monolithic form in many bone applications, although it has excellent bioactive features. Therefore, toughness improvement of biomaterials has been the focus of the research in biomechanics for many years. Several published reports highlight the mechanism behind the ductile particle toughening, which states that the ductile particles deform to bridge the faces of a propagating crack, thereby absorbing energy through plastic deformation of the particles and applying closure stresses in the crack tip region. In addition, the ductile particles may contribute to toughness by plastically deforming ahead of the crack tip as a result of the crack tip stresses, thus absorbing energy through plastic deformation of the constrained particles.

In a notable study, Clegg and Paterson (2004) reported on how to improve the toughening of HA bioceramics using platinum particles as reinforcement agents and their experimental analysis. Notice that the ductile phase of platinum is bioinert, so it is anticipated that it may not affect the biocompatibility of HA, rather it may enhance the mechanical behavior of HA. The composite compacts were fabricated from HA and dried ammonium hexachloroplatinate (ACP) powders by mechanical mixing followed by die pressing to 10 MPa in order to form a disc. The discs were then heated to 456°C to decompose the ACP and to produce a fine uniform dispersion of platinum particles throughout the HA matrix. Once the ACP was decomposed, the discs were subjected to die pressing to 80 MPa and then sintered for 4 h at high temperatures (1250°C, 1300°C, and 1350°C). The mechanical hardness of the composite system was determined by using a Vickers microhardness tester. The fracture toughness was estimated by measuring the length of cracks emanating from the ends of the hardness impressions. Figure 4.11 shows atypical picture of a crack formed by the hardness tester (Clegg and Paterson

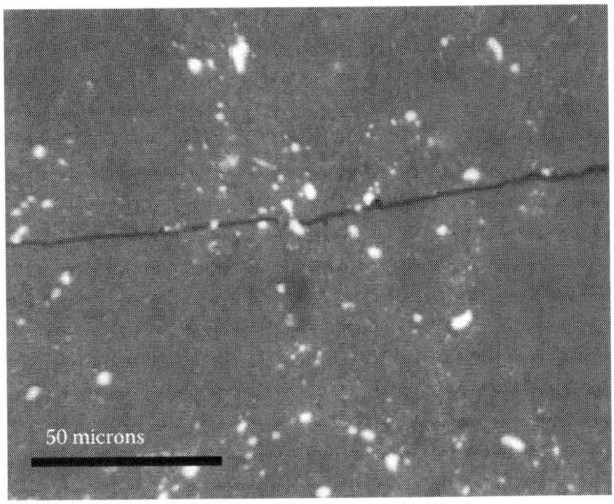

FIGURE 4.11
Micrograph shows crack formation produced by Vickers hardness impression. (Adapted from Clegg, R. E. and Paterson, G. D., Ductile particle toughening of hydroxyapatite ceramics using platinum particles. *Proceedings of the structural integrity and fracture*, Brisbane. 2004.)

2004). The crack propagation path was studied from the indentation analysis. As can be seen in Figure 4.11, the crack is passing through a platinum particle, which bridged the crack. However, it was noticed that the crack does not appear to be attracted to particles and several particles are just missed by the crack. The fracture toughness values estimated from the hardness testing are graphically illustrated in Figure 4.12 (Clegg and Paterson 2004). The results show that the inclusion of platinum particles into the HA matrix increased the fracture toughness values about twofolds higher than that of pure HA. The increase in fracture toughness correlated with the volume fraction of the reinforced platinum particles. This investigation thus demonstrated that HA bioceramics can be toughened by incorporation of the ductile particles as reinforcements.

In another interesting study, Delgado et al. (1999) reported the toughening of HA by incorporating zirconia biomaterial. The authors used magnesia partially stabilized zirconia (MgPSZ) as a reinforcement agent. The test specimens were made by mixing 20 wt.% of MgPSZ with HA in ethanol for 1 h, and die pressed under a uniaxial stress of 400 MPa to shape in the form of discs and 100 MPa was used to shape in the form of bars, followed by sintering at 1250°C for 4 h. The authors also made HA, as a control test specimen, under the same conditions without reinforcing the zirconia. The fracture toughness (K_{IC}) measurements performed using the single-edge notched bend (SENB) method was done using a three-point bending test. The fracture surfaces of the specimens were examined using SEM. The fracture toughness

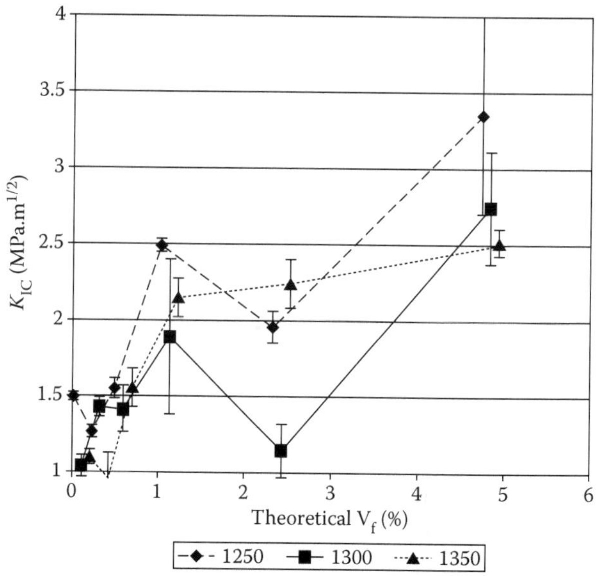

FIGURE 4.12
Fracture toughness (K_{IC}) of HA-platinum composite system as measured using Vickers hardness tester. (Adapted from Clegg, R. E. and Paterson, G. D., Ductile particle toughening of hydroxyapatite ceramics using platinum particles. *Proceedings of the structural integrity and fracture*, Brisbane. 2004.)

TABLE 4.4

Mechanical Test Data of HA Before and After Toughening with Zirconia

	Density	Hardness (H)	Young's Modulus (E)	Fracture Toughness (K_{IC})
Ceramic	(%)	(GPa)	(GPa)	(MPa m$^{1/2}$)
HA	96.27±0.43	4.14±0.28	213±26	0.72±0.07
MgPSZ-HA	94.35±0.52	2.94±0.20	112±17	1.73±0.09

Source: Adapted from Delgado, J. A. et al., *J. Mater. Sci. Mater. Med.*, 10, 715, 1999.

was also determined by indentation method using a Vickers hardness tester. Both results were compared.

Mechanical properties obtained by the indentation method for the samples of HA and MgPSZ-HA are shown in Table 4.4 (Delgado et al. 1999). It can be noticed from Table 4.4 that the fracture toughness values for the MgPSZ-HA are increased about 2.5 times higher than that of pure HA under the same experimental conditions. This is a very good sign of toughening of HA. The mechanical properties obtained by the three-point bending test are also given in Table 4.4. The fracture toughness and Young's modulus are found to be lower than those obtained from the indentation measurements. This is because of the porosity and the compacting defects of the test specimens, which can reduce the values measured in conventional tests. Notice that the microindentation tests are carried out on well-compacted surfaces of the specimen. The SEM micrographs of the fracture surfaces of the test specimens are shown in Figure 4.13 (Delgado et al. 1999). It shows a typical transgranular mechanism of fracture for the HA (see Figure 4.13a), whereas the toughened HA (MgPSZ-HA) exhibits less transgranular fracture mechanism (see Figure 4.13b) as compared to HA. This is because of the increased toughness of the MgPSZ-HA composite specimen. The increase of fracture toughness can be attributed to the transformation toughening of the MgPSZ particles and the presence of microcracking (see Figure 4.13c), which might have been promoted by the characteristic of thermal expansion coefficients of HA and MgPSZ. Based on the experimental results, the authors concluded that it is possible to toughen the HA bioceramics by incorporating MgPSZ as a reinforcement agent. These two experimental investigations, and others, clearly proved that toughening of biomaterials could be done using the right choice of reinforcement agents in order to improve the mechanical strength. The toughening mechanism may be extended to tailor the mechanical behavior of structural biomaterials to suit them in specific applications.

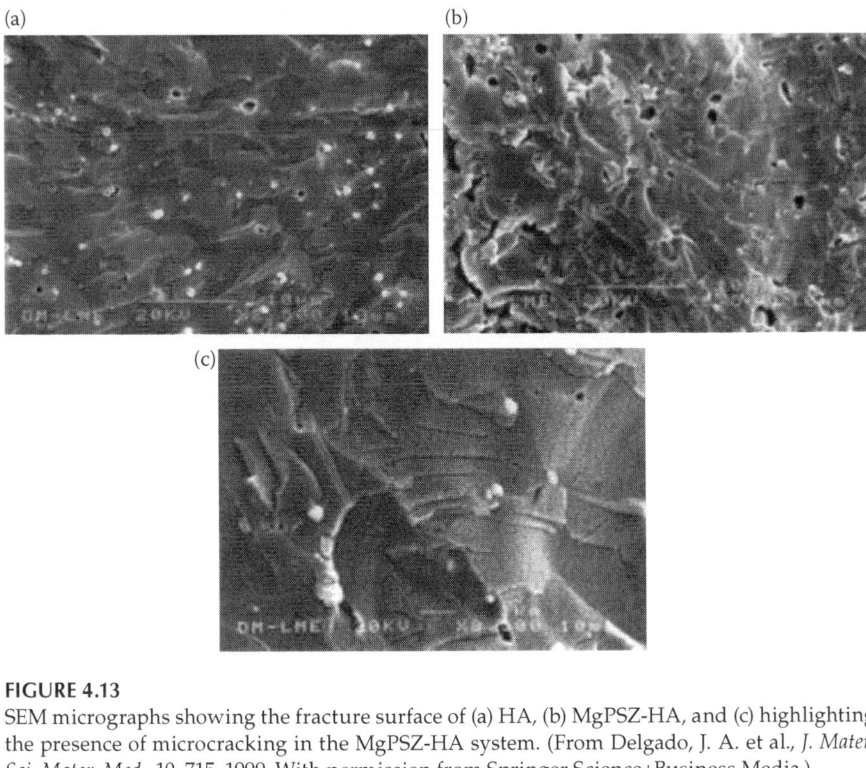

FIGURE 4.13
SEM micrographs showing the fracture surface of (a) HA, (b) MgPSZ-HA, and (c) highlighting the presence of microcracking in the MgPSZ-HA system. (From Delgado, J. A. et al., *J. Mater. Sci. Mater. Med.*, 10, 715, 1999. With permission from Springer Science+Business Media.)

4.9 Fatigue Mechanics

Fatigue refers to a mode of cracking or failure of a material that occurs due to repeated application of stress or strain. Fatigue is a special kind of failure in which fracture occurs not because of an instantaneous load that is applied. Rather, it is because a stress is applied for some period of time in which the cracks gradually grow until they finally reach a critical level. This concept is especially important when dealing with metallic implants because it is the most common cause of failure in load-bearing applications, in particular hip joints, bone plates, and dental implants. In an excellent article, Niinomi (2007) reviewed the fatigue characteristics of several metallic biomaterials, in which one can understand that fatigue of biomaterials is highly essential in order to understand the reliability of biomedical implants. It is established that the fatigue characteristics of biomaterials are closely related to their microstructural features. For example, the microstructure of metallic biomaterials changes according to their processing methodology and heat treatment employed in the process. Therefore, optimized processing conditions are essential to control the microstructural features of biomaterials that could eventually control their fatigue behavior. Figure 4.14 shows the fatigue characteristics of several metallic biomaterials (Niinomi 2007), demonstrating

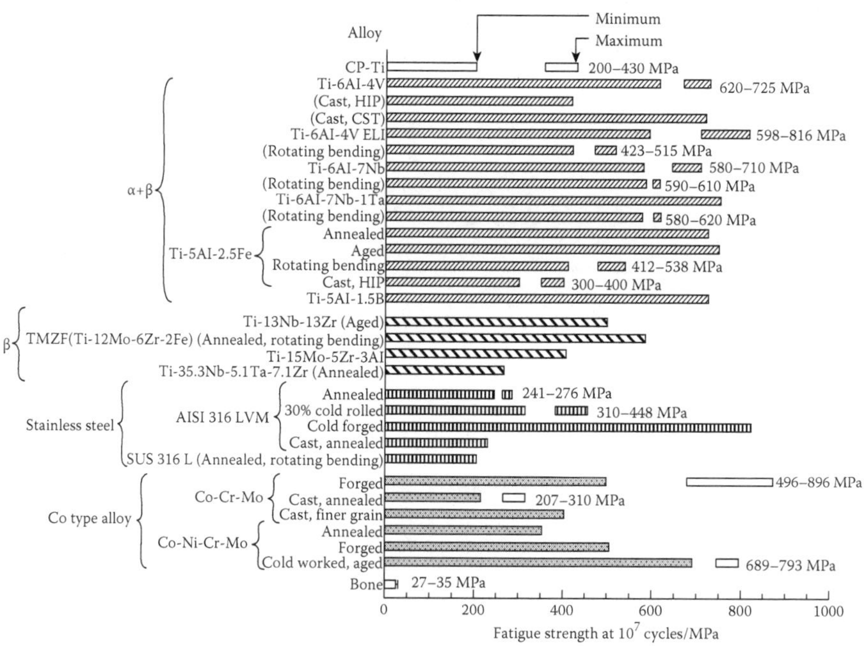

FIGURE 4.14
Fatigue strength of metallic biomaterials. (Reprinted from Niinomi, M., *Mater. Sci. Eng.*, A243, 231, 1998. With permission from Elsevier.)

that the fatigue strength of metallic biomaterials is higher than that of natural bone. Therefore, there is a need to manufacture composite biomaterials with a fatigue strength that closely mimics natural bone, so that the possibility of the occurrence of mechanical mismatching (stress-shielding) upon implantation could be minimized, and also would enhance the durability and longevity of implants, which leads to successful clinical results.

The fatigue behavior of a material is best represented by stress (S) cycles to failure (N) diagram (also called S–N curve). It is a quantitative measure used to determine the lifetime of biomedical implants. Higher stress level results in shorter fatigue life, while lower stress level allows longer fatigue life. The number of cycles that will cause failure at a certain stress level is known as fatigue life. Each and every implant material has their own fatigue limit. The significance of the fatigue limit is that if the material is loaded below this stress, then it will not fail, regardless of the number of times it is loaded. For instance, materials such as Cu and Al do not show a fatigue limit, therefore they will fail at any stress and number of cycles. Biomedical implants must have a high degree of fatigue resistance in order to prevent the implant's failure over the long life span. For load-bearing applications, it is anticipated that the implant must be capable of withstanding a maximum cyclic stress (5×10^7 cycles) and about 25 years of normal use without any sign of fatigue failure.

The fatigue life of a material can be expressed as the number of loading cycles required to initiate a fatigue crack and to propagate the crack to critical size. Therefore, it may be considered that fatigue failure occurs in three stages, namely crack initiation, crack propagation, and finally fracture. Among the many factors, dislocation density plays a major role in initiating fatigue crack formation. At this stage, dislocations accumulate near surface stress concentrations and form structures called persistent slip bands after a large number of loading cycles. Note that persistent slip bands are areas that rise above (extrusion) or fall below (intrusion) the surface of the component due to movement of material along slip planes. This leaves signs of tiny (micro in size) steps in the surface that serve as stress risers where micro size cracks could be initiated. These micro cracks further nucleate along the plane of high shear stress, which is often 45° to the loading direction. In order for fatigue cracks to initiate, three basic factors are necessary. First, the loading pattern must contain minimum and maximum peak values with significant variation. The peak values may be in tension or compression and may change over time, but the reverse loading cycle must be sufficiently great for fatigue crack initiation. Secondly, the peak stress levels must be of sufficiently high value. If the peak stresses are too low, no crack initiation will occur. Thirdly, the material must experience a sufficiently large number of cycles of the applied stress. Any material that undergoes a series of these steps encounters the crack formation and subsequent propagation, depending on the applied load.

Figure 4.15 shows several types of loading modes that could initiate a fatigue crack. Figure 4.15a shows sinusoidal loading mode roaming from a tensile stress to a compressive stress. For this type of stress cycle, the

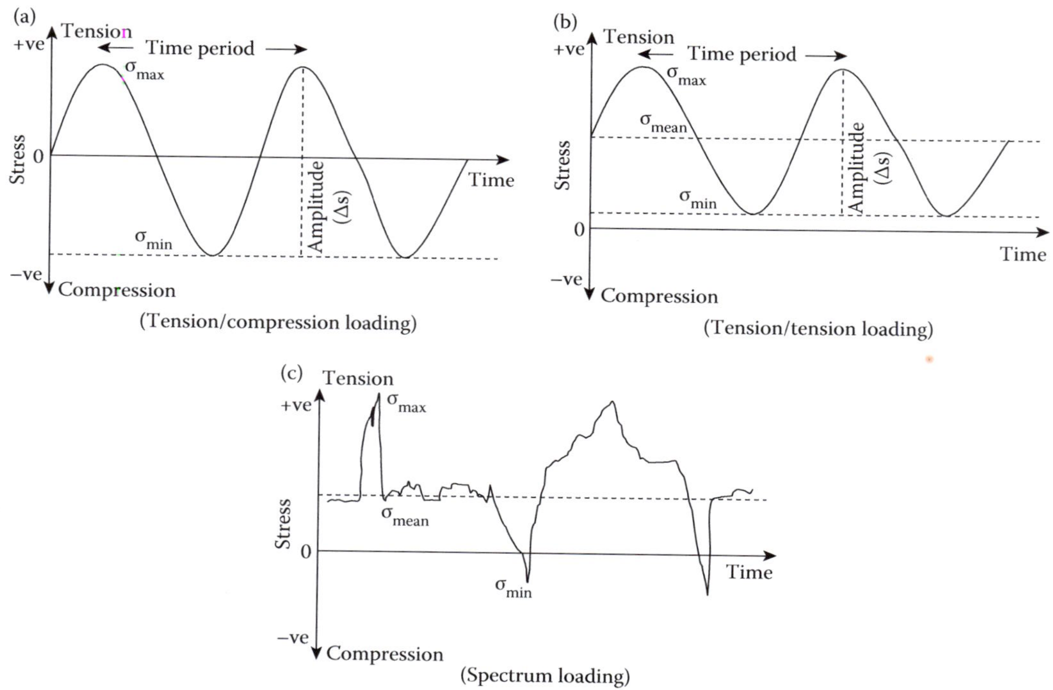

FIGURE 4.15
Types of loading that initiate a fatigue crack.

maximum tensile stress is the same as the maximum compressive stress, but the tensile stress is considered positive and the compressive stress is negative. Figure 4.15b shows sinusoidal loading mode from a tensile stress to a tensile stress. That is minimum and maximum stresses both in the tensile vicinity. Figure 4.15c shows spectrum-loading mode (also called variable-amplitude loading). In spectrum loading, only those cycles exceeding some peak threshold will contribute to fatigue cracking. It should be noted that determining the correct loading cycle for a part or a larger structure is one of the difficulties in fatigue analysis. Therefore, additional care should be taken while doing fatigue measurements, especially when dealing with biomaterials. The following section describes the fatigue analysis of biomaterials with illustrated experimental examples.

4.10 Fatigue Analysis of Biomaterials

Fatigue of biomaterials partly determines their long-term performance in the bodily environment under various mechanical stimuli. Although several factors contribute to fatigue behavior, surface conditions and environmental conditions greatly influence the fatigue failure of biomaterials. This is because the fatigue failure begins, in most cases, at the surface of the implant when in contact with body fluid, tissues, and other biological factors. The fact is that, in any biomaterials, surface layer (either coated layer or the material itself) bears most of the loads applied on them, and they are directly exposed to the bodily environment under different mechanical stimuli. Fatigue environments may be commonly categorized into two types, namely, strain controlled and stress controlled. Although most fatigue environments in the human body are a combination of these two levels, it is established that the very compliant nature of biological materials tends to place them toward the direction of strain-controlled fatigue. In a recent study, Lin et al. (2005) analyzed the fatigue behavior of different Ti-based alloys. The materials tested in this investigation include commercially pure Ti, Ti-7.5Mo, Ti-13Nb-13Zr, and Ti-6Al-4V. A servo-hydraulic-type testing machine was used for fatigue and other mechanical tests. A tension-to-tension stress mode was used for fatigue tests. The smooth plate specimens were subjected to uniaxial fatigue loading at room temperature in air at a frequency of 10 Hz with a stress ratio of $R = 0.1$. Table 4.5 shows ultimate tensile strength (UTS), YS at 0.2% offset, modulus of elasticity and elongation to failure of the four test materials (Lin et al. 2005). The results indicated that all three Ti alloys had significantly higher strength and lower elongation values than that of pure Ti. Among the three cast alloys, Ti-6Al-4V was found to have the highest YS and UTS values with the smallest elongation. The Ti-7.5Mo alloy had little higher UTS, comparable YS and a little lower elongation, as compared

TABLE 4.5

Tensile Test Data of Various Tested Ti-Based Materials

Material	Yielding Strength (MPa)	Tensile Strength (MPa)	Tensile Modulus (GPa)	Elongation (%)
c.p. Ti	527±46	641±52	105±7	19.7±1.3
Ti-6Al-4V	846±67	1137±17	117±7	7.1±1.9
Ti-13Nb-13Zr	656±22	945±14	77±3	17.3±1.3
Ti-7.5Mo	665±27	997±38	80±4	15.1±2.7

Source: Reprinted from Lin, C. W., Jug, C. P., and Chern Lin, J. H., *Biomaterials*, 26, 2899, 2005. With permission from Elsevier.

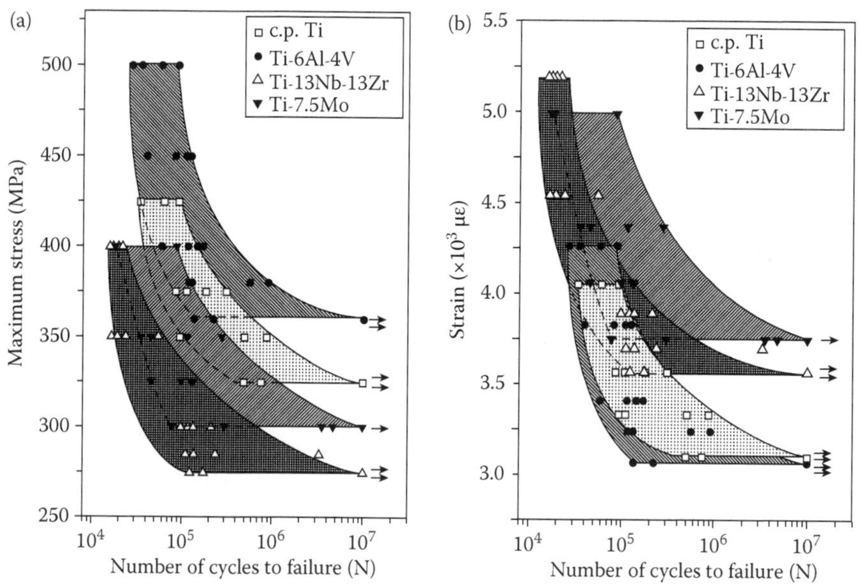

FIGURE 4.16

(a) S–N curves of various Ti-based materials and (b) strain-controlled fatigue data calculated from the respective S–N curves. (Reprinted from Lin, C. W., Jug, C. P., and Chern Lin, J. H., *Biomaterials*, 26, 2899, 2005. With permission from Elsevier.)

to Ti-13Nb-13Zr alloy. Ti-6Al-4V also had the highest tensile modulus among the four test materials. Unlike tensile strength, the tensile modulus of pure Ti was significantly higher than those of Ti-7.5Mo and Ti-13Nb-13Zr alloys.

The profiles of S–N curves of test materials are shown in Figure 4.16a, and the strain-controlled fatigue data calculated from S–N curves are depicted in Figure 4.16b (Lin et al. 2005). As shown in Figure 4.16a, Ti-6Al-4V and commercially pure Ti exhibited higher fatigue strengths than those of Ti-7.5Mo and Ti-13Nb-13Zr alloys. It can be noticed from the results that the strain-controlled fatigue performance of the test materials was entirely different from that of stress-controlled fatigue. As shown in Figure 4.16b, despite the commonly observed wide distribution in test data of cast materials, Ti-7.5Mo and Ti-13Nb-13Zr alloys demonstrated higher strain-controlled fatigue resistance than Ti-6Al-4V and commercially pure Ti. Among the four test materials, Ti-7.5Mo exhibited the best fatigue performance, while commercially pure Ti showed the worst fatigue behavior. The better strain-controlled fatigue performance of Ti-7.5Mo and Ti-13Nb-13Zr was not surprising, because of the fact that they had better strength/modulus combination than Ti-6Al-4V and commercially pure Ti. Based on the experimental results, the authors concluded that Ti-7.5Mo alloy demonstrated the best strain-controlled fatigue behavior as compared to other test materials. This study thus demonstrated the analysis of fatigue behavior of different types of Ti-based materials for use in biomedical applications.

4.11 Tribology

Tribology is the study of friction and wear aspects of two interacting surfaces in relative motion. As discussed earlier, the reliability of the biomedical implants mainly depends on their fracture and tribological behaviors. It is essential to evaluate the tribological behaviors of any load-bearing implants, in particular artificial hip joints, bone plates, and even dental implant materials, because they are often subjected to wear debris and surface degradation while in direct contact with host tissues upon implantation. The wear debris could cause adverse tissue reactions, such as inflammation, infection and associated pain, which may lead to substantial loss of new tissue generation around the implant and consequent loosening of the fixation and failure of the implant. A systematic study of tribological behaviors, such as friction and wear of biomaterials is therefore of great importance, which helps predict the reliability and long-term performance of the implants in the body environment.

4.11.1 Friction

Friction is a force that resists relative motion between two surfaces in contact with a fluid, body fluid for instance. The frictional force between two objects greatly depends on the magnitude of the perpendicular forces of the surfaces in contact, which is generally described as static or dynamic. The frictional force opposing to place an object into motion is called static friction. On the other hand, the frictional force tending to slow down the object in motion is called the force of dynamic friction (also known as kinetic or sliding friction). Dynamic frictional force is generally smaller than the static frictional force. The relationship between the static and dynamic frictional forces is illustrated in Figure 4.17. Friction is expressed in terms of static and dynamic

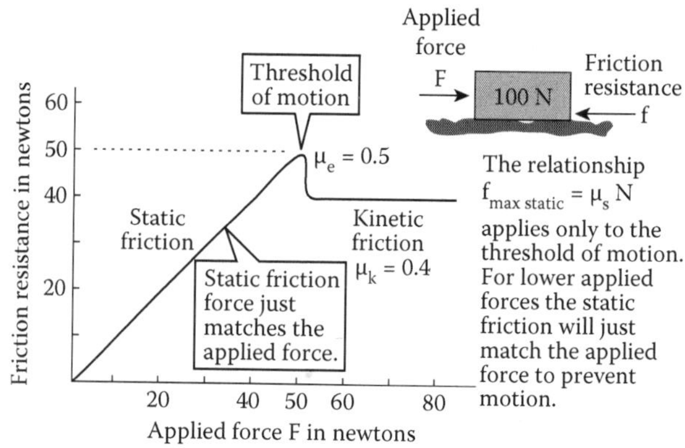

FIGURE 4.17
Relationship of static friction and kinetic friction. (Adapted with courtesy from http://hyperphysics.phy-str.gsu.edu/hbase/frict2.html.)

coefficients. The coefficient of friction (μ) is defined as the ratio of the sliding force to the total force pressing the two surfaces together. As stated above, the static friction can be written as

$$f_s = \mu_s F_n.$$

Here, f_s is the static frictional force, μ_s is the coefficient of static friction, and F_n is the normal force between the two surfaces. Note that the normal force acting on the object is generally associated with the force that the surface of one object exerts on the surface of another object in the absence of any frictional forces between the two surfaces. The normal force is always perpendicular to the two surfaces in contact. From the above equation, the coefficient of static friction can be derived as

$$\mu_s = f_s/F_n.$$

Here, μ_s is the coefficient of static friction, f_s is the static frictional force, and F_n is the normal force between the two surfaces. The force of static friction increases up to a maximum value (threshold), after which the object breaks loose and begins to move (see Figure 4.17).

Similarly, kinetic friction can be written as

$$f_k = \mu_k F_n.$$

Here, f_k is the kinetic frictional force, μ_k is the coefficient of kinetic friction, and F_n is the normal force between the two surfaces. From the above equation, the coefficient of kinetic friction can be derived as

$$\mu_k = f_k F_n.$$

Here, μ_k is the coefficient of kinetic friction, f_k is the kinetic frictional force, and F_n is the normal force between the two surfaces.

The coefficient of static and dynamic friction typically depends upon the surface conditions of the biomaterials. The coefficient of friction of some of the biomaterials is given in Table 4.6. The coefficient values are always expressed as one surface on another surface (e.g., amalgam-on-gold alloy). It should be noted that the higher the coefficient, the greater the force of friction. Also note that it is not possible to determine more accurate values of the coefficient of frictions due to changes in the surface conditions (e.g., smoothness/roughness) of the implants. That is why measurement of friction is a precise tribological characterization. There are several factors affecting the true frictional values of the biomaterials. For instance, surface layer conditions of the implants, such as surface contamination, surface coating, hardness, roughness, surface load, sliding velocity, vibration, temperature, humidity, and lubrication, are greatly influencing frictional values and thus they are critical when measuring friction. Therefore, one has to take special care to obtain accurate frictional values of the implants.

4.11.2 Wear

Wear can be defined as surface degradation and is often associated to material loss. Always think that wear will occur in materials whenever two surfaces move over each other, which could eventually gives progressive loss of material. Note that wear and friction are assumed very much the same thing and the terms are often misunderstood, but they are quite different. For instance, lowering the friction of biomedical implants does not necessarily lower the wear of the implant material. The wear properties of biomaterials certainly seems to be the least studied as compared to other mechanical behaviors. It is one of the important properties of biomaterials, which determines the durability and longevity of the implants. Wear of biomaterials results in particle debris and surface degradation, which is most often seen in orthopedic surgery. Among the several factors, friction, surface load, sliding distance, surface hardness, surface contamination, roughness, surface coating, temperature, humidity, and lubrication greatly influence the wear of biomaterials. Note that these factors also affect the frictional values of the biomaterials, as discussed earlier. Therefore, manufacturing wear-resistant biomedical implants that could lower the production of wear debris upon implantation is essential. This will prevent introducing foreign bodies (debris), associated with the implant's surface materials, into the host tissues.

Mechanical wear of biomaterials can generally be classified into four types: adhesion, abrasion, erosion, and fretting, which determines the durability of the implants. The first type, adhesive wear, is a common form of material loss in orthopedic surgery, especially when dealing with metallic

TABLE 4.6

Coefficient of Friction of Various Biomaterials

Material Couples	Coefficient of Friction	
	Dry	Wet
Amalgam On		
Amalgam	0.19–0.35	
Bovine enamel		0.12–0.28
Composite resin		0.10–0.18
Gold alloy		0.10–0.35
Porcelain	0.06–0.12	0.07–0.15
Bone On		
Metal (bead-coated)	0.50	
Metal (fiber mesh-coated)	0.60	
Metal (smooth)	0.42	
Bovine Enamel On		
Acrylic resin	0.19–0.65	
Amalgam	0.18–0.22	
Bovine dentin	0.35–0.40	0.45–0.55
Bovine enamel	0.22–0.60	0.50–0.60
Chromium–nickel alloy	0.10–0.12	
Gold	0.12–0.20	
Porcelain	0.10–0.12	0.50–0.90
Composite Resin On		
Amalgam	0.13–0.25	0.22–0.34
Bovine enamel		0.30–0.75
Gold Alloy On		
Acrylic	0.6–0.8	
Amalgam	0.15–0.25	
Gold alloy	0.2–0.6	
Porcelain	0.22–0.25	0.16–0.17
Hydrogel-Coated Latex On		
Hydrogel		0.054
Latex On		
Glass		0.470
Hydrogel		0.095
Metal (Bead-Coated) On		
Bone	0.54	
Metal (Fiber Mesh-Coated) On		
Bone	0.58	
Metal (Smooth) On		
Bone	0.43	

TABLE 4.6

Coefficient of Friction of Various Biomaterials (*Continued*)

	Coefficient of Friction	
Material Couples	**Dry**	**Wet**
Prosthetic Tooth Materials		
Acrylic on acrylic	0.21	0.37
Acrylic on porcelain	0.23	0.30
Porcelain on acrylic	0.34	0.32
Porcelain on porcelain	0.14	0.51

Source: Adapted with courtesy from http://www.lib.umich.edu/dentlib/Dental_tables/Coeffric.html.

implants. Adhesive wear occurs when two solid surfaces slide over one another under local stress. At low loads, an oxide layer usually forms on the contact surfaces, which prevents metallic bonding between the two surfaces, but results in a low rate of wear (often called oxidative wear). When the load is increased, the oxide layer breaks down and metallic bonding occurs between the two surfaces, which eventually causes rapid material loss and high wear debris, leading to premature implant failure. The second type, abrasive wear, refers to the loss of material that occurs when particles get between the two interacting solid surfaces. Abrasive wear can be of the sliding surfaces of a second material (called two-body wear) or can exist as particles between the two surfaces (called three-body wear). The consequences are severe surface scratches, particle debris, and dimensional changes of the implant, leading to loosening from the implanted position. This could eventually cause implant failure. The third type is erosion wear. Erosion is a material loss from the abrasive action of moving fluids on a solid surface. In other words, wear caused by suspended solid particles is referred to as erosion. Erosive wear is the dominant process in orthopedic implants because they are in direct contact with body fluid environment. The major difference between abrasion and erosion wear is that erosion involves the transfer of kinetic energy to the surface, whereas abrasive wear does not. This means that in erosion, material removal is a function of the particle velocity squared. The fourth type of wear is fretting. It is another kind of material loss, which occurs due to repeated cyclical rubbing between two solid surfaces in contact. As a result, loosening or removal of material from the original position takes place over a period of time. This type of material loss is often associated with a combination of adhesive and abrasive wear. This type of wear is also called fretting corrosion or oxidation. The following section describes how to analyze tribological behavior of biomaterials with illustrated experimental examples.

4.12 Tribological Analysis of Biomaterials

As discussed above, it is widely recognized that the friction and wear of metallic implants plays an important role in determining their long-term performance. Most of the load-bearing implants (e.g., hip joints) are made of two or more components using several biomaterials. These component biomaterials are in contact with each other's surface and even rub together after implantation because of local mechanical stimulus in the bodily environment. It is a simple logic that whenever two or more surfaces are in contact or rub together, there is a chance of friction; thus, the components may possibly wear over a period of time. When an implant is subjected to wear, nano/microparticles of the implants are leached out from their outer surface layer. The particle debris accumulated during wear remain in the surrounding tissues and act as foreign bodies, which could lead to adverse effects, such as inflammation, infection, pain, and even ostolysis. If this situation continues over time, then there is a possibility of implant loosening and ultimate failure. Therefore, the choice of biomaterials to manufacture medical implants or devices is of great importance.

There are numerous biomaterials currently available for use in the manufacture of biomedical implants. Among them, Ti, Ti-6Al-4V, CoCrMo, and stainless steel 316L (SS 316L) are clinically notable biomaterials. In an interesting study, Li et al. (2005) reported the tribological analysis of silicon carbide (SiC) with the aim of using it as a biomedical implant as an alternate to other currently used metallic implants, such as CoCrMo, Ti-6Al-4V, and 316L stainless steel. The authors undertook this study because the traditional orthopedic materials used for joint replacement, such as titanium, cobalt, chrome, and stainless steel, have a tendency to wear, and they believed that SiC might replace those materials owing to their tribological behavior. Interestingly, the experimental results showed that it has superior tribological properties to other metallic biomaterials tested in this study. The authors performed the tribological measurements on all the test materials, such as SiC, CoCrMo, Ti-6Al-4V, and 316L stainless steel. Friction, and wear analysis were carried out using a microtribometer. Figure 4.18 shows the comparison of the coefficient of friction, as a function of sliding distance, for all four test materials (Li et al. 2005). The results show that SiC has the lowest coefficient of friction (0.17), followed by CoCrMo, Ti-6Al-4V, and stainless steel. That is, an increase in the coefficient of friction was observed for the CoCrMo at a sliding distance of 2 m. In the case of Ti-6Al-4V and stainless steel, an abrupt increase in the coefficient of friction was observed from the beginning of sliding, and the coefficient of friction remained at higher values compared to SiC and CoCrMo test materials.

The surface scratches and wear damage were studied using SEM. The morphological characteristics of wear tracks and debris formed on the test materials are shown in Figures 4.19 and 4.20 (Li et al. 2005). The SEM

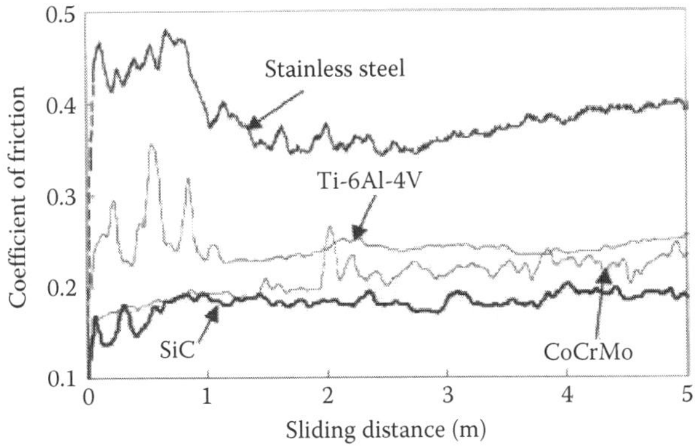

FIGURE 4.18
Coefficient of friction as a function of sliding distance for various test materials. (Adapted with courtesy from Li, X. et al., *J. Biomed. Mater. Res. Appl. Biomater.*, 72B, 353, 2005.)

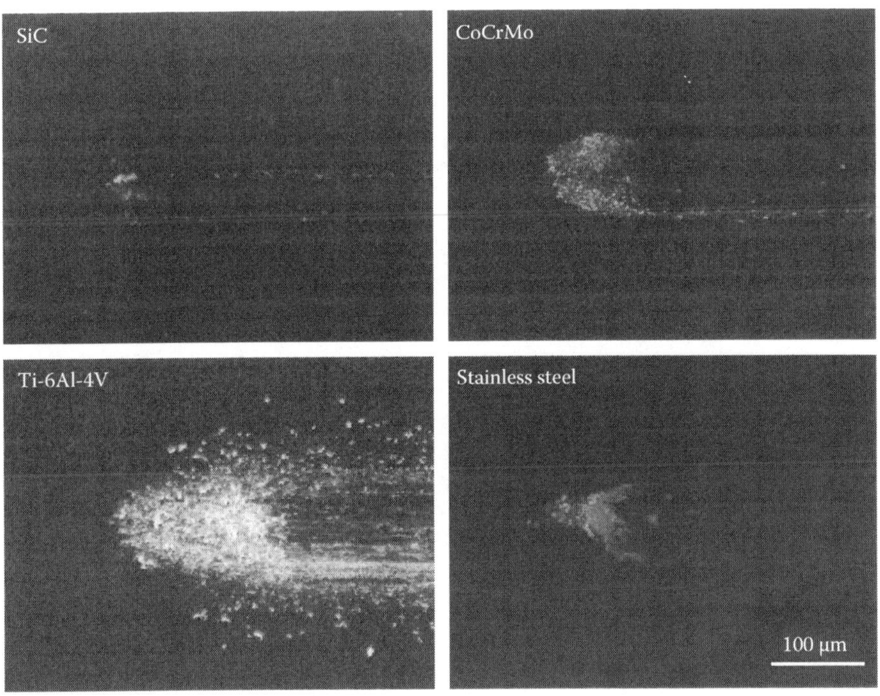

FIGURE 4.19
SEM images of wear tracks and debris formed on various test materials when slid against a WC ball after a sliding distance of 5 m. The end of the wear track is on the left-hand side of the image. (Adapted with courtesy from Li, X. et al., *J. Biomed. Mater. Res. Appl. Biomater.*, 72B, 353, 2005.)

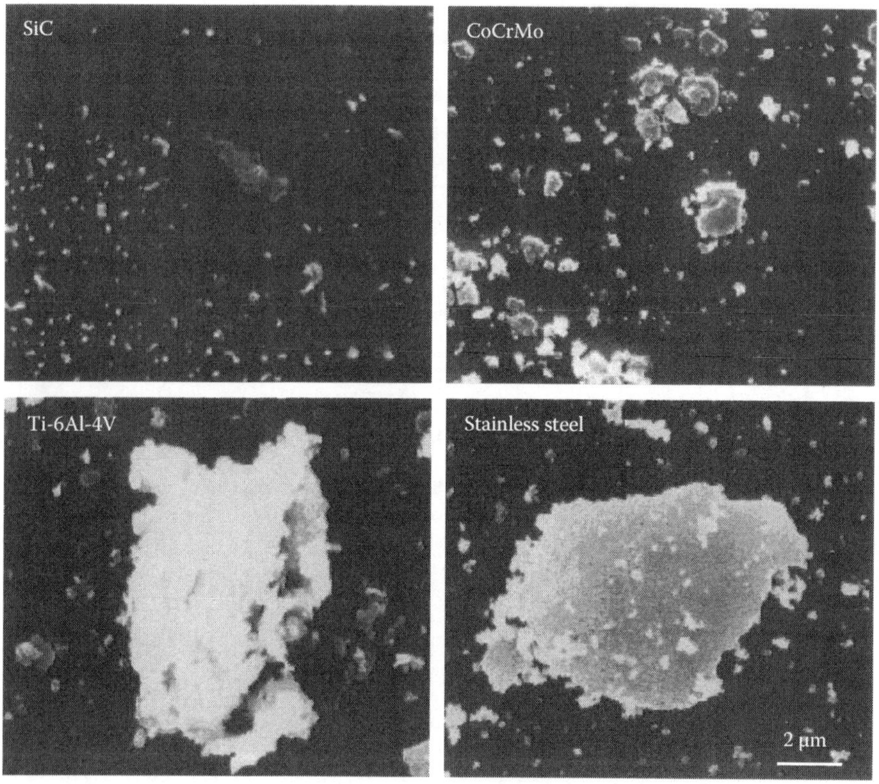

FIGURE 4.20
SEM images of wear debris particles formed on various test materials when slid against a WC ball. (Adapted with courtesy from Li, X. et al., *J. Biomed. Mater. Res. Appl. Biomater.*, 72B, 353, 2005.)

micrographs show that SiC has the smallest wear track and the least amount of debris as compared to other test materials (see Figure 4.19). The wear track and the amount of debris were found to be increased for CoCrMo, stainless steel, and Ti-6Al-4V. For Ti-6Al-4V and stainless steel, scratches with plastic flow of material were found within the wear tracks, owing to the sudden increase in the frictional coefficient. The size and morphology of the wear debris of all the test materials can be clearly seen in Figure 4.20. The micrographs show that the particle size of SiC wear debris is the smallest, followed by CoCrMo, Ti-6Al-4V, and stainless steel. The particle size of the wear debris is relatively uniform for SiC and CoCrMo, whereas Ti-6Al-4V and stainless steel has many large chip-like particulates, in addition to small particle clusters. The edges of these large chip-like particulates exhibit plastic deformation tearing characteristics. The wear debris, in particular the large chip-like particulates, greatly scratched the test materials, causing additional surface damage with a higher coefficient of friction. Based on the results obtained from the tribological and other mechanical behaviors, the authors suggested that SiC merits further evaluation for biomedical applications as an implant. All these data discussed in the tribological section clearly indicate that special attention must be paid in studying the friction and wear aspects of biomaterials in order to enhance their durability and longevity, which may provide a way to reduce or eliminate unwanted implant failure or other adverse tissue reactions caused by the production of metallic debris.

4.13 Case Study

Although biomaterials have long been used in load-bearing applications, such as hip replacement, postsurgical complications are often encountered due to mechanical mismatching or failure of implants. As we know, hip replacements are one of the most common orthopedic procedures. With reference to statistics, it is reported that the total number of hip replacements carried out in the year 2000 was about 152,000, which is an increase of about 33% compared to the year 1990 in the USA alone and it is expected to increase to about 272,000 by the year 2030 (Murugan 2005). When a hip replacement is performed, the damaged hip joint is removed. The hip joint is also called a ball-and-socket joint because the spherical head of the femur bone moves inside the cup-shaped hollow socket (called acetabulum) of the pelvis. The damaged ball-and-socket joint is then replaced with an artificial implant during surgery. An artificial implant has three parts: the stem, which fits into the femur; the ball, which replaces the spherical head of the femur; and the cup, which replaces the worn out hip socket. The selection of materials to be used in the implant depends on several factors, including the material's strength, the age and active condition of the patient, and the surgeon's preference. Although several materials, including metals, ceramics, and polymers, are available for use as hip replacement implant, HA-coated Ti-based metals have long been used as an artificial implant in hip replacement surgery, owing to their numerous excellent physical, mechanical, chemical, and biological properties, which facilitates stable and permanent fixation. However, occasionally, several mechanical complications, such as dislocation, loosening, wear, and fracture have been observed after surgery.

For example, in a notable publication, Sharma et al. (2004) reported on the fracture of HA-coated Ti femoral stem used in total hip replacement surgery. The authors reported three cases of fracture of the femoral stem prosthesis made of HA-coated Ti alloys. Three patients, aged between 51 and 66, had participated in the experimental studies. All of them had been implanted with a JRI femoral prosthesis made of wrought Ti alloy with plasma-sprayed HA coatings. The thickness of the coating sprayed on the metallic implant was found to be 150 μm and the bond strength of metal-HA was 60 MPa. Note that the thickness of the surface coating is critical to achieve the intended function of the implants. A few years postsurgery, the fracture sign of the femoral stem at the top of the distal tip due to fatigue failure was noticed (see Figure 4.21a and b) (Sharma et al. 2004). Most of the fracture surface exhibited low material deformation associated with the fatigue. An initiation site of crack propagation was observed at the surface. The presence of fine secondary cracks and fine striation marks found on the fracture surfaces also supported the mechanism of fatigue (see Figure 4.21c and d). Although the femoral component of the JRI hip replacement has a high success rate, there is occasional failure of the coated implants, as reported in this study. The results of this study showed that, in all three cases, the distal part of the prosthesis had bonded well to host tissue, but no sign of bonding of the proximal part was noticed. It is predictable that micromovements occurring in the proximal part might have caused fracture of the implant. The HA coating of a femoral component may become a significant problem if the proximal part of the femoral component fails to osteointegrate, causing excess loading on the distal part of the femoral component, which leads to fatigue failure of the implant. Notice that

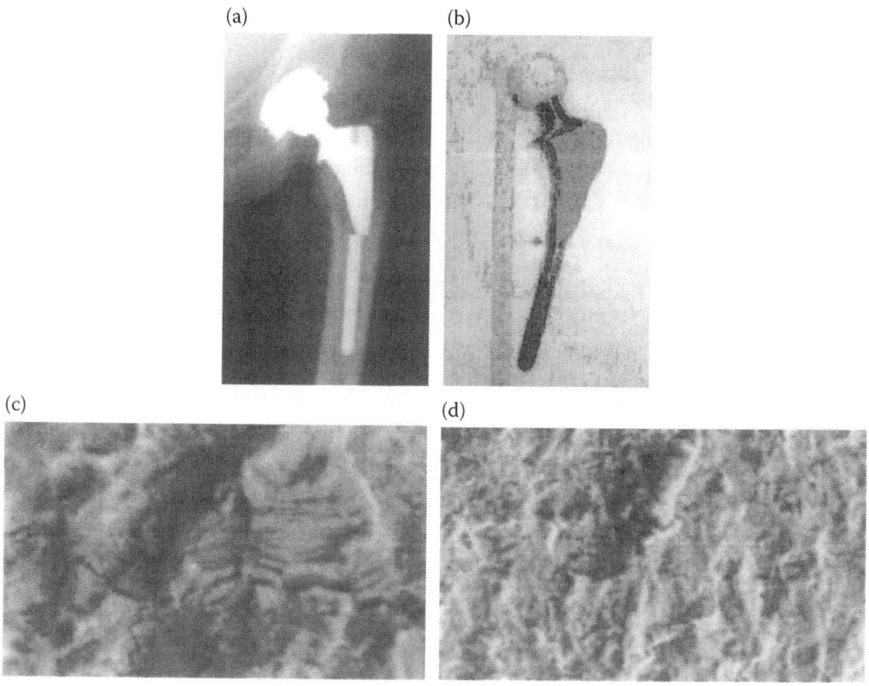

FIGURE 4.21
Clinical results: fracture failure of femoral stem with their surface morphology. (Adapted with courtesy from Sharma, D. K. et al., *Acta Orthop. Scand.*, 75, 768, 2004.)

this could be due to a stress-shielding phenomenon frequently seen in fully HA-coated implants as compared to proximally HA-coated metallic implants. The authors therefore suggested that attention must be paid in selecting the coated metallic implants for hip replacement applications.

4.14 Summary

Mechanical properties, in particular fracture toughness, fatigue, and wear, of biomaterials are very important for load-bearing applications, which determines the durability and longevity of biomedical implants. This chapter attempted to provide several mechanical behaviors of biomaterials required for achieving successful medical implants. As discussed in this chapter, there are several biomaterials available for manufacturing orthopedic and dental implants with favorable mechanical characteristics. Currently, however, there is no single material available for clinical purpose, which mimics the structure and function of the body's own material, tissue, or organ that require an artificial implant. This is because the structure and function of the human body parts are complex. Currently, there is a huge demand for structural biomaterials for load-bearing applications, in particular high strength/low modulus materials. The research on biomaterials is progressing with advanced technologies that may allow us to synthesize and design novel biomaterials with ideal mechanical characteristics to accomplish their specific task. So, success in this exciting endeavor requires a constant multidisciplinary approach from expertise in materials science, mechanical engineering, and cell biology.

Glossary

Crack: Break within a material but without complete separation of parts.

Crack propagation: A continuous growth of crack due to continuous applied force.

Deformation: Changes in shape and size of a material due to an external force.

Dislocations: A crystallographic defect or irregularity within a crystal system.

Elastic deformation: A temporary change in dimensions of a material under the action of force that is capable of recovering its original shape.

Failure: An ultimate separation or loss of material due to applied force.

Fatigue: A mode of progressive cracking or failure of a material that occurs when the material is subjected to cyclic loading.

Fatigue limit: The maximum stress that a material will endure without failure for an infinite number of cyclic loadings.

Fatigue strength: The maximum stress that can be sustained for a specific number of cyclic loadings without fracture.

Fracture: Separation of a material into two or more parts under the action of stress.

Fracture toughness: The ability of a material containing a crack to resist fracture.

Friction: The resistance to relative motion between two surfaces in contact.

Kinetic friction: A frictional force that acts to resist motion of an object that is already in a moving state.

Plane strain: A state of strain in which the strain is normal to the plane (x–y) and the shear strain is assumed to be zero.

Plane stress: A state of stress in which the normal stress and the shear stress directed perpendicular to the plane (x–y) is assumed to be zero.

Plastic deformation: A change in dimensions of a material under the action of force that are not recovered when the force is completely removed.

Slip: A process by which inelastic deformation is produced by dislocation.

Static friction: A frictional force that resists an object's beginning motion.

Tribology: The study that deals with the interaction of sliding surfaces in relative motion.

Wear: Loss or erosion of material from a solid surface by the action of another solid.

EXERCISES

4.1 What is deformation of materials? Explain their types with a specific example.

4.2 Define fracture and its types with examples of biomaterials.

4.3 Can necking phenomenon be observed in any kind of mechanical testing?

4.4 What are the different types of mode of loading in fracture toughening?

4.5 Can we improve the fracture toughness of biomaterials? If so, how?

4.6 Consider a thermoplastic polymeric material that has a fracture toughness value of 2×10^3 J/m^2 and a modulus of elasticity of 80 GPa. Find out the critical crack length under an applied stress of 300 MPa.

4.7 Derive the critical stress required for the crack propagation based on Griffith's theory.

4.8 What is the purpose of an S–N diagram and where is it used?

4.9 Distinguish static and kinetic frictional force and derive the coefficient of respective friction.

4.10 What is the clinical significance of wear in medical prostheses and how to test the wear of biomaterials or medical devices?

References

http://images.google.com/images?um=1&hl=en&q=implants+titanium.

http://hyperphysics.phy-str.gsu.edu/hbase/frict2.html.

http://www.lib.umich.edu/dentlib/Dental_tables/Coeffric.html.

Callister, W. D. 1994. *Materials science and engineering: An introduction*. New York: John Wiley.

Clegg, R. E. and G. D. Paterson. 2004. Ductile particle toughening of hydroxyapatite ceramics using platinum particles. *Proceedings of the Structural Integrity and Fracture*, eds. A., Atrens, J.N., Boland, R., Clegg, and J.R., Griffiths, 47–53. Brisbane.

Delgado, J. A. et al. 1999. Zirconia-toughened hydroxyapatite ceramic obtained by wet sintering. *J. Mater. Sci. Mater. Med.* 10:715.

Li, X. et al. 2005. Micro/nanoscale mechanical and tribological characterization of SiC for orthopedic applications. *J. Biomed. Mater. Res. Appl. Biomater.* 72B:353.

Lin, C. W., C. P. Jug and J. H. Chern Lin. 2005. A comparison of the fatigue behavior of cast Ti-7.5Mo with c.p. titanium, Ti-6Al-4V and Ti-13Nb-13Zr alloys. *Biomaterials* 26:2899.

Mayers, M. A. and K. K. Chawla. 1999. *Mechanical behavior of materials*. Upper Saddle River, NJ: Prentice Hall.

Meyers, M. A. and Chawla, K. K. 2009. *Mechanical behavior of materials*, 2nd Edition. Cambridge University Press, Cambridge, England.

Murugan, R. and S. Ramakrishna. 2005. Development of nanocomposites for bone grafting. *Comp. Sci. Tech.* 65:2385.

Niinomi, M. 1998. Mechanical properties of biomedical titanium alloys. *Mater. Sci. Eng.* A243:231.

______. 2007. Fatigue characteristics of metallic biomaterials. *Int. J. Fatigue* 29:992.

Parton, V.Z. 1992. *Fracture mechanics: From theory to practice*. Philadelphia, PA: Gordon and Breach Science.

Peterlik, H. et al. 2006. From brittle to ductile fracture of bone. *Nat. Mater.* 5:52.

Sharma, D. K. et al. 2004. Fracture o f fully hydroxyapatite-coated titanium femoral stem of a total hip replacement—a report of 3 cases. *Acta Orthop. Scand.* 75:768.

Zhang, C., Y. Leng, and J. Chen. 2001. Elastic and plastic behavior of plasma-sprayed hydroxyapatite coatings on a Ti-6Al-4V substrate. *Biomaterials* 22:1357.

Further Reading

Anderson, T. L. 1994. *Fracture mechanics: Fundamentals and applications*. Boca Raton, FL: CRC Press.

Fung, Y. C. 1993. *Biomechanics: Mechanical properties of living tissues*. Berlin: Springer.

Hayes, W. C. 1986. Bone mechanics: From tissue mechanical properties to an assessment of structural behavior. In *Frontiers in biomechanics*, ed. Y. C. Fung, 196–209. New York: Schmid-Schonbein.

Soboyejo, W. 2007. *Mechanical properties of engineered materials*. Boca Raton, FL: Taylor & Francis, CRC Press.

5

Nanoscale Phenomena

5.1 Introduction

The development of new materials always leads to advances in technology and creates innovative solutions to old problems. Nanomaterials and nanotechnologies are the current key fields with great challenges and possibilities. Nanomaterials, also called nanostructured materials, are single phase or multiphase materials with size less than 100 nm at least in one of the dimensions. For example, ultrathin coatings have one nanoscale dimension, nanotubes and nanowires have nanoscale in two dimensions, whereas nanoparticles (NP) are nanoscale in all three dimensions. A nanometer is one billionth of a meter or one thousandth of a micron and is equivalent to chopping a 1 cm length thread into ten pieces and then chopping one of the pieces into a million pieces, as schematically illustrated in Figure 5.1. The magnification required to visualize NPs would be equivalent to enlarging an apple to the size of the Earth. A comparison of nanofibers with human hair is shown in Figure 5.2.

Basically, nanotechnology is the process of manipulating matter at the atomic scale for practical use and it has begun to revolutionize materials used for traditional science and engineering applications. Nanotechnology is emerging at the crucial stage of convergence with biotechnology and information technology. Four generations of nanotechnology envisaged are as follows (Roco 2006):

- **Generation 1**: Passive nanostructures, including coatings, NPs and nanostructured metals, polymers, and ceramics designed to perform one task. Current era emerged around 2001.
- **Generation 2**: Active nanostructures, including transistors, targeted drugs and chemicals, actuators, and adaptive structures for multitasking. Next era.
- **Generation 3**: Nanosystems with interacting heterogeneous nanocomponents and various assembling techniques, networking at the nanoscale and new architectures. Should emerge around 2010.

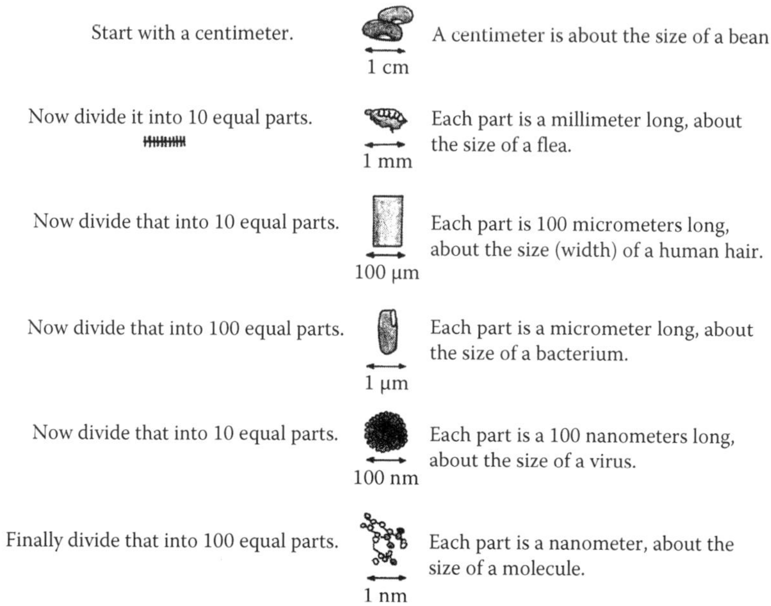

FIGURE 5.1
Comparison of sizes with related objects. (From http://snf.stanford.edu/Education/Nanotechnology.SNF.ppt#270,2,Slide 2. With permission.)

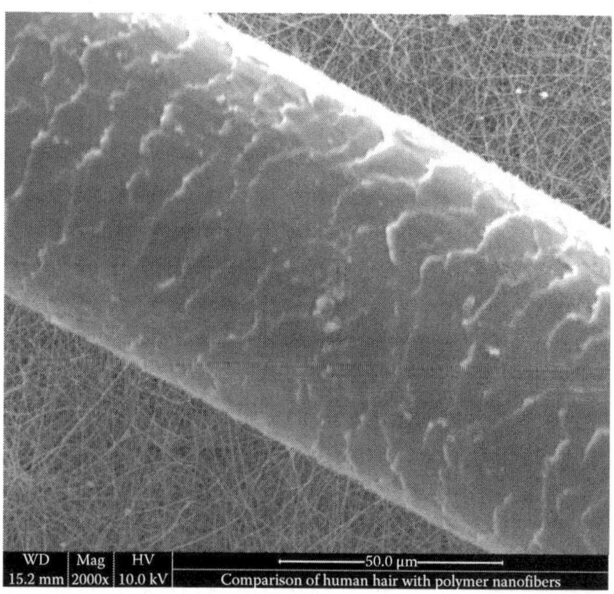

FIGURE 5.2
Comparison of nanofibers with a human hair.

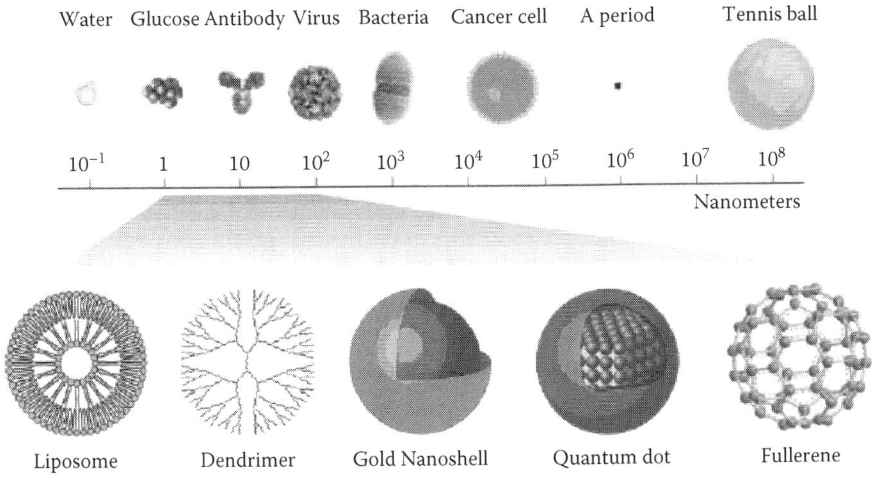

FIGURE 5.3
Comparison of nanoparticles compared with relative biological systems. (Reproduced from McNeil, S. E., *J. Leuko. Bio.*, 78, 585–94, 2005. With permission.)

- **Generation 4**: Integrated nanosystem, functioning much like mammalian cells, consisting of heterogeneous molecules that mimic the processes of life. May emerge around 2020.

The driving force for the use of nanotechnology in biomaterial applications is the similarity of the length scale in the biological structures, which range from proteins, DNA, and viruses (tens of microns), to cells and cellular structure (micron scale), as shown in Figure 5.3. In this chapter, synthesis, characterization, and properties, including the biological and environmental aspects of nanomaterials have been described.

5.2 Nanoscale Phenomena

Nanomaterials have been known and used by humans for centuries. For example, the decorative glaze found in medieval pottery contains NPs dispersed in a unique way in glaze to create unique colors that change with incident lighting and the ruby red color of the stained glass in churches is due to gold NPs trapped in the glass. Modern example of nanotechnology goes back to the late nineteenth century with the production of carbon black and its use in rubber. Although, the exact mechanisms were not known at the time, carbon black's nanoscale particles served to modify the behavior of rubbers. Due to the development of advanced characterization techniques at nanoscale and the novel synthesis routes for the large scale production and variety, the unique properties for a wide range of applications of nanomaterials has been realized.

The realization that nanomaterials would exhibit unique properties has become feasible with the synthesis of ultrafine-grained (UFG) materials by the in situ consolidation of nanoscale atomic clusters in the early 1980s (Gleiter 1981). The study of a new form of carbon (one of the building blocks of nature), called "Buckminster Fullerenes" (famously known as "Buckyballs"), in the mid-1980s has led to the entry of nascent nanotechnology into the mainstream research. The subsequent investigations have resulted in the discovery of "carbon nanotubes" (CNT). The CNTs are tube-like structures of carbon atoms, which are basically sheets of graphite rolled up with their edges connected to form a cylinder. The concurrent developments in analytical tools capable of resolving atomic, molecular, and crystallographic structures in the last 20 years also contributed significantly to the development of nanotechnology.

5.2.1 Properties at Nanoscale

The promising aspect of nanotechnology is its ability to create nanostructured materials that will have novel properties on the bulk materials (macroscale). The properties of the nanomaterials neither correspond to the free atoms or molecules it is composed of nor the bulk material with identical composition, but on many relevant phenomena occurring at the nanoscale, mainly due to the following changes in its international structure:

- Increased surface area of grains
- Increased volume of grain boundaries
- Increased amount of surface atoms
- Formation of discrete electronic energy levels (quantum effect)

The surface area of NPs increases with a decrease in size. This is because a NP of 1-nm size will have 100% of its atoms on its surface, while a 3-nm size NP of spherical shape will have 50% of its atoms on its surface, as indicated in Figure 5.4 (Klabunde 1996). As the grain size decreases, the boundary region between the grains increases. So, nanomaterials, which are basically of smaller grain size, have a large amount of grain boundary area. For a grain size of a single atom, then it would be a perfect disorder of amorphous state. In conventional micron grain size materials, impurities preferentially diffuse to the grain boundary region and may lead to intergranular fracture. Since nanophase material has a large amount of grain boundaries to diffuse, there may be homogenization of impurities and hence less susceptibility to failure.

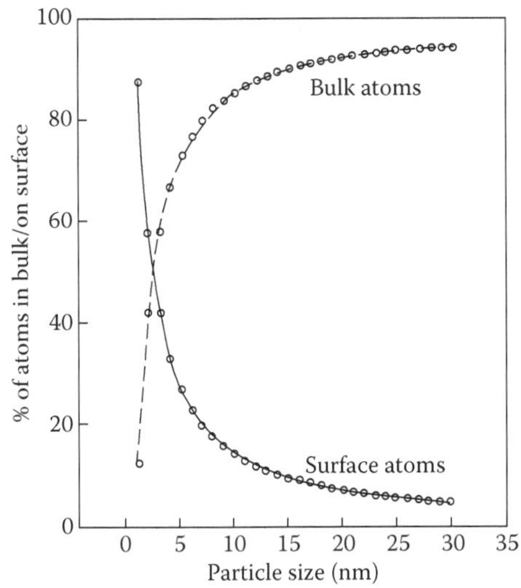

FIGURE 5.4
Percentage of bulk and surface atoms as a function of particle size (based on calculations). (Reprinted from Klabunde, K. J. et al., *J. Phys. Chem.*, 100, 12142–53, 1996. With permission from The American Chemical Society.)

The empirical Hall–Petch equation predicts that strength increases with decreasing grain size as

$$\sigma_y = \sigma_o + kd^{-1/2},$$

where σ_y is the yield strength, σ_o is the lattice yield stress (minimum stress required to move a dislocation), k is a constant (slope of the Hall–Petch plot), and d is the grain size. The hardness of the material also has a similar dependence with grain size. So, the mechanical properties, like strength and hardness, of polycrystalline nanomaterials increases with decreasing grain size. As the increase in strength is due to the piling up of the dislocations at grain boundaries, the increase in the total surface area of the grains increases the dislocation density at the surface, which in turn increases the strength of the nanomaterials. However, when the grain size is less than the dislocation spacing, the above relation is no longer valid and the strength decreases with decrease in grain size, as shown in Figure 5.5. This is attributed to grain boundary sliding due to high defect density. But the decrease in strength improves the formability of nanomaterials, especially ceramics. Superplasticity has also been exhibited by many nanostructured materials relatively at lower temperatures than conventional grain size materials (Padmanabhan 1996).

The large number of surface atoms of nanocrystals provides many active sites for reactions, thereby increasing its chemical and catalytic reactivity.

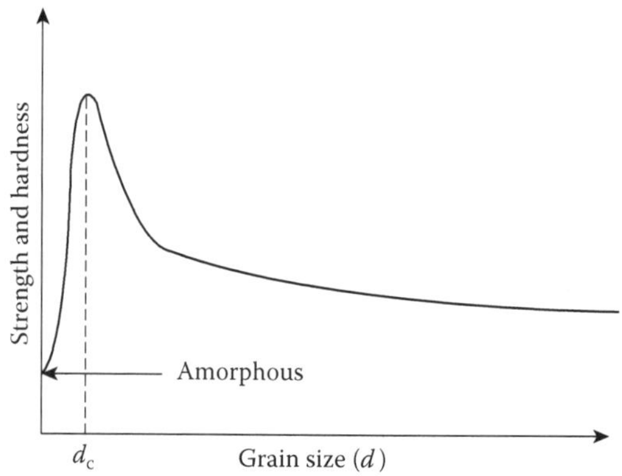

FIGURE 5.5
Strength and hardness vs. grain size. (From Lane, R. et al., *AMPTIAC Q.*, 6, 31, 2002. With permission.)

The thermal properties of the nanostructured materials also change due to enhanced diffusivity at the grain boundaries. Decrease in melting point and thermal conductivity has been observed for nanostructured metals and ceramics.

Many properties of the bulk materials are fundamentally determined by its band structure, which consists of continuous electronic energy levels. However, when the size of the nanocrystals is smaller than about 10 nm, the continuous energy bands collapse into discrete, atomic-like energy levels. This is due to the confinement of electronic wave functions within the particle boundary because of the comparable dimensions, for example, electrons "feel" the presence boundaries and respond to changes in particle size by adjusting their energy. This phenomenon is known as the quantum-size effect, and the nanocrystals are called quantum dots (QDs). The discrete energy levels lead to a discrete absorption spectrum of QDs, in contrast to the continuous absorption spectrum of a bulk semiconductor. So, QDs can be developed to emit and absorb a specific wavelength of light by changing the NP diameters, as shown in Figure 5.6. For example, the nanocrystals of cadmium selenide, which has been extensively studied, will appear yellow around 1.5 nm size, red around 4 nm, and black for larger sizes.

The magnetic properties of NPs also exhibit unusual behaviors resulting from the size effects and interactions with surrounding particles. Several small ferromagnetic particles form only a single magnetic domain, giving rise to superparamagnetism, unlike bulk magnetic materials consisting of multiple magnetic domains. Reducing the size of the magnetic materials changes the electronic properties by reducing the symmetry of the system and by introducing a quantum confinement.

The novel properties of nanomaterials, as summarized in Table 5.1, thus seems to mainly depend on grain size and size distribution, chemical

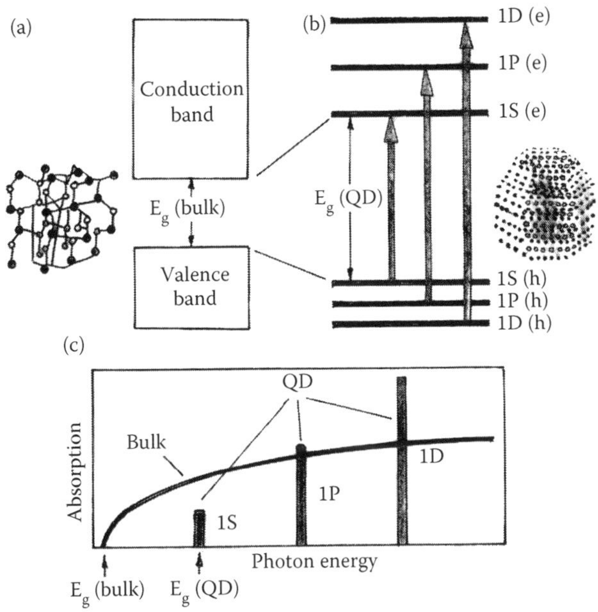

FIGURE 5.6
Schematic representation of energy bands of bulk CdSe (a) and energy levels of QD CdSe (b) and their absorption spectrums (c) corresponds to the absorption spectrum. (From http://quantumdot.lanl.gov/pages/Publications/Klimov_LAscience.pdf. With permission.)

composition, presence of interfaces (grain boundaries, free surface), and interactions between the constituent domains.

5.3 Processing of Nanostructured Materials

Nanostructured materials have structural features that are less than 100 nm at least in one dimension. These features are usually produced by processing ("nanostructuring") in one of two general ways: (i) top-down process/one-step approach and (ii) bottom-up process/two-step approach.

The top-down methods directly convert bulk materials into submicron- or nanoscaled materials by structural decomposition (Figure 5.7), thus it is also called "one-step approach." These techniques exhibit significant advantages compared to bottom-up processes: bulk nanomaterials are achieved in fully dense shape without involving nanopowders, and without grain coarsening as during nanopowder consolidation. By contrast, the bottom-up approach starts with atoms, ions, or molecules to build the nanoscale phase (Figure 5.7), which are subsequently consolidated as bulk materials (two-step process). Both approaches can be carried out in gas, liquid, supercritical fluids, and solid states of metals (Hu 1999).

TABLE 5.1

List of Novel Properties and Relevant Applications of Nanomaterials

Property	Enhancement Factors	Applications
Chemical	Increment of their surface area that increases the chemical activity	Catalysts for noxious and toxic gases; fuel cells using bimetallic nanoparticles
Mechanical	Reduction in grain size increases fatigue life. Possess good formability and machinability. Porous and extremely lightweight materials	Tougher and harder cutting tools, rocket engines, thrusters, and vectoring nozzles; ductile, machinable ceramics some with superplastic behavior; better insulation materials, like aerosols and smart (ability to respond to change in their Surroundings) windows, which darken when the sun is too bright and lighten themselves otherwise
Optical	Quantum confinement of electrical carriers, efficient energy and charge transfer over nanoscale distances and a highly enhanced role of interfaces	Casings to improve shielding against electromagnetic interference. Glues for use in optoelectronics
Electrical/ electronic	Due to their large grain boundary (surface) area, they can hold considerably more energy, optical absorption band can be introduced or an existing band can be altered	High energy density batteries that require far less frequent recharging and last much longer. Large electrochromic display devices
Magnetic	Coercivity and saturation magnetization increases with a decrease in the grain size and an increase in the specific surface area	High-power rare-earth magnets for quieter submarines, automobile alternators, land-based power generators, ultrasensitive analytical instruments, and magnetic resonance imaging (MRI)
Biological	Improved permeability, enhanced adsorption of proteins	Permeability through biological barriers, improved biocompatibility, targeted drug delivery

Source: Based on http://www.engr.utexas.edu/che/nano; http://www.nanomat.com/nano-app.htm. With permission.

5.3.1 Top-Down Methods

Plastic deformation is well known to alter the microstructure and properties of metallic materials. For example, during heavy rolling or drawing, microstructure refinement takes place and this leads to an improvement in strength, although with reduced ductility. The severe plastic deformation (SPD) technique produces UFG microstructures that exhibit both high strength and good ductility in various bulk metallic materials. Basically, large amounts of defects, mostly dislocations, are created in the material, which then self-assemble into nanoscale grains (also called cells, subgrains), sometimes under external

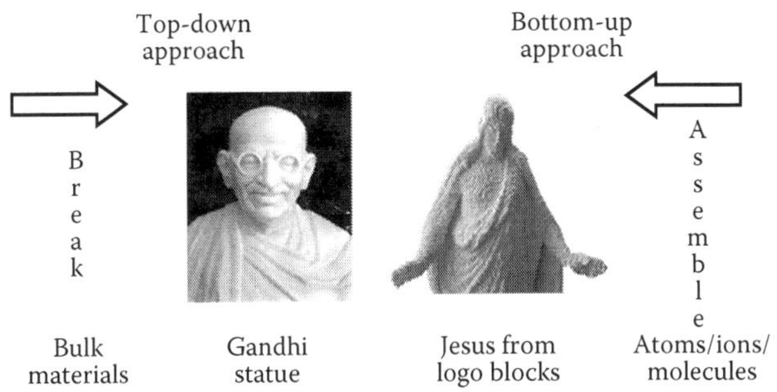

FIGURE 5.7
Schematic diagram of top-down and bottom-up approaches for nanomaterials synthesis. (Modified from Hu, E. and Shaw, D., *Nanostructure science and technology: R&D status and trends in nanoparticles, nanostructured materials, and nanodevices,* National Science and Technology Council, Washington, DC, 1999.)

TABLE 5.2
Top-Down Methods for the Synthesis of Nanostructured Materials

Method	Process Description
Equal channel angular pressing	Material is passed through a die a few times with two channels of intersection at 90°–120°
Severe plastic torsion straining	Disk-shaped sample is compressed to high pressures and one of the die is moved relative to the other
Multiple forging	Repeated forging of the material at elevated temperatures with change of the axis of the applied stress
Accumulative roll-bonding	Repeated rolling of similar or dissimilar metals sheets
Repetitive corrugation and straightening	Repeated bending and straightening of metallic sheets
Friction stir welding	Sample cooled to liquid nitrogen temperature were friction stir welded
Multipass coin-forging	Repeated pressing of metal sheet between sine wave-shaped dies with rotation of the sample followed by flat forging
Constrained groove pressing	Uses wedged-shaped dies in the above process
Surface mechanical attrition	Shot peening of metallic surfaces with a larger number of steel balls at ultrasonic frequency for a short time
Ball milling	Material undergoes severe mechanical deformation by ball milling

heating. The self-assembly of dislocations lowers the free energy such that the density is lower within the subgrain and higher at its boundary The various mechanical/thermal methods used for the preparation of nanostructured materials by the top-down approach are listed in Table 5.2.

The equal channel angular pressing (ECAP) route produces UFG structures by deformation of bulk samples by pure shear and has the ability to produce large samples (60 mm diameter and 200 mm length) for further

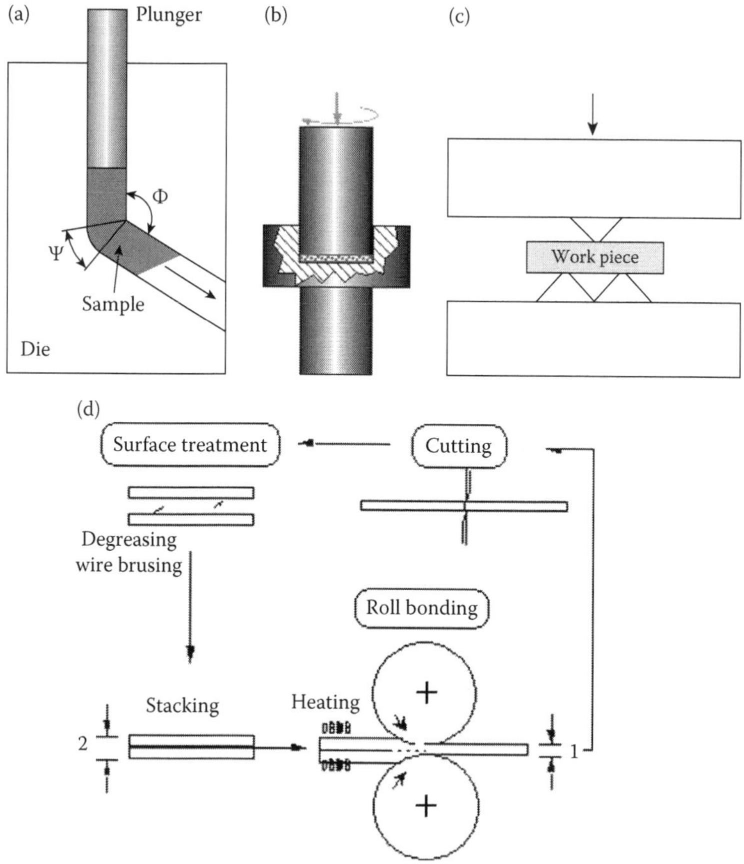

FIGURE 5.8
Schematic diagram of equal channel angular pressing (a), severe pressure torsion straining (b), repetitive corrugation and straightening (c), and accumulative roll bonding (d). (Reprinted from http://www.nanospd.org/Resources/SPDTechniques.htm. With permission from International Steering Committee for NanoSPD. Reprinted from Tsuji et al., *Scripta Mater.*, 40, 795, 1999. With permission from Elsevier.)

processing by more conventional means (Valiev et al. 2003). Further thermomechanical treatments can effect in novel properties, like increased strength combined with good ductility, which are not possible through conventional methods. The schematic diagram of ECAP route is shown in Figure 5.8, in comparison with severe pressure torsion straining (SPTS), repetitive corrugation and straightening, and accumulative roll-bonding routes. Nanostructured metallic materials with grain sizes below 100 micron can only be produced by SPTS and accumulative roll-bonding techniques. Although SPTS can be used for powders, it has a limitation on sample size for further mechanical testing. The accumulative roll-bonding technique

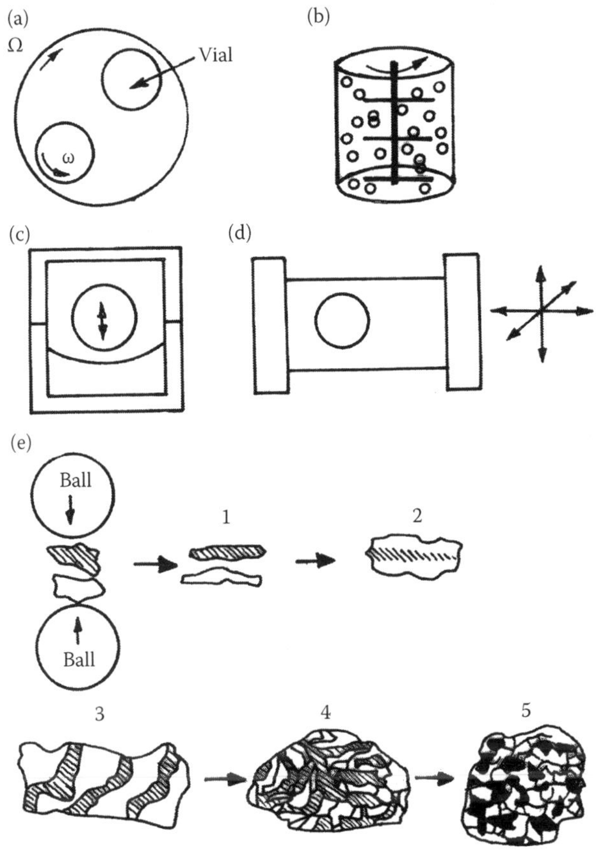

FIGURE 5.9
Various types of milling machines used for processing nanostructured materials: (a) planetary mill, (b) attrition mill, (c) 1D vibrating mill, (d) 3D vibrating mill, and (e) schematic diagram of the evolution of mechanical alloying of powder particles. (Reproduced from Gaffet, E. et al., *J. Mater. Chem.*, 9, 305–14, 1999. With permission from The Royal Society of Chemistry.)

may not be viable for a large-scale production as it involves many repetitive process cycles (Koch 2003).

Ball milling has also been used to produce nanostructured materials and can be divided into two types: mechanical milling and mechanical alloying (Lane 2002). In the first process, also called mechanical attrition, high-energy ball milling is used to grind and refine the grains of elements and compounds to nanoscale size. The second type, also called reaction milling, involves material transfer leading to *in situ* solid-state chemical reactions between precursor materials during milling. A schematic diagram of the behavior of powder particles during mechanical alloying is shown in Figure 5.9, along with various milling apparatus (Gaffet 1999). Although all the solid elements can be ball milled to have nanosize grains, the balance between the defect/dislocation density introduced by milling and its recovery by thermal process limits the minimum grain size attainable in mechanical milling. The minimum grain size achievable thus depends on both the process parameters and material properties. Generally, extended milling times result in more uniform grain sizes.

Large quantities of nanostructured metallic material with grain sizes less than 100 nm can be easily produced by this simple and straightforward milling process. However, severe contamination from the milling media (balls and vial) and environment, nonuniform particle sizes due to short milling times, and nonhomogeneous chemical composition due to incomplete milling reactions are serious problems with the ball-milling process. The effects of environmental contamination can be minimized by performing the milling in the presence of liquid nitrogen, which is also referred to as cryogenic milling. Also, by optimizing the milling temperature and other milling parameters, *in situ* consolidation of the nanoscale powder to solid spheres can be achieved (Zhu 2003). Another commonly used approach to produce bulk nanostructured metals is crystallization of a metastable amorphous structure formed by nonequilibrium processing, such as rapid solidification or mechanical alloying. The presence of the residual amorphous phase may affect the inherent properties of the nanostructured materials.

5.3.2 Bottom-Up Methods

The "bottom-up" approach represents the concept of assembling a nanomaterial from basic building blocks of atoms or molecules via chemical reactions. This approach provides the possibility of creating exact materials with the desired property. The various techniques developed for the production of nanostructured materials by this approach can be grouped into physical methods that involve reactions in gas phase and chemical methods that involve reactions in liquid phase as

- Physical methods
    - Gas-phase condensation
    - Metal evaporation
    - Spray pyrolysis
    - Laser ablation
    - Plasma synthesis
- Chemical methods
    - Sol-gel synthesis
    - Self-assembly
    - Electrolytic deposition

- Chemical vapor deposition
- Laser pyrolysis

The inert gas condensation (IGC) is the straightforward method to consistently produce nanoscale metallic materials (Gleiter 1989). In this process, the metal is quickly heated above its melting point in a vacuum chamber, which produces adequate vapor of atoms. A background gas, which is mostly inert, is continuously introduced and removed from the chamber at low pressures. This gas flow moves the metal vapor away from the heating zone and because of condensation, the vaporized atoms agglomerate to form very small clusters of nanoscale size (Figure 5.10). These clusters are carried by convection current to the walls of a tube cooled by liquid nitrogen, which are then scraped, collected, and compacted as a pellet in the chamber itself. As ultrahigh vacuum (UHV) is used in this process, the nanomaterial formed is highly pure without any contamination. Nanostructured oxides and other compounds of the evaporated metal can be formed by introducing a suitable reactive gas in the cold gas stream (Siegel 1991). Electron beam heating, laser ablation, sputtering, or plasma methods are also used for the evaporation of the materials (Figure 5.9) (Hahn 1997).

Alternatively, a few droplets of the precursor solution of the metal are sprayed into a flame and the evaporation of the solvent leads to the

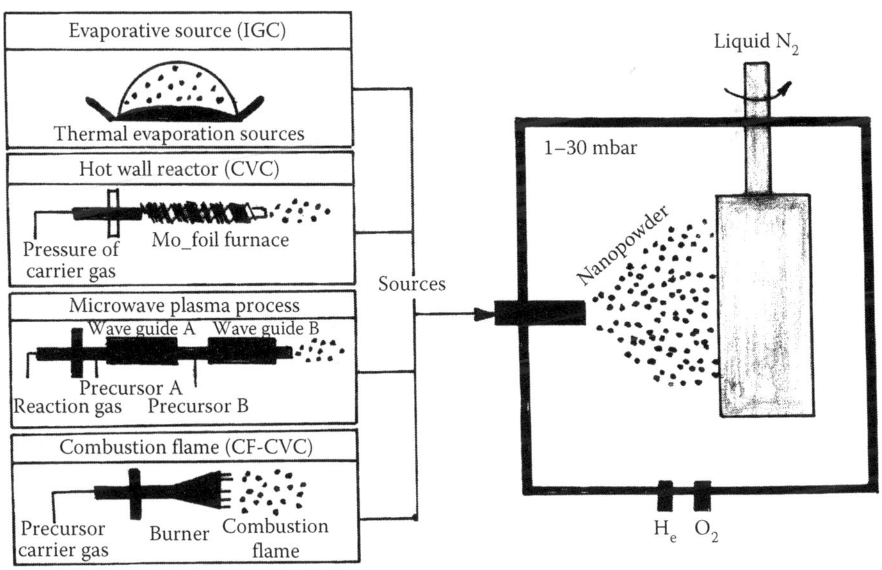

FIGURE 5.10
The gas phase synthesis technique of nanocrystalline materials. (Reprinted from Hahn, H., *Nanostruct. Mater.*, 9, 3–12, 1997. With permission from Elsevier.)

homogenous nucleation and growth of the particles. The rapid cooling results in the formation of NPs. The flame spray pyrolysis (FSP) processes are attractive as they do not require vacuum, inert atmosphere, or high temperatures. Also, a wide variety of precursor can be used so that a broad spectrum of functional metal, metal oxide, and mixed metal oxide NPs can be synthesized. Although thermal plasma and lasers are also used as the heating source, ultrasonic spray pyrolysis is a relatively new method for fabrication of submicrometric metallic particles. The FPS process has been used for the commercial production of NPs (Swihart 2003).

The self-assembly of molecules into macroscopic components is now emerging as a promising synthetic strategy to form nanostructured materials and by definition, self-assembly is a process in which molecules (or parts of molecules) spontaneously form ordered aggregates/components without external intervention (Whitesides 2002). A schematic diagram of the self-assembly process at the liquid–air interface during the early stages of an evaporating drop leading to the formation of nanocrystals is shown in Figure 5.11. The direct observation of monolayer islands of Au nanocrystals on the top surface of the drop and its growth as a compact structure by self-assembly using an optical microscope is also shown in Figure 5.11 (Bigioni 2006). Self-assembly is a thermodynamically favorable spontaneous process. The interactions through which self-assembly occurs are generally weak (i.e., comparable to thermal energies) and noncovalent, such as van der Waals, Coulomb, hydrophobic, capillary force, and hydrogen-bonding interactions. This is because to generate ordered structure by self-assembly, it must be possible for the components to adjust their positions or must be reversible once it is formed. So, the interactions are of the order of the forces tending to disrupt them. Weak covalent interactions (π–π interactions coordination bonds) are also increasingly being accepted as appropriate for self-assembly. The mobility and complimentarity among the components are also crucial for self-assembly process. Normally, self-assembly is carried out in solution or at an interface to provide the required movement of the components.

Although, self-assembly concepts were initially developed with molecules, now the concepts have the potential to self-assemble components of any size and any ordered states of matter that probably cannot be generated by any other type of process. By self-assembly, it is possible to assemble nanometer-scale components into ordered zero-dimensional (0D) nanoparticles, one-dimensional (1D) nanorods, nanowires, nanotubes, and nanobelts, two-dimensional (2D) monolayers and thin films and its extension to three-dimensional (3D) super lattice nanostructures. For example, self-assembly of Au nanocrystals, nanorods, AB or AB_2 2D superstructures and ... polypyrrole 3D assembled nanostructures have been developed (Wang ... Functional organic molecules are often used as capping agents to ...ze and passivate the NPs, but they also affect the assembly process ...sulting superstructure. As nature self-organizes the biomolecules, ...peptides and proteins, to form well-defined structures with specific

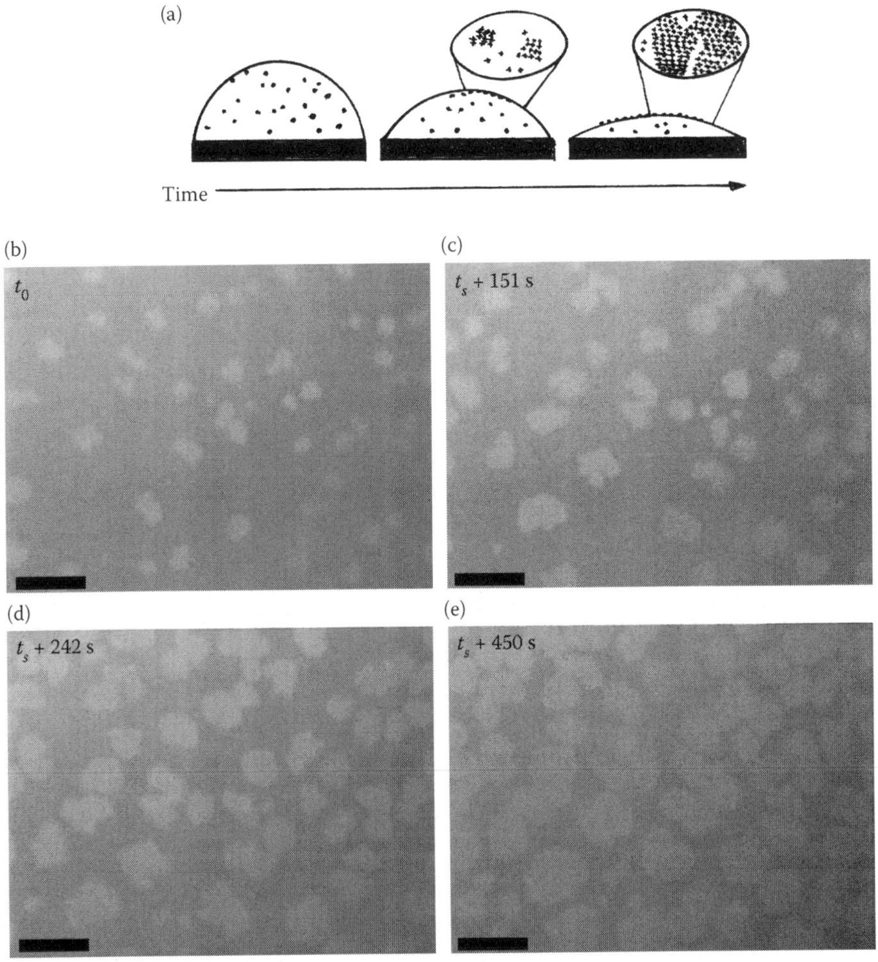

FIGURE 5.11
(a) Schematic diagram of the self-assembly process at the liquid–air interface during the early stages of drying, illustrating the formation of nanocrystals. (b–e) Optical micrographs of the growth sequence of 6-nm caped gold nanocrystals forming monolayer islands by self-assembly on the top surface of an evaporating drop. Scale bars are 50 μm. (Reprinted from Bigioni, T. P., Lin, X. M., Nguyen, T. T., Corwin, E. I., Witten, T. A., and Jaeger, H. M., *Nature Mater.*, 5, 265–70, 2006. With permission from Macmillan Publishers Ltd.)

functions, this knowledge of the self-assembly process has been exploited in the design of novel nanostructured biomaterials (Zhang 2005). Amphiphilic molecules such as surfactants, lipids, block copolymers, polysaccharides, and DNA are used. PuraMatrix is a commercially available nanofiber scaffold formed by self-assembly of peptide Lego molecules (as it resembles the toy Lego bricks with both pegs and holes to precisely assemble) and has been used for bone tissue applications. The unusual combination of high recognition, selectivity, and polyanionic character are the motivation to use DNA molecules, and large-scale uniaxial gold nanorods has been formed by DNA-assisted assembly. The controlled growth of viruses and bacteria can be exploited to assemble NPs, mainly magnetic and semiconductor nanomaterials, to form fibers and wires.

The nanostructured materials can also be assembled by biomimetic, template-assisted, and external-field assisted processes. The biomimetic route, also referred to as the bio-inspired route, is based on the understanding or perhaps mimicking of the ways in which biological materials (e.g., bone, tooth, shells, skin, cartilage, tendons, silk) are assembled and then apply the processes to develop new materials by the self-assembly route. The main characteristic of biominerals is that the organic matrix is first arranged and the inorganic nanophase, which reinforces the matrix, grows within the organic template (Dujardin 2002). So, the production of nanostructures by the biomimetic route mostly focuses on the self-assembly of hybrid organic and inorganic building blocks. Nanostructured materials with some characteristics of enamel have been formed by biomimetic synthesis of the fluorapatite-gelatin hybrid system (Bush 2001).

By self-assembly route, it may be difficult to have control over the size, shape, and structure of the assemblies for device applications. So, templates with predetermined structures on patterned surfaces could be used to direct the self-assembly of nanocomponents in the confined spaces, which will eventually produce assemblies with required size, shape, and structure (Wang 2005). Microfabrication methods, such as photolithography, can provide surface patterns at nanometer scale. Both the top-down and bottom-up approaches are thus integrated in the template-assisted assembly route. The membrane-mimetic compartments, like vesicles and microemulsions, are also often used as confined reaction media for the synthesis of inorganic NPs. The self-assembly at the liquid/water interface by Langmuir–Blodgett film techniques frequently results in more complicated structures. Due to the weak nature of the noncovalent interactions, external fields such as electric, magnetic, electrophoretic, pressure, and shearing fields have been applied for the assembly of nanoscale components into large blocks.

The sol-gel synthesis method is a wet chemical method that has been extensively used for the formation of nanostructured materials compared to any other solution-based synthesis methods. It basically involves the formation of hydroxide compound gels from organometallic precursors, which are heated in a controlled manner to obtain the final product (Lane 2002). The sol-gel method has been extensively used in the formation of nanostructured materials as it can be used for

- Synthesis of almost any materials
- Cosynthesis of two or more materials
- Both metals and ceramics synthesis at low temperatures (<600°C)

- Extremely homogeneous and ultrahigh purity (99.9999%) materials synthesis
- Precise control of physiochemical, mechanical, and microstructure properties
- Commercially viable larger production of the final products

Collectively, chemical synthesis methods are advantageous as they allow tailoring of the assembly of atomic or molecular precursors, enhancing the control over mixing of constituent phases at the molecular level for the required stoichiometry. They are also easily upgradeable for the production of bulk quantities of nanoscale materials. Although they have been extensively used for the synthesis of nonmetallic materials, some of the methods are extended for the formation of nanostructured metallic materials. For example, chemical reduction of liquid polyols containing the dissolved metallic salts, using microwaves has been used for the formation of metallic nanophases (Komarneni et al. 2004). However, nanostructured metals by the two-step approach often have defects, such as porosity and cracks, which lead to very low ductility of the materials. The one-step approach, in comparison, can produce 100% dense and defect-free nanostructured metals, which exhibit superior mechanical properties.

5.4 Characterization Techniques

The current developments in nanotechnology have been made possible by the simultaneous advancement in instrumentation to observe measure and manipulate the individual nanomaterials and nanostructures at atomic-level resolution. The characterization of nanomaterials includes measurements such as size and size distribution, shape and morphological features (surface roughness, porosity, etc.), state of dispersion, surface area and surface chemistry, physical and chemical properties. The characterization techniques can generally be classified as single-particle or ensemble techniques. The single-particle techniques isolate and collect data from individual particles. A common example of a single-particle technique is electron microscopy. In ensemble techniques, response from a statistically significant number of particles is measured simultaneously. Laser light scattering technique is a commonly employed ensemble technique. In general, morphological and surface information, such as shape and aspect ratio, as well as texture and roughness parameters, can only be obtained with the single-particle techniques. The parameters for each particle are recorded to generate a statistical distribution for the entire set of particles. However, the complete characterization of nanomaterials is important for understanding its properties and their effects to develop applications. Basic information on the principals of characterization methods, which are generally agreed to be the minimal characterization required for nanomaterials, is discussed.

5.4.1 X-Ray Diffraction and Scattering Methods

The wavelength of x-rays are in the same order as the dimensions of the nanostructures and hence, provide a variety of techniques for the structural characterization of nanomaterials, such as high-resolution x-ray diffraction (HRXRD), x-ray reflectometry (XRR), and small-angle x-ray scattering (SAXS). All the techniques are also virtually nondestructive. The x-ray diffraction (XRD) method has long been widely used for the determination of crystallinity, crystal structures, cell parameters, phase identifications, preferred orientation, and residual stress in materials. Therefore, it has also been used to characterize most of the above parameters of NPs, nanowires and tubes, and nanostructured materials. In XRD, a collimated x-ray beam is incident on the sample and the intensity of the elastically scattered (diffracted) beam due to the periodic arrangement of atoms in the sample is measured as a function of the diffracted angle "2θ". The interplanar spacing "d" between atomic planes in the crystalline material is then calculated from Bragg's law:

$$2d\sin\theta = \lambda,$$

where "λ" is the wavelength of the x-rays used and, from d, other structural parameters are subsequently obtained. Interestingly, a decrease in crystallite size causes broadening of the diffraction peak and from the full width at half maximum (FWHM) height of the diffraction peak, the nanocrystallite size $t_{(hkl)}$ perpendicular to a crystallographic plane (hkl) can be evaluated according to the Scherrer formula, $t_{(hkl)} = K\lambda/B\cos\theta_{(hkl)}$, where t is the crystallite size (nm); K is the shape factor ($K = 0.9$); λ is the wavelength of the x-rays ($\lambda = 1.54056$ Å for Cu-Kα radiation); B is the FWHM (rad) and $\theta_{(hkl)}$ is the Bragg's diffraction angle (°). This simple technique is thus very useful in characterizing not only NPs, but also for measuring the film thickness of highly textured thin films. Since peak broadening is also caused by inhomogeneous strains due to residual stress in the crystallite, careful analysis of the peak shapes should be done to obtain the contribution due to the crystallite size of the peak width. The NPs are also often twinned, which gives particle sizes different from the true size obtained by direct techniques such as electron microscopy.

In SAXS, a highly collimated x-ray beam is passed through the sample and the scattered x-rays at small angles are measured, as shown schematically in Figure 5.12 (Svergun 2003). The scattering occurs in all directions and is dominated by coherent scattering, which interferes and produces diffraction effects. The resulting pattern has been found to provide structural

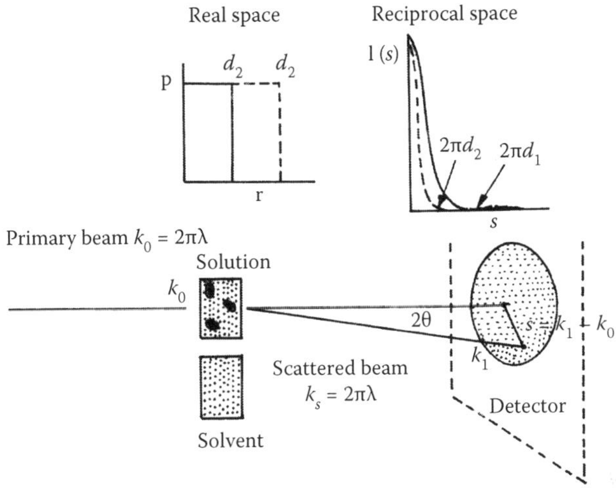

FIGURE 5.12
Schematic diagram of the SAXS method and comparison of the experimental data with the Fourier transformation from real to reciprocal space. (From Svergun, D. I. and Koch, M. H. J., *Rep. Prog. Phys.*, 66, 1735–82, 2003. With permission.)

information on the inhomogeneities of the electron density within 100 nm. As nanostructured materials differ in atomic density in the interior of the grains and the interface region, the surface-to-volume ratio of the internal structure of NPs can be determined by SAXS. This method yields not only information on the sizes and shapes of NPs, but also on its internal structure. However, it may be difficult to reconstruct the exact microstructure from the SAXS pattern, since all phase information is lost in a scattering and only scattering intensity can be measured. Also, the SAXS results are essentially the Fourier transform of the electron density, which must be deduced in order to resolve the morphology, as shown in Figure 5.12.

5.4.2 Electron Microscopy

Transmission electron microscopy (TEM) is one of the most powerful techniques to provide valuable information on size, shape, and morphology of NPs. In TEM, highly accelerated electrons (100 KeV to 1 MeV) are focused on a thin specimen of the sample or NPs held on a thin amorphous carbon or polymer films, and the transmitted electrons, after penetrating through the sample, are either deflected or undeflected depending upon the scattering processes experienced by electrons during the passage. Elastic scattering gives rise to diffraction patterns with the deflection of the transmitted electron beam. As an electron can be focused on any region of interest, it is called selected-area diffraction (SAED) and can be used to characterize the crystal structure of individual NPs, nanorods and wires,

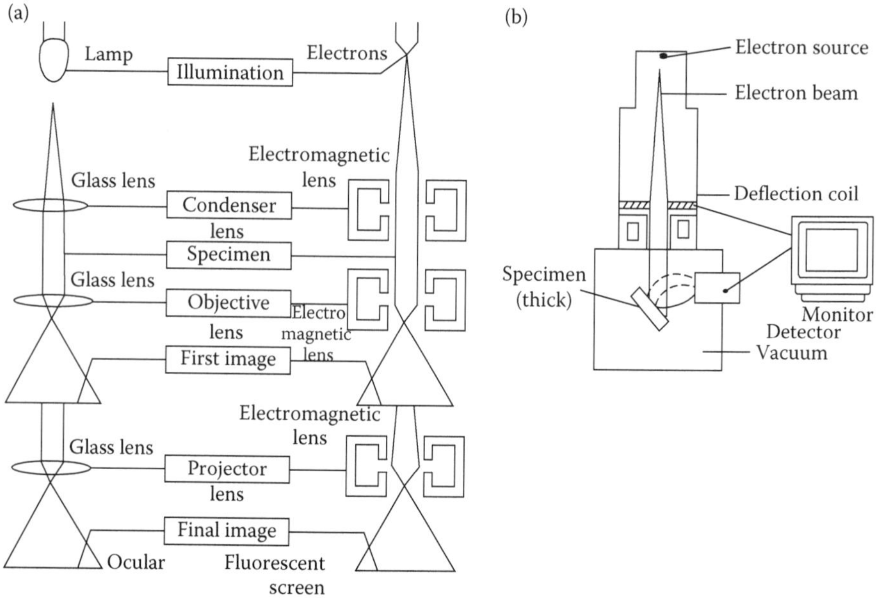

FIGURE 5.13
Comparison of a projector with TEM (a) and schematic diagram of a SEM (b). FEI Company, All you want to know about electron microscopy. (From www.feicompany.com.)

and different regions of the nanostructured materials. Inelastic scattering with the sample electrons at heterogeneities such as dislocations, defects, density variations, grain boundaries, second-phase particles, etc., causes complex absorption and scattering effects, leading to intensity variation of the undeflected transmitted electron beam. A comparison of the TEM with the optical microscope is shown schematically in Figure 5.13. By using TEM, either imaging the sample or structural analysis of the sample can be carried out. The greatest advantage of higher magnification above million times and higher resolution of few nm is due to the small effective electron wavelength. For example, the wavelength of 100 KeV electrons is 0.37 nm. The higher the accelerating voltage, the better the resolution of materials. The TEM thus provides direct information on the size and shape of nanoparticles at very high resolution. However, enough particles should be examined to have a realistic representation of the sample. Nowadays, automated image analysis software is used for this purpose. The major limitation of TEM is its limited depth of resolution and it provides only two-dimensional images. But chemical information of the nanomaterials can be carried out by analyzing the energy of the x-rays emitted (EDAX) or by measuring the energy loss of the primary beam (EELS).

Scanning electron microscopy (SEM) is one of the most versatile methods for characterizing nanostructured materials. In the SEM, an electron beam with a very fine spot size of ~5 nm (energy from a few hundred eV to 50 KeV) is scanned across the specimen surface (instead of transmitted, as in TEM). During penetration and passage through the sample, a variety of interactions occur and this results in the emission of electrons and photons from the sample, which is used for imaging and characterization of the sample. Some of the SEM modes widely used to characterize nanostructured materials include secondary and backscattered electrons, x-ray mapping, electron beam induced current, electron channeling, electron backscattered diffraction, and Auger electron microscopy.

The secondary electrons are produced due to inelastic scattering of the incident electron beam and are used for routine morphological imaging. Basically, they are collected by a secondary electron detector and are used to modulate the intensity of a display system, such as a cathode ray tube. The image is built up pixel by pixel as the beam is scanned across the sample and is displayed. The backscattered electron image is formed by detecting the elastically scattered high-energy primary electrons. The resolution of the SEM is limited by the size of the electron beam spot being scanned (not by the wavelength of electron beam) and is much less than that of a TEM. Using high-resolution SEM, nanomaterials can be imaged at resolutions approaching 0.3 nm at 30 KeV. The chemical composition of the nanostructured materials are routinely characterized using the characteristic x-rays or Auger electrons from the sample under electron beam.

5.4.3 Scanning Probe Microscopy

Scanning probe microscopy (SPM) is a group of techniques that directly provides three-dimensional real-space images and allows locally measured properties of nanostructured materials at atomic resolution. In all the SPM techniques, an atomically sharp tip (typically of 3–50 nm dimension with one or a few atoms) is scanned at a few Angstroms above the surface or moved on the sample and the interaction between the tip and the sample is measured as shown in Figure 5.14. Alternatively, the surface is scanned under the probe. The tip is mounted on a cantilever and the scan may cover a distance of around 100 microns in the x and y directions and about 4 μm in the z direction. The different types of SPM techniques are characterized by the probe and its interaction with the sample surface and are no longer restrained by the wavelength of electron or light.

One of the first tools used for the investigation of nanomaterials was the scanning tunneling microscope (STM) in 1981. The STM formed the basis for the family of scanning probe tools. The STM uses an atomically "sharp" tip (typically pyramidal in shape and coming to a point that is literally one or two atoms across), which is moved over a sample's surface a few Angstroms from making contact. The tip is then scanned across the surface in a regular pattern (much as one would mow a lawn) and the electrical current (called tunneling current), which traverses the gap between the tip and the sample, is monitored. By keeping the height of the tip constant and measuring the

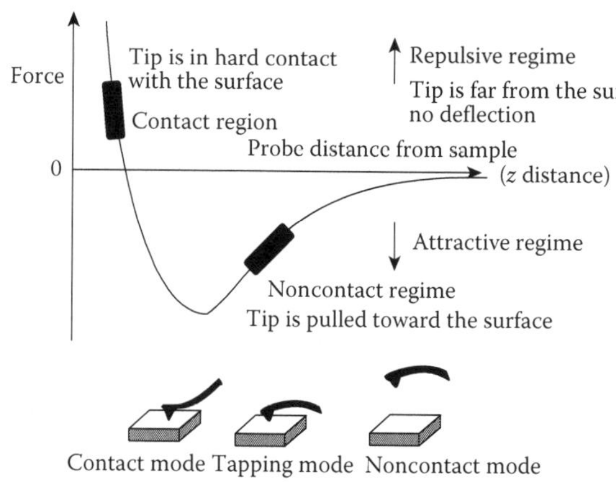

FIGURE 5.14
Schematic diagram of SPM, force–distance curve, and typical AFM micrograph. (From http://www.aleajactaest.org/data/events/1stALEA/Biodegradation_HSAzevedo_1stAleaJactaESTTutorialCourse_Ischia_July2005.pdf.)

changing electrical current (more when close to the sample, less when farther away), or by keeping the current constant and measuring the deflection of the tip, a topographical map can be generated of the sample's surface. The device relies upon the small amount of electric current, which crosses the gap between the tip and the sample ("tunneling").

The other most widely used member of the SPM family is the atomic force microscope (AFM). Similar to the STM, it uses an atomically sharp tip, but instead of carefully moving it just Angstroms from the sample, the AFM actually drags its tip along the sample's surface. (This exaggerates the interaction at this scale—the atomic forces actually prevent atoms from "dragging," they are simply pushed into very close proximity.) The tip is mounted on a cantilever-like spring. The overall forces between the tip and the sample surface deform the cantilever elastically. By measuring the deflection of the cantilever, the interatomic forces exerted can be calculated using the spring constant of the cantilever. Thus, the AFM can be operated in several modes depending on the tip–surface interactions, as shown by the force–distance curve in Figure 5.14. In the contact mode, the tip experiences a strong repulsive force, while in the noncontact mode, the tip is not touching the sample, but is quite close to the sample and experiences a weak attractive force. The scanning force microscopy (SFM) measures the interaction forces as the tip is moved toward the sample surface and does not record any morphological features. The interaction forces, such as van der Waals forces, capillary forces, and frictional forces, can be measured. By modifying the tip, the various local properties of the nanostructured materials can be revealed. For example, by coating the tip with a magnetic material, the local magnetic properties can be determined by magnetic force microscopy (MFM). Similarly, local electrostatic properties using electrostatic force microscopy (EFM) and local thermal distribution using scanning thermal microscopy can be revealed. The local variation in the frictional properties of the surface can be qualitatively characterized by measuring the twist of the cantilever rather than deflection in the lateral force microscopy.

The cantilever tip can be driven in a vibrating mode near its resonant frequency and the amplitude or phase changes can be measured in dynamic force mode (DFM) AFM. As the tip is oscillated closer to the sample than the noncontact mode, the tip intermittently touches (taps) the surface (Figure 5.14), also commonly referred as "tapping mode" or intermittent-contact mode. Tapping the surface has the advantage of improved lateral resolution with less damage to the tip–surface interactions. By oscillating the tip at high frequencies in the repulsive regime, the local elastic properties of the sample can be measured from the slope of the force–distance curve, as in the force modulation method. At high oscillation frequencies, the interaction time between the tip and the surface is reduced; therefore, soft materials can be studied, as the tip touches the surface very gently. The phase shift of the oscillating tip relative to the driving signal can be used to characterize the local variation in properties, such as friction, adhesion, viscoelasticity, etc., along with the morphology by simultaneously using DFM mode.

In near-field scanning optical microscopy (NSOM), the AFM tip is used to transmit light from an external source at nanoscale and scanned very close to the sample. As both the dimension of the tip and its distance from the surface are much smaller than the optical wavelength, NSOM gives images at very high resolution approaching 1 nm beyond the diffraction limit ($\lambda/2$) of optical microscopy. Thus, SPM can be used to characterize the surfaces of any solid materials from insulators, semiconductors to conductors, as well as transparent and opaque materials. It also has the advantages of being applicable in any environment, such as air, high vacuum, liquids, or high pressures. In addition, SPM has minimal sample preparation requirements compared to other techniques.

5.4.4 Light Scattering Techniques

Scattering of light is a natural phenomenon that occurs everywhere, for example, the blue color of the sky and the brilliant colors seen at sunrise and sunset are due to light scattering by atmospheric particles. Basically, scattering occurs (part of the radiation in all directions) whenever there is a discrete variation in the refractive index within the medium of travel, such as solid particles in a liquid. By measuring the scattered light intensity, information on the scatter at nanoscales can be extracted. In static light scattering (SLS), also known as multiangle laser scattering (MALS), Rayleigh, or classical scattering technique, the particles suspended in a liquid are illuminated with a coherent light source, such as lasers, and the time-averaged intensity of the scattered light by a field of particles is measured. The size distribution is obtained by modeling the scattering profile and an optical model such as Mie scattering expressions is widely used, which expresses the scattering pattern produced by various sized spherical particles by solving the Maxwell's equation exactly for spherical boundary conditions. Smaller particles generate wide-angle, low-intensity signals, whereas larger particles generate diffraction patterns at small scattering angles with high intensity, as schematically shown in Figure 5.15. Also, the intensity greatly decreases with increasing scattering angles. So, for a more reliable characterization of small particles, polarization measurements of the scattered light have been used, as its intensity depends on the polarization state of the incident light. But particles with a diameter less than 100 nm are too small to be reliably detected by scattering. However, the SLS technique is relatively fast compared to other methods that provide similar information.

In dynamic light scattering (DLS), also known as quasi-elastic light scattering (QELS) technique, the time-dependent fluctuations in the intensity of the scattered light is measured. The Brownian motion (movement in random direction) of the particles causes rapid fluctuations in the intensity of light scattered due to interference (Figure 5.15), as the distance between the particles is varying, as a function of time around a mean value at a particular observation angle (varying from 10° to 90°). Basically, the frequency of

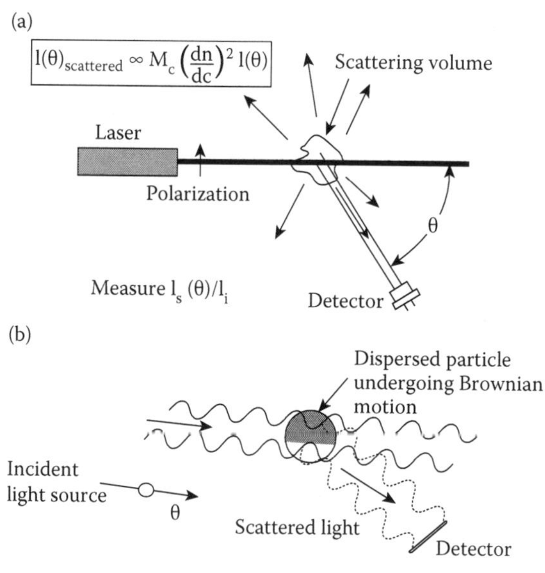

FIGURE 5.15
Schematic diagram of a typical MALS system. (a) (**I**$_s$) scattered intensity, (**I**$_i$) incident intensity, (**M**) molar mass, (**c**) concentration, (**dn/dc**) polarizability, and (**P**) angular scattering factor; (b) Doppler shift due to Brownian motion of particle. (Reproduced from http://www.biochemist.org/bio/02802/0025/028020025.pdf © 2006. With permission from The Biochemical Society; http://www.future.org.au/news/November/seeing_the_light.html.)

the scattered light by the moving particle is shifted due to Doppler broadening and the shift in the light frequency is related to the size of the scattering particle. As smaller particles cause a greater shift in frequency due to higher average velocity than larger particles, this difference in frequency of the scattered light is used to determine the particle size distribution. The time dependence of the scattered intensity is obtained by typically capturing two successive images and measuring the degree of correlation between the images. For this reason, this technique is also called photon correlation spectroscopy (PCS). From the intensity fluctuations, the velocity of the Brownian motion, called translational diffusion coefficient, is calculated, which is converted into a hydrodynamic radius (particle size) using the Stokes–Einstein equation. The DLS can be used for determining the average particle size between 3 and 3000 nm and its main advantage over rival techniques is that size information can be obtained in the order of a few seconds to a few minutes.

5.4.5 Gas Adsorption Measurements

The measurement of the amount of adsorbed inert gas, such as nitrogen, argon, krypton, or carbon dioxide, on a solid surface is a powerful and most commonly used technique to characterize the surface area, particle size, and porous structure of nanostructured materials. The gas adsorption takes place under suitable temperature and pressure conditions in order to reduce the surface energy due to an imbalanced attractive force on surface atoms, and adsorption may be classified as either physical adsorption or chemisorption. The physical adsorption involves weak molecular forces, such as van der Waals forces, and by reducing the partial pressure, the physically adsorbed gases can be easily removed from the solid surface. The formation of a chemical bond provides the driving force in chemisorption and chemisorbed gases are usually difficult to remove. The gas adsorption measurements probe not only the surface area of the NPs, but the entire surface including irregularities and pore interiors, as shown schematically in Figure 5.16. The gas adsorption isotherm is a plot that describes the equilibrium relation between the amounts of adsorbed gas with the partial pressure of the gas at constant temperature. The BET "Brunauer, Emmett, Teller" adsorption isotherm is frequently used to calculate the total surface areas of solids by physical adsorption of gas molecules. It involves adsorption of a monolayer of nitrogen gas molecules on the surface of the particles (Figure 5.16) and then heating to vaporize the monolayer to measure the amount of nitrogen adsorbed. The surface area is thus determined from adsorption measurements, and by assuming spherical shape and unimodal distribution of the NPs, the surface area can be easily converted into particle size. The sample is pretreated at an elevated temperature in vacuum or flowing gas to remove any contaminants prior to the measurements.

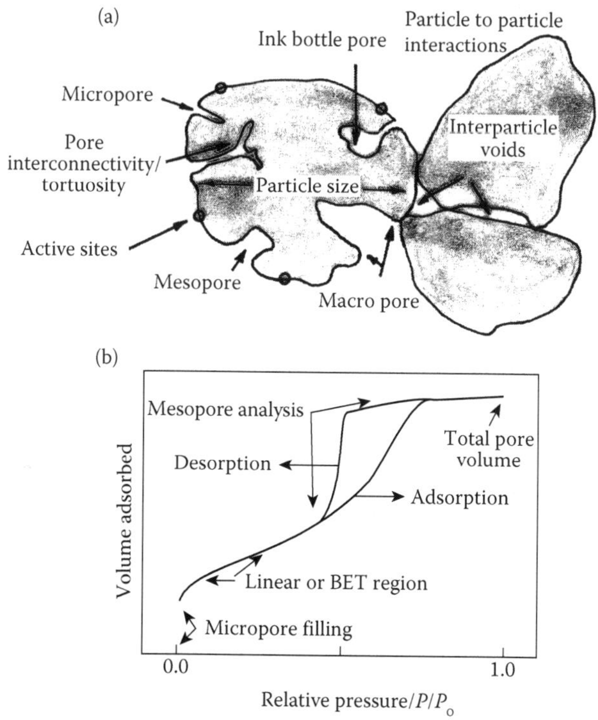

FIGURE 5.16
Schematic diagram of the surface irregularities and pore interiors of nanoparticles (a) and adsorption isotherm (b). (From http://www.npl.co.uk/mnt/meetings/28sep05/presentations/mike_tucker.pdf. With permission.)

5.5 Environmental and Safety Aspects of Nanomaterials

Any new emerging technology may affect the social, economic, and environmental aspects of our world in ways that are entirely unanticipated. Often the crisis becomes known only after the product of the technology is commercialized and widely used, such as the problems caused by asbestos, chloroflurocarbons, leaded gasoline, DDT, and many other substances. The consequences can go beyond human suffering and environmental harm, to regulatory battles and costly cleanup efforts. But, unlike other new technologies, there is a long history of nanomaterials being safely used in applications such as reinforcement of silicone rubber, control of paint rheology, and coatings of glossy inkjet paper. However, materials approaching nanometer length scale can have interactions with biological and environmental systems. Although it is possible that some nanomaterials may have the capacity to affect behavior at the cellular, subcellular, and protein levels to generate toxicity, currently there is no conclusive data indicating that these effects will become a major problem. The public is yet to view nanotechnology as a noteworthy hazard in contrast to the debates on nuclear power and genetically altered food (Nel 2006), despite science fiction novels and news media projecting a scary scenario of "grey goo" condition (i.e., self-replicating nanoscale robots consuming all materials including plants and animals). However, there is a real concern on the requirement of the safety issues, for the full potential of nanotechnology to be exploited. Also, an understanding of nanotoxicity and safety evaluations of nanotechnology may facilitate the safe manufacturing and implementation of the engineered nanoproducts.

NPs form the basis for nanomaterials, which encompass many forms. Earlier studies on the toxicity of NPs were focused on the atmospheric exposure to particulate matter (PM), which may be naturally occurring or generated as a by-product of reactions, such as vehicle exhaust, road dust, smokestacks, forest fires, windblown soil, volcanic emissions, and sea spray (HEL 2002). The size spectrum of contaminants in air and water is shown in Figure 5.17. The ultrafine particulates (with diameter <100 nm) are predominately polluted from vehicle emissions as a by-product of the combustion of fossil fuels and have the highest content of potentially toxic hydrocarbons. They are mainly inhaled and deposited in the respiratory tract of humans. Relatively, they can penetrate deeper into lung tissue and are potentially more dangerous than fine or coarse PM. The pulmonary toxicity of PM is relatively well studied and its exposure is correlated with the increased risk of asthma, chronic bronchitis, airway obstruction, and decreased gas exchange. Recent studies show that PM is also a cardiovascular risk factor associated with heart attacks, heart rhythm disturbances, and sudden death (Brook 2004). However, the ultrafine PM from combustion consists of a core of carbon coated with a layer of chemicals, including hydrocarbons,

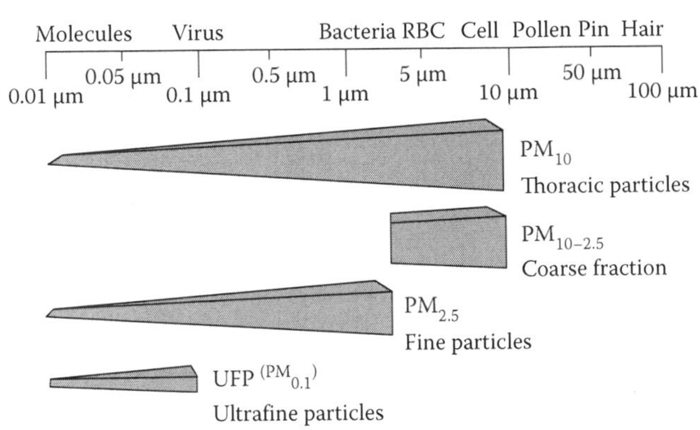

FIGURE 5.17
Size distribution of particulate matter in air pollution in comparison with some biological contaminants. (From Brook, R. D. et al., *Circulation*, 109, 2655–71, 2004.)

metals, nitrates, sulfates, etc. (Figure 5.18), and all of them may contribute to its toxicity (Nel 2005).

The engineered NPs, by contrast, are homogenous and can be formed in various sizes and shapes (e.g., spheres, fibers, tubes, rings, planes). As discussed earlier, the decrease in size of an engineered NP can modify the physiochemical and structural properties of the corresponding bulk materials. This creates the opportunity for increased interaction with biological tissues and increased uptake, which can lead to toxic effects. The various possible mechanisms through which an NP may interact with biological tissues are schematically shown in Figure 5.19 and a few are highlighted below:

- Decrease in particle size increases its surface area with more atoms on the surface and hence with a potential number of reactive groups on the surface
- Discontinuity in crystal planes may be created, which increases surface defects and also modifies the electronic structure with alters the electronic properties
- Formation of specific surface groups that can modify the surface properties to be hydrophilic, hydrophobic, lipophilic, lipophobic, catalytically active or passive

These properties can result in the generation of reactive oxygen species (ROS) and oxidative stress, which forms the basis of the current mechanisms for the explanation of the toxic effects of NPs. For example, the interaction of the NP with molecular dioxygen can increase the ROS through electron capture, leading to the formation of toxic superoxide radical (O_2^-). Oxidative

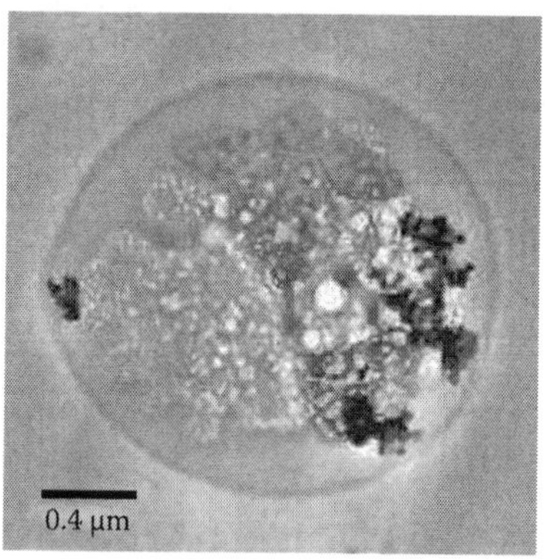

FIGURE 5.18
TEM micrograph of an ultrafine particle collected from air pollution. (From Nel, A., *Science*, 308, 804–6, 2005. With permission.)

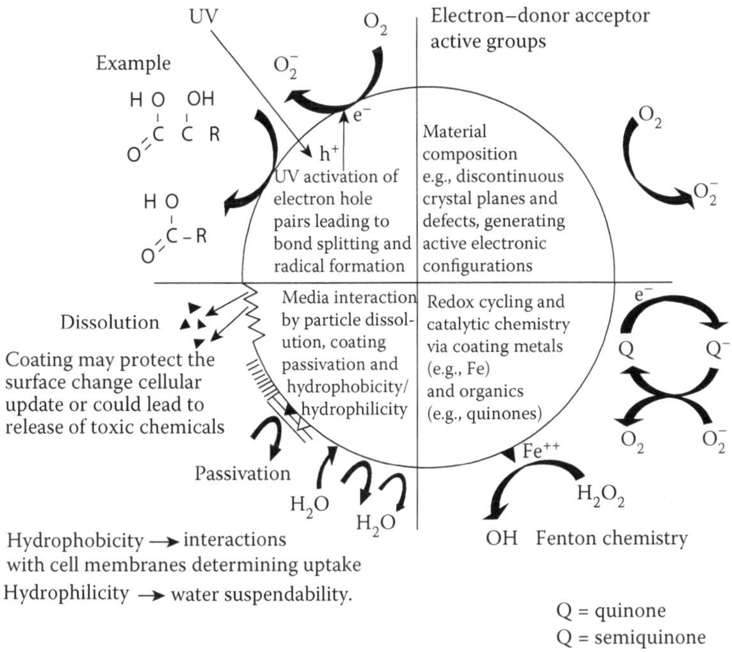

FIGURE 5.19
Possible mechanisms for nanoparticle interaction with biological tissues. (Reprinted from Nel, A. et al., *Science*, 311, 622–27, 2006. With permission from AAAS.)

stress refers to the depletion of antioxidant defenses, such as glutathione and antioxidant enzymes. Although ROS is also generated under normal conditions at a low frequency, it is easily neutralized by the above antioxidants, while exposure to NP results in the increase of ROS generation, leading to the accumulation of oxidized glutathione causing the oxidative stress (Nel 2006).

The biological activity of particles increases as the particle size decreases. Thus, there are many more potential routes of exposure to NP, including skin, gastrointestinal tract (GIT), and systematic administration for diagnostic and therapeutic purposes, as shown in Figure 5.20. The skin is the largest organ of the body and is a primary route for exposure to NP during manufacturing and through the use of skincare products. The NP of zinc oxide and titania are used in sunscreens and in cosmetics for their UV absorption properties. Regular dermal exposure to these NPs can lead to its penetration of the stratum corneum barrier of the skin and gaining access to the epidermis. This could lead to either exaggeration of the immune system by direct recognition of NP, or initiation of an autoimmune response due to self-protein interactions with NP, or trafficking of NP to lymph nodes (Oberdorster 2005; Nel 2006).

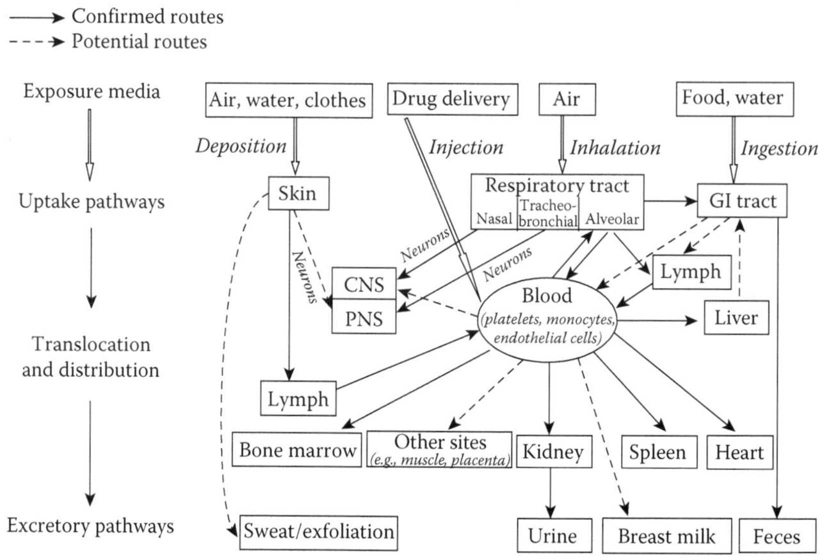

FIGURE 5.20
Biokinetics of nanoparticles illustrating many possible uptake and translocation routes. (*Particle Fibre Toxi.* 2:8 from http://www.particleandfibretoxicology.com/content/2/1/8, 2005.)

The GIT is potentially one of the most important portals of entry for NP exposure through ingestion of water, food, or drugs. Although most of them are removed via feces, some being resistant to gastrointestinal degradation can result in their efficient uptake via the GIT, which can pass through the mucosal lining and epithelial barrier of the intestine. They either accumulate at the base of the intestinal lymphatics or distribute to other organs such as the cardiovascular system, liver, spleen, bone marrow, central nervous system, and endocrine organs (Powell 2000; Moghimi 2001). Exposure to NP may also lead to its transfer to the brain, involving neuronal pathways from deposits on the nasal olfactory mucosa via the olfactory nerve in the nose. Thus, NP can overcome the blood–brain barrier (BBB), which is comprised of tightly bound endothelia that serve to retard brain entry of most high molecular weight and/or hydrophilic drugs. The surface charge properties of carbon NPs have been shown to affect the integrity and permeability of the BBB and exhibit chemical effects within the brain (Lockman 2004).

NPs are mostly chemically coated to avoid aggregation and to have desired properties. The coatings may also influence the interactions with cells and enhance its uptake by cells. Similarly, the NP aggregation may also cause toxicity and, in particular, the intracellular aggregation of NP may induce cell death similar to diseases caused by protein aggregation (sickle cell disease). The fullerenes have a tendency to form aggregates, which are water-soluble and bacteriocidal. These properties raise concern in the ecosystem, as bacteria form the basis of the food chain in many ecosystems. The surface properties of NP may also favor adsorption of molecules and proteins, which cause conformational changes of the protein due to adsorption. The denatured or degraded adsorbed protein on the NP surface may lead to changes in the functions, which can facilitate transport of toxins into the cells. Antibiotics may crossreact with native denatured proteins inducing autoimmunity. Industrial workers who breathe particulate matter and patients with orthopedic implants, which generate fine particulate wear debris, have a significant high risk of autoimmune disorders.

Overall, the NP may be more toxic than the conventional large size particles due to the following features:

- High surface area
- Enhanced chemical reactivity
- Easier penetration into cells

Although single-cell wall nanotubes are found to be more toxic than multiwall nanotubes, the effect of the shape of NPs on toxicity is still unknown (Jie 2005). Also, in many cases, the NP will be a component of nanostructured materials, such as nanocomposites and surface coatings. In such cases, the potential for direct exposure will be minimal except during processing or from their fragments during degradation. It is obvious that size alone may not be a critical factor in deciding the toxicity of NPs. So, complete characterization of NPs is needed in screening for potential adverse effects, which are not usually considered for conventional grain size materials in toxicity evaluation studies. Hence, the following key elements/aspects are included in the toxicity screening of NPs:

- Physiochemical characterization
- *In vitro* testing methods
- *In vivo* assays

The physiochemical properties to be tested for toxicity include size, shape of crystal structure, composition, porosity, and surface properties, as listed in detail in Table 5.3. The portal of entry toxicity and target organ toxicity are to be evaluated in the *in vitro* test methods, while for *in vivo* assays, a two-tier approach is prescribed for evaluating pulmonary, oral, dermal, and injectable exposures. The various potential target cells and markers for evaluation are listed in Table 5.3.

TABLE 5.3

Recommended Tests for Toxicological Evaluation of Nanomaterials

Physiochemical Characterization		*In Vitro* Tests		*In Vivo* Assays	
Physical	**Chemical**	**Portal of Entry**	**Cell Types**	**Tier 1**	**Tier 2**
		Lung			
Size	Composition	Skin	Epithelium	Pulmonary exposure	Pulmonary exposure
Size distribution	Surface area	Mucosa	(Intestinal, buccal, vaginal)		
Shape	Surface charge	Endothelium	Macrophages	Oral exposure	
Crystal structure	Surface contamination	Blood	Immune cells	Skin exposure	
Porosity	Surface chemistry	Liver	Fibroblasts	Injection	
Agglomeration state		Spleen	GALT		
		Central & peripheral nervous system	Red blood cells		
		Heart	Platelets		
		Kidney	Hepatocytes		
			Kupffer cells		
			Lymphocytes		
			Neuronal cells		
			Astroglial cells		
			Cardiomyocytes		

Source: Oberdörster G. et al. Principles for characterizing the potential human health effects from exposure to nanomaterials: elements of a screening strategy, Particle Fibre Toxi. 2:8 (Open Access article with the electronic version online at: http://www.particleandfibretoxicology.com/content/2/1/8), 2005; Nel, A. et al., *Science*, 311, 622–27, 2006.

5.6 Summary

The developments and commercialization of nanotechnology are still at an early stage. Thus, it provides an important opportunity to get nanotechnology right in time to apply the lessons from the mistakes of other technologies by identifying the risks, steps for remedy, and shape the technology's trajectory. Also, an understanding of nanotoxicity could be potentially exploited, such as a new chemotherapy for cancer to target microchondria and initiate cell death and as new diagnostic and therapeutic applications because of its potential for rapid and widespread distribution within the body.

Glossary

Antioxidants: Chemicals that protect against oxidation, which causes rancidity in fats and damage to DNA.

Aspect ratio: The width-to-height ratio of an object such as fibers.

Bacteria: One-celled living organisms, typically about one micron in diameter. Bacteria are among the oldest, simplest, and smallest types of cells.

Bulk technology: Technology based on the manipulation of atoms and molecules in bulk, rather than individually; most present technology falls into this category.

Cancer: Disease of multicellular organisms characterized by the seemingly uncontrolled multiplication and spread within the organism of apparently abnormal forms of the organism's own cells.

Capillaries: Microscopic blood vessels that carry oxygenated blood to tissues.

Carcinogen: Agent capable of causing cancer.

Cell: A membrane-bound unit, typically microns in diameter and contains a nucleus holding all the genetic information of the organism.

Crystal lattice: The regular three-dimensional pattern of atoms in a crystal.

Dislocation: A linear crystallographic defect characterizing the region of discontinuity in the crystal lattice of the materials.

Dissolution: Deterioration in an organism such that its original structure cannot be determined from its current state.

DNA (deoxyribonucleic acid): Molecules of long chains consisting of four kinds of nucleotides; the order of these nucleotides encodes the information needed to construct protein molecules.

Enzyme: A protein that acts as a catalyst in a biochemical reaction.

Grain boundary: Outside area of a grain that separates it from other grains and is a region of misfit between the grains, usually one to three atom diameters wide.

Nano: A prefix meaning ten to the minus ninth power, or one billionth.

Nanotechnology: Technology based on the manipulation of individual atoms and molecules to build structures to complex, atomic specifications.

Neoplasm: Tissue mass arising from abnormal, uncoordinated proliferation of cells.

Neuron: A nerve cell, such as those found in the brain.

Nucleotide: A small molecule composed of three parts: a nitrogen base (a purine or pyrimidine), a sugar (ribose or deoxyribose), and phosphate. They serve as the building blocks of nucleic acids (DNA and RNA).

Nucleus: In biology, a structure in advanced cells that contains the chromosomes and apparatus to transcribe DNA into RNA.

Precursor: A substance that is transformed into another following a reaction.

Ribosome: A molecular machine found in all cells, which builds protein molecules according to instructions read from RNA molecules. Ribosomes are complex structures built of protein and RNA molecules.

RNA (ribonucleic acid): A molecule similar to DNA. In cells, the information in DNA is transcribed to RNA, which, in turn, is "read" to direct protein construction.

Synapse: A structure that transmits signals from a neuron to an adjacent neuron (or other cell).

Toxicity: The ability of a substance or mixture of substances to cause a harmful effect on humans or animals.

Tumor: Swelling, used to refer to neoplasms.

Tunneling current: Current due to the transport of electrons across the gap between the tip and the sample without changing its energy. It occurs due to the overlap of wave functions, which is forbidden in classical mechanics, and exponentially decays with an increase in the gap.

Twin: Lattice planes that have adjacent planes with orientation as mirror images.

Virus: A small replicator consisting of little more than a package of DNA or RNA that, when injected into a host cell, can direct the cell's molecular machinery to make more viruses.

EXERCISES

5.1 What are called nanostructured materials and how will you classify them based on their dimensions?

5.2 Why nanomaterials are expected to have unique properties than conventional materials?

5.3 How does the strength of nanoparticles vary with their size?

5.4 Why do quantum dots emit and absorb light at specific wavelengths?
5.5 What are the advantages of top-down methods to produce nanostructured materials?
5.6 How will you produce metallic materials with ultrafine-grained microstructures?
5.7 What are the limitations of the milling process to produce nanostructured materials?
5.8 Why may bottom-up approach methods be called a two-step process for the production of nanostructured materials?
5.9 How are nanomaterials produced by the inert gas condensation method?
5.10 Why do you anticipate weak interactions for the self-assembly process?
5.11 How is human bone formed by the self-assembly process?
5.12 How can the XRD method be used to measure the nano-crystallite sizes and why, often, it may not be the true size of nanoparticles?
5.13 What type of information can be obtained by using TEM for the characterization of nanomaterials?
5.14 How can the surface of a nanostructured metallic conductor be characterized by a SPM technique?
5.15 What type of modes can be used for the operation of the AFM based on the force–distance curve?
5.16 How can the scattering of light be used to measure the size of nanoparticles?
5.17 What do you mean by adsorption isotherms and how can it be used to calculate nanoparticle size?
5.18 Why do you expect engineered nanoparticles to have increased biological activity?
5.19 Which mechanism has been proposed for the possible toxic effects of nanoparticles?

References

Bigioni, T. P., Lin, X. M., Nguyen, T. T., Corwin, E. I., Witten, T. A., and Jaeger, H. M. 2006. Kinetically-driven self assembly of highly-ordered nanoparticle monolayers. *Nature Mater*. 5:265–70.

Brook, R. D. et al. 2004. Air pollution and cardiovascular disease: A statement for healthcare professionals from the expert panel on population and prevention science of the American Heart Association. *Circulation* 109:2655–71.

Dujardin, E. and S. Mann. 2002. Bio-inspired materials chemistry. *Adv. Mater.* 14:1–14.

Gaffet, E. et al. 1999. Some recent developments in mechanical activation and mechanosynthesis. *J. Mater. Chem.* 9:305–14.

Gleiter, H. 1981. Deformation of polycrystals, mechanisms and microstructures. In *Proceedings of the Second Riso International Symposium on metallurgy and materials science*, eds. N. Hansen, A. Horsewell, T. Leffers, and H. Lilholt, 15–22, Risø National Laboratory, Risø, Roskilde, Denmark.

———. 1989. Nanocrystalline materials. *Prog. Mater. Sci.* 33:223–315.

Hahn, H. 1997. Gas phase synthesis of nanocrystalline materials. *Nanostruct. Mater.* 9:3–12.

Hu, E. and D. Shaw. 1999. Synthesis and assembly. In *Nanostructure science and technology: R&D status and trends in nanoparticles, nanostructured materials, and nanodevices*, ed. R. W. Siegel, E. Hu, and M. C. Roco, 15–33. Washington, DC: National Science and Technology Council.

Jia, G. et al. 2005. Cytotoxicity of carbon nanomaterials: Single-wall nanotube, multiwall nanotube, and fullerene. *Environ. Sci. Technol.* 39:1378–83.

Klabunde, K. J. et al. 1996. Nanocrystals as stoichiometric reagents with unique surface chemistry. *J. Phys. Chem.* 100:12142–53.

Koch, C. C. 2003. Top-down synthesis of nanostructured materials: Mechanical and thermal processing methods. *Rev. Adv. Mater. Sci.* 5:91–99.

Komarneni, S. et al. 2004. Microwave-polyol process for metal nanophases. *J. Phys.: Condens. Matter* 16:S1305–12.

Lane, R., B. Craig, and W. Babcock. 2002. Materials ease: Materials engineering with nature's building blocks. *AMPTIAC Q.* 6:31–36.

Lockman, P. R. et al. 2004. Nanoparticle surface charges alter blood-brain barrier integrity and permeability. *J. Drug Target* 12:635–41.

McNeil, S.E. 2005. Nanotechnology for the biologist. *J. Leuko. Bio.* 78:585–94.

Moghimi, S. M., A. C. Hunter, and J. C. Murray. 2001. Long-circulating and target specific nanoparticles: Theory to practice. *Pharmacol. Rev.* 53:283–318.

Nel, A. 2005. Air pollution-related illness: Effects of particles. *Science* 308:804–6.

Nel, A. et al. 2006. Toxic potential of materials at the nanolevel. *Science* 311:622–27.

Oberdörster G. et al. 2005. Principles for characterizing the potential human health effects from exposure to nanomaterials: elements of a screening strategy, Particle Fibre Toxi. 2:8 (Open Access article with the electronic version online at: http://www.particleandfibretoxicology.com/content/2/1/8).

Padmanabhan, K. A. and H. Hahn. 1996. Microstructure, mechanical properties and possible applications. In *Proc. Symp. on synthesis and processing of nanocrystalline powder*, 21–32. Warrendale, PA: Minerals, Metals and Materials Society.

Powell, J. J. et al. 2000. Immune potentiation of ultrafine dietary particles in normal subjects and patients with inflammatory bowel disease. *J. Autoimmun.* 14:99–105.

PuraMatrix: http://www.puramatrix.com/.

Roco, M. C. 2006. Nanotechnology opens new frontiers in science, engineering. http://news.uns.purdue.edu/html3month/2006/0601.O.Roco.nano.html.

Tsuji, N., Saito, Y., Utsunomiya, H., and Tanigawa, S. 1999. Ultra-fine grained bulk steel produced by accumulative roll-bonding (ARB) process. *Scripta. Mater.*, 40:795.

Siegel, R. W. 1991. Cluster-assembled nanophase materials. *Ann. Rev. Mater. Sci.* 21:559–78.

Svergun, D. I. and M. H. J. Koch. 2003. Small-angle scattering studies of biological macromolecules in solution. *Rep. Prog. Phys.* 66:1735–82.

Swihart, M. T. 2003. Vapor-phase synthesis of nanoparticles. *Curr. Opin. Coll. Inter. Sci.* 8:127–33.

Taniguchi, N. 1974. On the basic concept of nanotechnology. In *Proc. Intl. Conf. Prod. Eng. Tokyo*, Part II. Tokyo: Japan Society of Precision Engineering, 18–23. Tokyo: JSPE.

Valiev, R. Z. et al. 2003. SPD-processed ultra-fine grained Ti materials for medical applications. *Adv. Mater. Proc.* December:33–34.

Wang, D. et al. 2005. Nanostructured systems from low-dimensional building blocks. In *Nanofabrication towards biomedical applications*, ed. C. S. S. R. Kumar, J. Hormes, and C. Leuschner, 55–93. Weinheim: Wiley–VCH.

Whitesides, G M., and M. Boncheva. 2002. Beyond molecules: Self-assembly of mesoscopic and macroscopic components. *Proc. Nat. Acad. Sci.* 99:4769–74.

Zhang, S. 2005. Designing novel materials and molecular machines. *Econ. Perspect.* 22–25, eJournal.

Zhu, X. K. et al. 2003. Synthesis of bulk nanostructured Zn by combinations of cryomilling and powder consolidation by room temperature milling: Optimizing mechanical properties. *Scr. Mater.* 49:429–33.

Further Reading

Gogotsi, Y. ed. 2006. *Nanomaterials handbook.* Boca Raton, FL: CRC-Taylor & Francis.

Gonsalves, K. E., S. P. Rangarajan, and J. Wang. 2000. *Handbook of nanostructured materials and nanotechnology*, Volume 1, *Synthesis and processing*. San Diego, CA: Academic Press.

Köhler, M. and W. Fritzsche. 2005. *Nanotechnology: An introduction to nanostructuring techniques*. Weinheim: Wiley.

Kumar, C. S. S. R. ed. 2006. *Biological and pharmaceutical nanomaterials.* Chichester: John Wiley.

———. 2006. *Nanomaterials – Toxicity, health and environmental issues*. Weinheim: Wiley-VCH.

Poole, C. P. and F. J. Owens. 2003. *Introduction to nanotechnology*. New York: Wiley.

Reich, S., C. Thomsen, and J. Maultzsch. 2004. *Carbon nanotubes: Basic concepts and physical properties*. Weinheim: John Wiley.

Theodore, L. 2005. *Nanotechnology: Basic calculations for engineers and scientists.* Hoboken, NJ: Wiley.

Theodore, L. and R. G. Kunz. 2005. *Nanotechnology: Environmental implications and solutions*. Hoboken, NJ: Wiley.

Wang D., Gill, M. P., Lu, G., and Lu, Y. 2005. Nanostructured systems from low-dimensional building blocks, In: Nanofabriction Towards Biomedical Applications, eds. C.S.S.R. Kumar CSSR, J. Hormes, and C. Leuschner, 55–93. Weinheim: Wiley-VCH.

Wolf, E. L. 2004. *Nanophysics and nanotechnology: An introduction to modern concepts in nanoscience*. New York: Wiley.

6

Metallic Biomaterials

6.1 Introduction

Metals account for about two thirds of all the elements in the periodic table and have free electrons that distinguish them from nonmetals. Metals have very good strength, ductility, high melting points, thermal and electrical conductivity, and toughness. These properties are due to metallic bonding, which can be thought of as consisting of a three-dimensional array of positively charged ion cores immersed in a cloud of free electrons. The delocalized electrons (free electrons) are responsible for their excellent electrical and thermal properties. Further, the nondirectional character of the interatomic bonding allows plastic (permanent) deformation of the metal with increasing strength for a particular shape and usage. The properties of a metal can be improved by alloying; an alloy is a mixture of a pure metal with one or more other elements. For example, brass is an alloy of copper and zinc metals, while steel consists of iron alloyed with nonmetallic carbon. Alloying can result in three different metallic systems: solid solutions in which one metal in low concentration (solute) substitutes the atomic position of the other (solvent); interstitial solid solution in which a smaller atom, like carbon, fits between the spaces of the existing atom; and intermetallic compound in which a new compound is formed with a new atomic arrangement.

6.2 Metallic Biomaterials

Metals and alloys are most widely used as biomaterials due to their excellent mechanical properties. Most of the metallic biomaterials are used as passive substitutes exclusively for load-bearing implants, such as total hip and knee prostheses, fracture healing aids as bone plates, pins and screws, and plates, spinal fixation wires, and dental implants, as shown in Table 6.1. Some metals are used for more active roles in medical devices, as parts of artificial heart valves, vascular stents, pacemaker leads, catheter guide wires, and cochlear implants (Table 6.1).

TABLE 6.1

Examples of Various Metallic Materials and Their Biomedical Applications

Applications	Stainless Steel	Co-Cr Alloys	Ti and its Alloys	NiTi Alloy	Gold Alloys	Hg-Ag-Sn Amalgams
Bone and joint replacement		X	X			
Fracture fixation "plates" etc.	X		X	X		
Dental implants (fillings and posts)		X	X			
Dental restorations		X		X (orthodontic wires)	X	X
Stents	X			X		
Surgical instruments	X					
Parts of other devices, e.g., artificial hearts (heart valves), pacemakers, catheters		X				
Pacemaker encapsulation			X			

TABLE 6.2

Properties of Metallic Implants

Characteristics	Stainless Steel	Co-Cr Alloys	Ti and Ti-6Al-4V
ASTM code	F138 (CW), 139	F75, F562, F799	F67, F136
Commercial name	316L	MP35N	cpTi, Ti6Al4V
Major metals present	Fe, Cr, Ni	Co, Cr, Mo	Ti, Al, 4V
Density (g/cm^3)	7.9	7.8	4.4
Young's modulus (GPa)	200	230	127
Yield strength (MPa)	207–689	241–1586	170–827
UTS (MPa)	540–1000	900–1540	825–900
Hardness (Hv)	350	240	310–350
Elongation (min%)	12	10	8
Fracture toughness (MPa)	~100	~100	~80

Source: Compiled from Black, J., *Biological performance of materials: Fundamentals of biocompatibility*, Marcel Dekker, New York, 1999; Davis, J. R., *Handbook of materials for medical devices*, ASM International, Materials Park, OH, 2003; Park, J. B. and Kim, Y. K., *Biomaterials: Principles and applications*, CRC Press, Boca Raton, FL, 2003; Ratner, B. D. et al., In *Biomaterials science: An introduction to materials in medicine*, San Diego, Elsevier Academic Press, 2004. With permission from Taylor & Francis Group.

Metallic biomaterials can be conveniently grouped into three major metal groups: iron-based stainless steels, cobalt-based alloys, and pure titanium and titanium alloys, as listed in Table 6.2. Both the steels and cobalt alloys have corrosion resistance due to alloying addition of chromium, which renders the alloy passive. Titanium itself develops passivity and results in corrosion resistance of its alloys. The major advantages of using certain metals and alloys for biomedical applications, are their biocompatibility, appropriate mechanical properties, and reasonable cost.

6.2.1 Stainless Steels

Metals like Fe, Cr, Co, Ni, Ti, Ta, Nb, Mo, and W can only be tolerated in minute amounts in the blood. Leaching of metals is also possible in the body, which leads to corrosion, poisoning, and weakening of the implant. So, alloying is done to improve the properties of the metallic materials. Steels are alloys of iron with very low carbon content ($\leq$0.2 wt.%), as shown in Figure 6.1, and stainless steels have a significant amount of chromium (17–20%). Alloying with the addition of chromium results in corrosion-resistant steel by forming a strongly adherent chromic oxide film (~2 nm thick) on the alloy surface. In the presence of oxygen, this oxide film forms and heals itself. The alloy contains a small percentage of molybdenum (2–4%) to improve the resistance to pitting corrosion and is popularly known as 316L stainless steel. The three-digit designation corresponds to the American Iron and Steel Institute (AISI) numbering system for stainless steels and the 300 series are austenitic (face-centered cubic crystal structure), whereas the

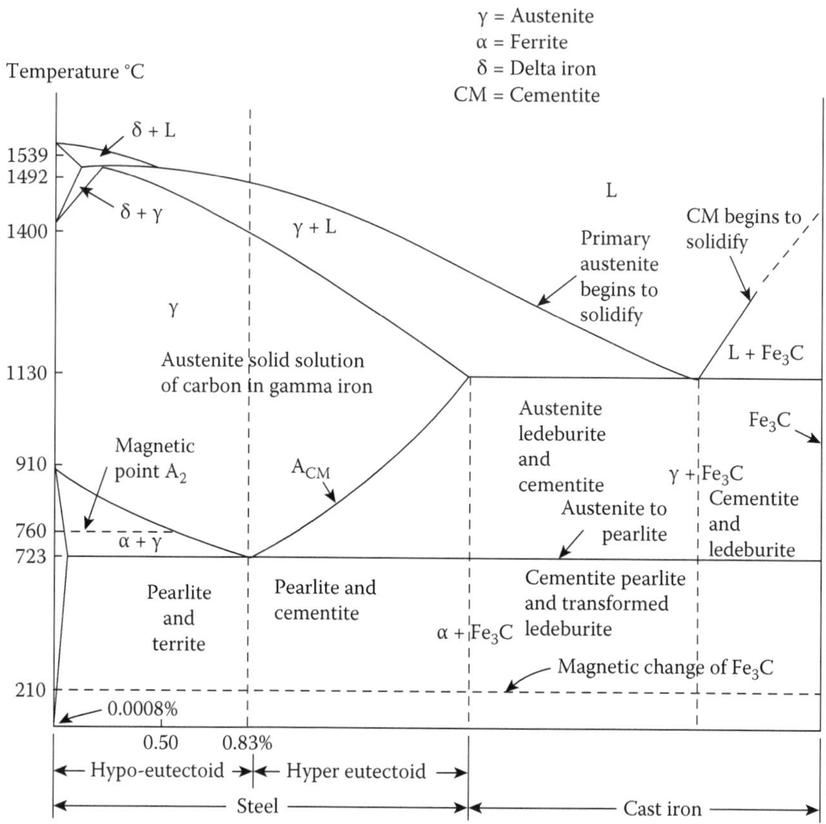

FIGURE 6.1
Iron–carbon phase diagram. (Extracted from Pollack, H. W., *Materials science and metallurgy*, 4th ed. Englewood Cliffs, NJ: Prentice Hall, 1988.)

400 series are either ferritic (body-centered cubic structure) or martensitic (body-centered tetragonal structure) stainless steels. The letter "L" indicates very low carbon content of 0.03% than 0.08% in 316 and the reason for the low carbon content is to improve corrosion resistance (Table 6.3). Carbon content more than 0.03% can lead to the formation of carbides, such as $Cr_{23}C_6$, along the grain boundaries and such steels are called "sensitized" (weakened). Formation of grain-boundary carbides can result in the depletion of chromium in the regions adjacent to the grain boundary and also reduce the formation of the protective chromium oxide. Therefore, these steels are prone to failure through corrosion-assisted fracture at the sensitized regions.

The 316L steel also has nickel and minor amounts of manganese, silicon, sulfur, and phosphorous. The nickel is added to stabilize the stronger austenitic phase to counter the tendency of formation of the weaker ferrite phase by chromium addition. The American Society for Testing and Materials (ASTM) designates this steel as F138/139 (F138 covers bar and wire and F139

TABLE 6.3

Chemical Composition of Metallic Implants

ASTM Designation	Al	C	Co	Cr	Fe	Mo	Mn	N	Ni	O	P	S	Si	Ti	V	W	Others
F138, 139	–	0.03[b]	–	17.0–19.0	[a]	2.25–3.00	2.0[b]	0.10	13.0–15.0	–	0.03[b]	0.01	0.75[b]	–	–	–	0.50 Cu
F1314	–	0.03[b]	–	20.5–23.5	[a]	2.0–3.0	4.0–6.0	0.2–0.4	11.5–13.5	–	0.025	0.01	0.75[b]			–	0.50 Cu, 0.1–0.3 Nb, 0.1–0.3 V
F1586	–	0.08	–	19.5–22.0	[a]	2.0–3.0	2.00–4.25	0.25–0.50	9–11	–	0.025	0.01	0.75	–		–	0.25 Cu, 0.25–0.80 Nb
F2229		0.08	–	19.0–23.0	[a]	0.5–1.5	21–21	0.9 min	0.1	–	0.03	0.01	0.75	–	–	–	0.25 Cu
F75	0.3	0.35	[a]	27–30	0.75	5.0–7.0	1.0	0.25	1.0	–	0.02	0.01	1.0			0.2	0.01 B
F799	–	0.35[b]	[a]	26–35	0.75	5–7	1.0[b]	0.25[b]	1.0[b]	–	–	–	1.0[b]	–	–	–	
F90	–	0.05–0.15	[a]	19–21	3.0	–	1–2	–	9–11	–	0.04	0.03	0.4	–	–	14–16	
F562	–	0.025	[a]	19–21	1.0	9.0–10.5	0.15	–	33–37	–	0.015	0.01	0.15	1.0		–	
F67	–	0.01[b]	–	–	0.3–0.5	–	–	0.03–0.05	–	0.18–0.40	–	–	–	[a]	–		
F136	5.5–6.5	0.08[b]	–	–	0.25[b]	–	–	0.05[b]	–	0.13[b]	–	–	–	[a]	3.5–4.5		

Source: Compiled from Black, J., *Biological performance of materials: Fundamentals of biocompatibility*, Marcel Dekker, New York, 1999; Davis, J. R., *Handbook of materials for medical devices*, ASM International, Materials Park, OH, 2003; Park, J. B. and Kim, Y. K., *Biomaterials: Principles and applications*, CRC Press, Boca Raton, FL, 2003; Ratner, B. D. et al., In *Biomaterials science : An Introduction to Materials in Medicine*, San Diego, Elsevier Academic Press, 2004. With permission from Taylor & Francis Group.

[a] Balance.

[b] Maximum amount.

covers sheet and strip, ASTM 1992). As per ASTM specifications, 316L is a single-phase austenite alloy and should not have ferritic or carbide phases. So, 316L is vacuum melted and this special production method improves the pitting corrosion resistance and provides a ferrite-free microstructure. The recommended grain size for 316L is about 100 micron or less (ASTM grain size number $n = 5$ in the relation $N = 2^{n-1}$, where N is the number of grains counted in one square inch area at 100 × magnification) and should be relatively uniform throughout the specimen.

This group of austenitic stainless steel is nonmagnetic and cannot be hardened by heat treatment. So, 316L is used in the cold-work (30%) condition with markedly increased yield, ultimate tensile, and fatigue strength relative to the annealed state. The typical microstructure of the annealed and cold-worked 316L stainless steel without any ferritic and carbide phase is shown in Figure 6.2. The variations of the mechanical properties of the 316L alloy on cold working (for greater strength) and on heat treatment (annealing to obtain softer materials) is also listed in Table 6.4.

The martensitic stainless steels are ferromagnetic and have high hardness. Thus, they are ideally suited for dental and surgical instruments like dental burs, dental chisels, orthodontic pliers and scalpels, bone curettes, chisels, and gouges, etc. The ferritic stainless steels cannot be strengthened by heat treatment, while cold working significantly lowers its ductility. So, they have very few applications as fasteners and handles in medical devices.

Stainless steel may also corrode inside the body under highly stressed and oxygen-depleted regions, such as the contacts under the screws of a bone fracture plate. So, 316L stainless steels are used for temporary implant applications as bone screws and plates, intramedullary nails and rods. The corrosion resistance, wear resistance, and fatigue strength of the alloy is improved

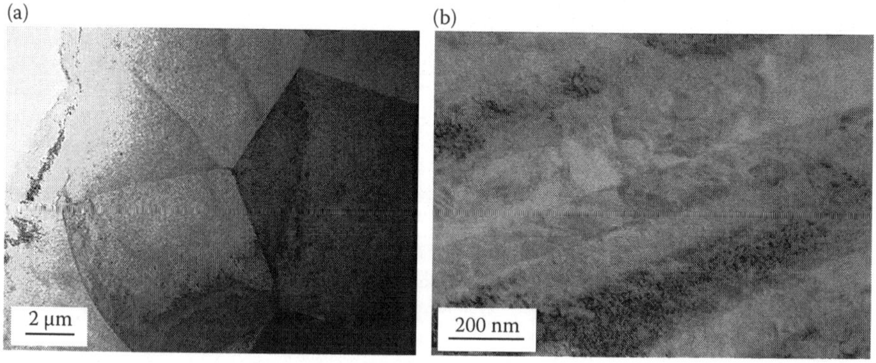

FIGURE 6.2
Typical microstructure of annealed (a) and cold worked (b) 316L stainless steel. (Courtesy of Angenete J. 2004. *A TEM investigation of the influence of nitrogen and cold working on the microstructure of solid solution annealed austenitic stainless steel (316L)*, 02-24 Figures 3 and 5, NanoAnalys, SKI Report 29, by Magnus Hansson and SeijiYamamaoto, Goteburg, Sweden.)

TABLE 6.4

Mechanical Properties of Austenitic Stainless Steels

	F138		F1314		F1586		F2229	
Properties	**Annealed**	**Cold Worked**	**Annealed**	**Cold Worked**	**Annealed**	**Medium Hard**	**Annealed**	**Cold Worked[a]**
Yield strength (MPa)	172	690	380	862	430	700	586	1227
UTS (MPa)	485	860	690	1035	740	1000	931	1496
Elongation (min%)	40	12	35	12	35	20	52	19
Fracture toughness (MPa)	~100	~100	–	–	–	–	–	–

Source: Compiled from Davis, J. R., *Handbook of materials for medical devices*, ASM International, Materials Park, OH, 2003; Park, J. B. and Kim, Y. K., *Biomaterials: Principles and applications*, CRC Press, Boca Raton, FL, 2003. With permission from Taylor & Francis Group.

[a] 30%.

by surface modification methods, such as anodization, passivation, and ion implantation (Bordiji 1996).

Other stainless steels, such has nitrogen-strengthened alloys (ASTM F1314, F1586, and F2229), which have better corrosion resistance and mechanical properties than 316L have also been developed (Table 6.4). The ASTM 1314 and ASTM F2229 fall into the 200 series austenitic stainless steels. The F1314 was one of the first nitrogen-strengthened stainless steels developed for fracture fixation applications and the F2229 is essentially a nickel-free alloy developed in response to nickel-allergy problems associated with the other alloys. The ASTM F1586 is another variant of the standard grade 316 and has been used for bone screws and plates and spinal fixation components. The nitrogen content and chemical composition of these alloys are listed in Table 6.3. The nitrogen-strengthened alloys produced by the special electro-slag refining (ESR) route have pitting corrosion equivalent (PRE) values above 30 compared to 26 for 316L and also exhibit higher tensile strength, impact strength, fatigue strength, and yield strength than 316L (Davis 2003).

6.2.2 Cobalt-Chromium Alloys

Cobalt forms a solid solution with chromium up to 35% Cr addition (alloy crystal structure remains the same as Co), which enhances the corrosion resistance of the Co-Cr alloy by an order of magnitude greater than that of stainless steels. Molybdenum is also added to produce finer grains for higher strengths. The Co-Cr alloys are difficult to machine and hence, they are cast or wrought processed into the required shape. So, the Co-Cr alloys are divided into two basic types: castable Co-Cr-Mo (ASTM F75) alloy and Co-Ni-Cr-Mo (ASTM F90 and F562) alloys, which are wrought processed. The grain size of the wrought alloys is invariably finer than that of the comparable cast alloys and so the strength of the wrought alloys is better than cast alloys. The cast alloys have long been used for dental applications and recently for artificial joints. The relatively new wrought alloy is used for stems of heavily loaded joints, such as knee and hip. Four types of Co-Cr alloys (ASTM F75, F799, F90, and F562) are used as medical implants and the chemical composition of the alloys are listed Table 6.3 (Davis 2003).

The ASTM F75 alloy is cast into various shapes by investment casting. Basically, the alloy is melted and then poured into the ceramic molds of intricate shapes of stems, oral implants, and dental bridge work. The mold is obtained by coating (investing) the wax model of the required shape by ceramic mold materials and then melting the wax. So, the process is also called "lost wax process" (Horton 1988). The casting process can result in nonequilibrium cooling, leading to a variation in composition, large grain size and with casting defects such as inclusions, which are detrimental to the implant properties. The F799 alloy, which is a modified F75 alloy, is mechanically processed by hot forging at 800°C after casting and this results in the doubling of the fatigue, yield, and ultimate strengths of the alloy compared to as-cast F75 alloy. The F99 alloy is also called thermomechanical Co-Cr-Mo alloy and has minor variations in composition to that of F75. Powder metallurgical techniques have also been used to avoid casting problems and to improve the mechanical properties (Brunski 2004). The F75 alloy powder is compacted and sintered simultaneously by hot isotatic pressing (HIP). This results in a much finer grain and also very uniform distribution of carbides. Thus, the HIP F75 alloy has better mechanical properties than the cast equivalent.

The F90 is a wrought alloy and has tungsten and nickel elements added to improve its machinability and fabrication. The mechanical properties of the annealed alloy is similar to that of F75 alloy, but on cold working (44%), the properties doubled by more than that of F799 alloy. The F562 alloy, originally called MP35N, is also a wrought alloy and contains significant amounts of nickel and relatively higher amounts of molybdenum. The F562 alloy contains approximately 35% of cobalt and nickel, followed by a significant amount of chromium and molybdenum elements.

The "MP" indicates the multiphasic nature of the alloy, which is formed by thermal treatments and forging to improve its mechanical properties. Due to the higher amount of cobalt, part of the fcc structure of the matrix transforms to hcp structure by cold working. The presence of both phases impedes the dislocation motion and strengthens the alloy. On further age treatment at 430°C–600°C, Co_3Mo precipitates are formed, which also strengthen the alloy by precipitation hardening. The superior fatigue and ultimate tensile strength of the wrought F562 alloy also makes it strongest among the metallic materials available for implant applications that require long service without failure, such as hip joint stems (Park 2003).

6.2.3 Titanium and Titanium-Based Alloys

Low specific gravity (lightness), good corrosion resistance, and excellent biocompatibility are the outstanding features of titanium for implant applications. The formation of a stable, thin, coherent titanium oxide (TiO_2) on the surface of the titanium and its alloys provides superior corrosion resistance compared with stainless steel and Co-Cr alloys. The oxidized film, if scratched or damaged, is capable of rehealing and restoring itself in the body under physiological conditions and is also believed to be responsible for osseointegration of titanium implants *in vivo*. Titanium is an allotropic material that changes from the hexagonal close-packed structure (hcp, α-Ti) to the body-centered cubic structure (bcc, β-Ti) at 882°C. The required phase, microstructure, and subsequent properties of titanium alloys can be controlled by the addition of interstitial elements, such as oxygen, nitrogen, and carbon and alloying elements. For many years, both unalloyed commercially pure (cp) titanium (ASTM F67) and the Ti-6Al-4V titanium alloy (α-β alloy, ASTM F136) have been widely used as an implant material in bone surgery in the fields of osteosynthesis, oral implantology, and in joint prosthesis. Recently, metastable β alloys with lower elastic modulus and better biocompatibility compared to α-β alloys have been developed for orthopedic implant applications.

cpTi (98.9–99.6) is essentially α-phase titanium and is well known for not causing any allergic reactions. The oxygen content strongly affects the ductility and strength of cpTi. There are four grades of cpTi based on the oxygen content (0.18–0.40%), and the mechanical properties of various grades are listed in Table 6.5. Higher impurity content leads to higher strength, but reduces the ductility of cpTi (Brunski 2004). For biomedical applications where high strength is not required, but excellent corrosion resistance is the main requirement, such as pacemaker cases, housing for ventricular-assisted devices, implantable infusion drug pumps, screws and staples for spine surgery, unalloyed titanium (ASTM F67 grades) is used (Davis 2003). cpTi is also used for dental implants, maxillofacial, and craniofacial implants.

Alloying with aluminum stabilizes the α phase and because the α-phase alloys are single-phased, they cannot be heat treated for precipitation hardening. The addition of vanadium stabilizes the β phase and with controlled amounts of β-stabilizers, the high strength β phase can also be stabilized at room temperature. So, Ti-6Al-4V ELI (ASTM F136) alloy is a two-phase (α-β) alloy and can be strengthened 30%–50% more by solution treatment and aging than the annealed conditions. ELI refers to extra-low interstitial and is a variant of the Ti-6Al-4V (ASTM F1472) alloy. The interstitial content significantly affects the yield, tensile, and fatigue strengths of titanium. Generally, the alloy is processed to have a microstructure of fine-grained α phase (formed during aging) with isolated β precipitates (formed during annealing) at the grain boundaries (called mill annealed). This microstructure has a high fatigue life/endurance (Brunski 2004). The main advantage of titanium-based alloys as a bone implant material is their favorable strength-to-density ratio. Stainless steel and Co-Cr alloys have densities of approximately 8.8 and 7.8 g/cm^3, respectively. But titanium has a density of only 4.5 g/cm^3. Although the strength of the cpTi and Ti-6Al-4V alloy is comparable to that of 316 stainless steel or Co-Cr alloys, the specific strength (strength per density) of the titanium implants exceeds any other implant material; thus, they are widely used for hip and knee replacement arthoplastry. Vanadium has been reported to be toxic and to leach out from the implants, causing adverse tissue effects. The ASTM listed two more α-β alloys for medical applications without vanadium content as indicated in Table 6.5, which are similar to the Ti-6Al-4V alloy from a metallurgical perspective (Davis 2003). The Ti-6Al-7Nb (ASTM 1295) has been used for femoral hip stems, bone plates, and spinal components. The Ti-3Al-2.5Fe (ASTM 2146) has excellent cold formability and is used for tubing and intramedullary nails.

Compared with the elastic moduli of either stainless steel or Co-Cr alloys, Ti and Ti-6Al-4V have much lower (approximately half) moduli that are still almost an order of magnitude higher than that of bone. The β alloys, which have greater amounts of β stabilizers than the α stabilizers, have also been developed for orthopedic applications. These are vanadium-free alloys with

TABLE 6.5

Chemical Composition and Mechanical Properties of Ti and Its Alloys

Properties	α Microstructures				α–β Microstructures			β Microstructures		
ASTM Specification	**F67 Grade 1**	**Grade 2**	**Grade 3**	**Grade 4**	**F136**	**F1295**	**F2146**	**F1713**	**F1813**	**F2066**
Alloy	cpTi[a]	cpTi[a]	cpTi[a]	cpTi[a]						
Major elements (wt%)	0.2Fe, 0.18O	0.3Fe, 0.25O	0.3Fe, 0.35O	0.5Fe, 0.40O	6Al, 4V	6Al, 7Nb	3Al, 2.5V	13Nb, 13Zr	12Mo, 6Zr, 2Fe	15Mo
Tensile strength (MPa)	240	345	450	550	860			1030		
Yield strength (MPa)	170	275	380	485	860	795	585	900	1000	655
Elastic modulus (GPa)	–	–	–	–	110	105	100	~81	~79	~78
Elongation (min%)	24	20	18	15	10–15	10	15	45/10–16	18–22	22
UTS (MPa)					930	860	690	1000	1050	795

Source: Compiled from Davis, J. R., *Handbook of materials for medical devices*, ASM International, Materials Park, OH, 2003; Park, J. B. and Kim, Y. K., *Biomaterials: Principles and applications*, CRC Press, Boca Raton, FL, 2003. With permission.

[a] 0.03 N, 0.10 C, 0.015 hydrogen.

niobium, zirconium, molybdenum, tantalum, and iron as major alloying elements. All the elements exhibit excellent biocompatibility, thus the β alloys offer enhanced biocompatibility with reduced elastic moduli. The Ti-Nb-Zr-Ta (TNZT) alloys have the lowest elastic moduli among all the metallic implants used (Davis 2003).

The disadvantages of titanium for medical use include relatively low shear strength, poor wear resistance, and difficulties in fabrication. The very high friction and wear rates are the result of the persistent oxide on the surface, which remains intact under low loads and slow sliding wear. However, if the passive film is broken under high shear stresses and not regenerated promptly, then exposed metal leads to cold welding with the articulating surface. This leads to the continuous removal and reformation of the passive layer, resulting in the gradual consumption of the material. Eventually, surface roughness increases and abrasive wear occurs, with the hard oxide debris acting as abrasives (Long 1998). Hence, titanium is not used for articulating joints, but is used as the structural components in orthopedic implants, such as the femoral stem. However, various surface engineering techniques, like coating methods, surface modifications, and ion implantation, have been tried to improve the tribological properties of titanium.

6.2.4 Shape Memory Alloys

The ability of a material to recover to a preset shape upon heating (above the transformation temperatures) and to return to a certain alternate shape upon cooling is known as the shape memory effect (SME). The SME was first discovered in an equiatomic alloy of nickel and titanium (TiNi or NiTi, Nitinol). The NiTi alloy exhibits the SME near room temperature. This alloy is soft and easily deformable in its lower temperature form (martensite), but it resumes its original shape and rigidity when heated to its higher temperature form (austenite). So, the SME is based on the diffusionless martensitic phase transformation. The NiTi alloy also exhibits superelastic behavior, i.e., the alloy can also be strained several times more than conventional metal alloys without being plastically deformed, within a given temperature range. This superelastic property is also based on martensitic transformation (Duerig 1990). A schematic diagram illustrating the SME and superelastic behavior of NiTi alloy is shown in Figure 6.3. The shape memory alloys (SMA) is the group of alloys that exhibit SME and only a few alloys, such as NiTi, Cu-Zn-Al, and Cu-Al-Ni, have been found to recover substantial amounts of strain or generate significant force on changing shape.

The unique properties (Table 6.6) of thermal SME and the superelasticity of NiTi provide the possibilities for new applications that no other implant material has offered before. The idea behind SME applications is to introduce the smaller deformed structure of the alloy of the low-temperature phase into the body, where its shape changes into a different and much larger structure from the body heat. The thermal shape change effect can be utilized to have

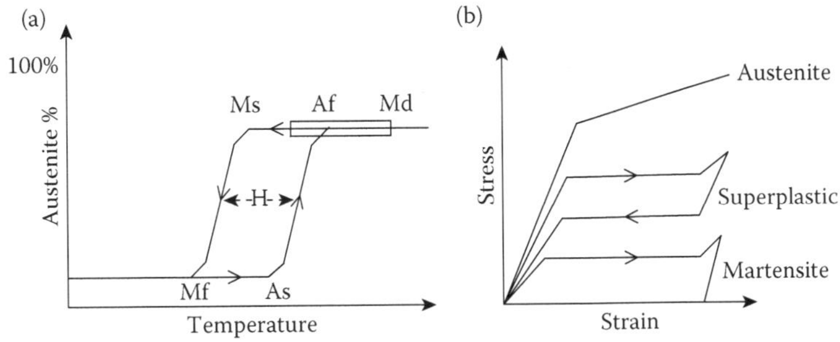

FIGURE 6.3
Typical transformation versus temperature curve (a) of NiTi shape memory alloy and stress vs. strain curve (b) of different phases of NiTi shape memory alloy at constant temperature (As = austenite start, Af = austenite finish, Ms = martensite start, Mf = martensite finish and Md = highest temperatures to strain-induced martensite, H = hysteresis). (From Duerig, T. W. et al., *Engineering aspects of shape memory alloys*, Butterworth-Heinemann, London, 1990. With permission from Elsevier.)

a beneficial impact within the body, such as to restrict, dilate, push apart, or pull together body components. The superelastic behavior has been used in orthodontic archwires. NiTi has the ability to absorb huge amounts of strain energy and release it as the applied strain is removed. Further, it provides a constant force over a large strain range, which enhances tooth movement with greater patient comfort. The elasticity of NiTi is approximately 10 times that of steel and upon release of the stress or strain, the orthodontic SMA wire springs back to its original shape. In addition, it is not too stiff or harsh for the tooth, unlike stainless steels. The NiTi also has excellent torqueability and kink resistance, which are important for medical guidewires. Some other promising biomedical applications of SME alloys include

- Vascular stents to provide reinforcement to the walls of the blood vessel
- Vena cava filters that anchor in veins and filter the clots
- Orthopedic staples to compress the parts of the broken bone and promote healing
- Guide wires that are resistant to kinking and permanent bending due to superelasticity
- Surgical tools that can be contorted to designated shapes and then made to return to their initial form
- Tools for minimally invasive surgery and advanced techniques, including angioplasty and laparoscopic surgery (Mantovani 2000)

The NiTi alloys also exhibit good biocompatibility and corrosion resistance *in vivo* despite a high content of nickel, which is toxic. The strong intermetallic bond between nickel and titanium seems to eliminate the risk of reaction,

TABLE 6.6

Properties of Tantalum, Gold, and Shape Memory Alloys

Name/Properties	Shape Memory Alloys	Gold and Gold Casting Alloys				Tantalum
Principle Alloying elements (wt.%)	49–51 Ni[a], 51–49 Ti[a]	Au	11.5 Ag, 78.1 Au, 9.9 Pt	10.0 Ag, 76.0 Au, 10.5 Cu, 2.4 Pd, 1.0 Zn	25.0 Ag, 56.0 Au, 11.8 Cu, 5.0 Pd, 1.7 Zn	99.9
Density (g/cm³)	6.45	19.32	18.4	15.6	13.8	16.0
Young's modulus (GPa)	~83 (aus.) ~28–41 (mart.)	45 (tensile)		–	–	186–191
Yield strength	~195–690 (aus.) ~70–140 (mart.)		420	270	350	140
UTS (MPa)	895					205
Elongation (min%)	–		15	30	30	20–30

Source: Compiled from Davis, J. R., *Handbook of materials for medical devices*, ASM International, Materials Park, OH, 2003; Mantovani, D., *JOM*, 52, 36–44, 2000. With permission.

[a] at.% (aus., austenite; mart., martensite).

even in patients with nickel sensitivity. A titanium-based metal that does not contain nickel has also been developed.

6.2.5 Dental Amalgam Alloys

Dental amalgams are popular dental alloys made by mixing liquid mercury with powdered alloys of silver (~65%), tin (~29%), copper (~6%), zinc (2%), etc., and the resulting pasty material is packed in the dental cavity. The reaction of mercury with the Ag-Sn intermediate phases (mainly Ag_3Sn) leads to the setting of the amalgam in about a day and the final content of mercury is about 45–55% (Park 2003). The amalgam develops adequate compressive strengths to restore the chewing surfaces, which are subjected to heavy forces. Since there is no adhesion between the tooth and the amalgam, the dimensional stability of the amalgam during the setup and its ability to reproduce the contour of the cavity is crucial for its long-term stability. The presence of mercury, a known toxic material, has aroused controversy on the use of amalgams and a mercury-free amalgam based on gallium (commercial brand name "Galloy") has been tried (McComb 1998).

6.2.6 Noble and Other Metals

The noble metals, such as gold, platinum, palladium, iridium, rhodium, and silver, exhibit very good resistance to corrosion and oxidation (though Ag isn't that high) and are used as biomaterials mainly for dental applications. Gold and gold alloys are most widely used for dental restoration application due their excellent durability, stability, and high corrosion resistance. For centuries, pure gold has been used for filling dental cavities. The gold foils (~60 μm thick), gold powder (particle diameter, 15 μm) wrapped in gold foil, or some combination of these forms are built up in the cavity and joined by pressure (cold-welded). These fillings are very stable and leak-free, but have the disadvantage of high thermal conductivity. As pure gold is soft, this type of restoration is limited to areas that are not stressed.

Gold casting alloys, which are based on the gold-silver-copper alloy system, are used for dental restoration applications and typically contain between 60 and 80% gold with enough palladium, platinum, or silver (to bring the noble-metal content to at least 75%), with the balance being copper and zinc. Alloying with copper and a small amount of platinum improves the strength, while the zinc addition lowers the melting point and scavenges the oxides formed during melting. Use of silver compensates for the copper color. The alloy is cast into the mold of the impression of the dental cavity. Gypsum silica is used as mold material to withstand the high temperature of the molten gold alloy and the impression of the cavity is prepared using wax. Another class of gold casting alloys based on the gold-palladium-platinum alloy system has been used for bonding with porcelain dental materials. Composition of the alloys is optimized to match the thermal expansion of porcelain and to avoid discoloring the porcelain, but to form strong reaction-bonded joints. For crowns and cusps, harder alloys with relatively less amounts of gold are used (Park 2003). The compositions specified by the American Dental Association (ADA) for the high-noble alloys are listed in Table 6.6.

The precious metals also exhibit resistance to electrochemical corrosion and low-threshold potentials for electrical conductivity. They are used as alloys for medical electrodes in neural prostheses, such as cardiac pacemakers, spinal cord stimulators, and phrenic nerve stimulators (PNS). The electrodes transmit a current for electrical simulation in the required areas of the nervous system for control of respective organs (Davis 2003). One of the commonly used electrodes is made up of platinum and platinum-iridium alloys (10–30% Ir). Silver exhibits antimicrobial properties and is mostly used as silver salts and complexes that release silver ions. It is also used as suture wires, cranial support plates, and tracheostomy tubes.

Tantalum is well known for its superior biocompatibility and has been used in clinical applications for more than 50 years. It exhibits excellent corrosion resistance to most of the acids, aqueous salt solutions, and organic chemicals as that of a glass. It has a very high density (>16 g/cm^3), but only limited strength (Table 6.6). cpTi (99.90%) has been used on non-load-bearing implant applications as suture wires for skin closure, tendon, and nerve repair; clips for ligation of vessels; staples for abdominal surgery; and foils and sheets for nerve anatomoses, canioplasty, and reconstructive surgery (Davis 2003).

Alternatively, tantalum has been coated on a vitreous carbon skeleton structure to create a metallic configuration that is very similar to trabecular (cancellous) bone, and the new porous metal structure called "Trabecular Metal™" (Zimmer Inc.) has been successfully used for hip and knee replacements (Medlin 2003). The carbon content is typically 1% by weight and from a biocompatibility point of view, the composition is that of tantalum. Trabecular Metal typically has an interconnected pore volume of 75–85% with an average pore size of 400–600 micron. This means more pathways for bone ingrowth, but with sufficient mechanical strength compared to other porous implants. The tantalum coating has also been used for x-ray marking due to its high density and has been applied to a variety of implants.

6.3 Nanostructured Metallic Implants

Metals and alloys are composed of grains, which consist of many atoms. The grains vary in size from tens of microns (a micron is a millionth of a meter) to one or more millimeters, and are often invisible to the naked eye. The physical properties of bulk metallic materials are influenced by its grain structure. Metals with grain sizes below one micron are known as nanostructured metals and typically consist of crystalline or quasicrystalline particles/grains

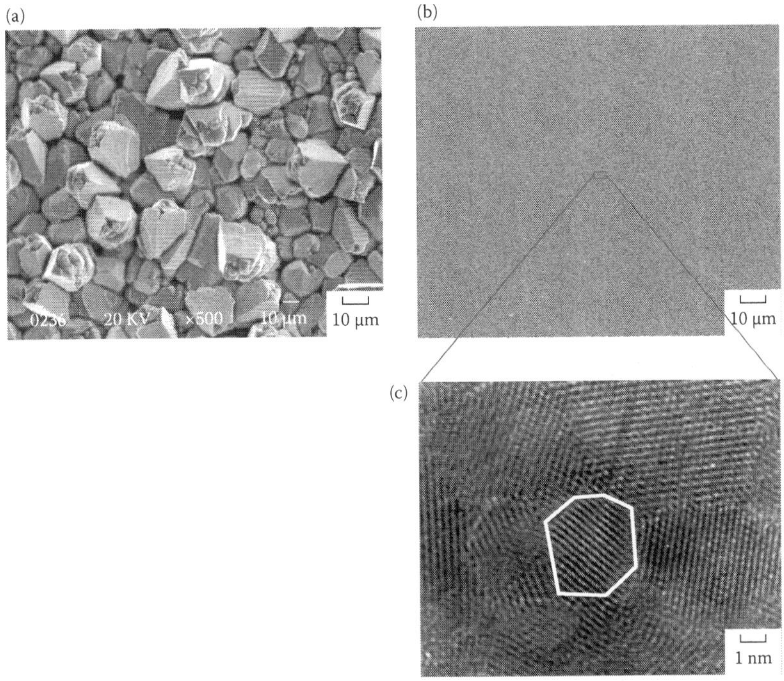

FIGURE 6.4
Electron micrograph of (a) micrograin, (b) and (c) nanograin structures. (Courtesy of Integran Technologies Inc.)

with sizes ranging from 1 to 100 nm. As the grain size decreases, there is a significant increase in the volume fraction of grain boundaries or interfaces. The transmission electron micrographs illustrating the grain structure of both conventional and nanocrystalline metals are shown in Figure 6.4.

Medical implants, such as orthopedic and dental implants and heart valves, are made of titanium, cobalt and stainless steel alloys. The average life time of orthopedic implants, such as total hip replacements (THR), is only about 12–15 years. This means, even those who undergo hip replacement surgery at the age of 65 years will require at least one revision surgery and still younger patients may need many revision surgeries throughout their life time. The main reasons for the failure of the implants are

- Incomplete bone growth on the implant surface resulting in lack of bonding of the implant to juxtaposed bone
- Wear debris that are formed at the articulating surfaces of the implants gets stuck at the surrounding tissue causing bone cell death
- Differences in the mechanical properties of the implant and the surrounding tissue leading to stress shielding, which causes loosening of the implant (Sato and Webster 2004)

Also, most of the currently used implants have smooth surfaces that promote the formation of undesirable fibrous soft tissue, which may not properly integrate the implant with the surrounding tissue. Therefore, to have successful integration of orthopedic implants with the surrounding bone, the surface features of the implant must stimulate rapid bone formation.

Bone is a nanophase material composed of collagen protein that has nanometer features, and nanophase hydroxyapatite. Similar to collagen, the other proteins of the extracellular matrix of the bone also possess features such as size, folding, and patterns at the nanoscale. This clearly suggests that osteoblasts (bone-forming cells) are adapted to features at the nanoscale and hence, a nanostructured implant can promote new bone formation. Reduction in grain size of the material from conventional micron size to nanometer size is also accompanied by changes in the properties, such as

- Increased number of grain boundaries
- Increase of grain boundary volume (Kenneth et al. 1996)
- Higher surface area
- Higher surface roughness
- Higher wettability characterized by lower contact angles

The increase in the wettability and other surface features, in particular the high surface roughness, enhances the adsorption of proteins on the implant from bone marrow, blood, and other tissues. The initial adsorption of proteins, which mediate the cell attachment, enhances the osteoblast functions on the implant surface, and leads to the earlier integration of the implant with the tissue. Though the influence of nanoparticulate wear debris on increasing the cell viability has to be well established, the presence of nanoparticles has also been shown to convert the toxic effects on cell viability by conventional particles (Gutwein and Webster 2004). The applications of some novel nanostructured metallic materials for biomaterial applications are expanded in the following sections.

The effects of nanophase metallic materials on cellular functions have been studied. The osteoblast cells were seeded on pure Ti (F67, grade 2), Ti6Al4Mo (F136), and Co28Cr6Mo (F799) compacts (Webster and Ejiofor 2004). The compacts were formed from their respective metallic particulates of either submicron or nanosize (largest size < 2.5 μm) particulates and conventional micron size (smallest size > 7.5 μm) particulates by compression at room temperature. The morphology of Ti and Ti alloy particles was spongy, while that of Co-Cr alloy particle was spherical. Increased nanometer size surface roughness and large amounts of interparticulate voids were revealed on nanophase compacts compared to conventional compacts. Enhanced osteoblast adhesion was observed on nanophase compacts of all three metallic systems compared to the conventional phase metallic compacts. The osteoblast attachment and cell protrusions occur primarily at the particle boundaries. Hence, a greater amount of interparticulate voids seem to promote osteoblast adhesion on nanophase compacts compared to conventional phase metallic systems. Interestingly, the osteoblast attachment is more on Ti compared to Ti6Al4Mo and Co28Cr6Mo nanophases, but the net effect is nearly the same on all three metallic system, which have different compositions and elements.

The influence of nanotexturing of titanium (cpTi) and titanium alloy (Ti-6Al-4V) on the expression bone matrix proteins by the cultured osteoblast cells was evaluated (Oliveria and Nanci 2004). The nanotextured surfaces were created by chemical deoxidation and controlled reoxidation using an H_2SO_4/H_2O mixture. Bone sialoprotein (BSP), fibronectin (FN), osteopontin (OPN), and type-I collagen are associated with initial events in bone formation. As early as 6 h after seeding osteogenic cells, nanotextured surfaces exhibited a higher proportion of cells with peripheral distribution of OPN and overexpression of both OPN and BSP both intra and extracellularly for a three-day culture period. The early deposition of these two multifunctional matrix proteins may influence the kinetics of osteoblast differentiation and the subsequent rate of bone formation.

Gold nanoparticles strongly absorb light in the near-infrared (800–200 nm) region, while both blood and soft tissues are highly transparent in this region. So, by simply shining a laser light, the gold particles can be selectively heated if embedded in soft tissues (Chen et al. 2005). Thus, gold nanoparticles–laser light interaction can be used to perform a variety of biomedical applications, from local treatments to emit signals for imaging. For example, they can be tuned to destroy cancer tumors by local heating. They can be modified by attaching a range of biomolecules such as antibodies, and targeted to specific tissue or tumors. Also, they can be adopted to carry drugs, genes, or even cradle restorative stem cells. For example, they can be used for the treatment of cancer either by targeting them to attach to the cancer to locate by imaging techniques to destroy the cancer by selective local heating nor delivery of drugs with laser. Alternatively, they are used to locate the damaged areas on arteries and then deliver stem cells to build new blood vessel. Biologically active molecular networks consisting of phage (viruses that infect only bacteria) directly assembled with gold nanoparticles, have been fabricated recently to build a matrix that can support stem cells (Souza et al. 205). These networks have both the physical and biological features within a single entity and can be used as biological sensors, cell-targeting agents, and as scaffolds to grow needed tissue *in vitro* or *in vivo*.

Collectively, these examples clearly indicate the potential of nanostructured metallic materials to directly signal the adsorption of the required matrix proteins, favor the adhesion correct cells, and ensure the early integration with tissues. Nanostructured titanium with very low elastic modulus, but with very high strength, is also commercially available (Reade Advanced Materials, USA; Metallic LLC, USA). Using the high strength titanium, it is now possible to design hollow implants similar to bone, including mechanical properties. Overall, the future seems to be for nanostructured metallic implants with improved biological performance.

6.4 Case Study

In the human skeletal system, the joint that is located at bone junctions is an important component and may be involved in transmitting the load from bone to bone by muscular action and is normally accompanied by the relative motion of the respective bones. The hip joint links the pelvis and the upper thigh bone or femur (longest bone in the human body) and permits a relatively large range of rotary motion by a ball-and-socket-type joint, i.e., ball-shaped femur head fits into cup-like cavity known as acetabulum, within the pelvis. The articulating surface of the joint is covered with a layer of smooth cartilage (a fairly soft, white substance about 1/8 inch thick) containing body fluids that lubricate and cushion the joint, allowing the bones to move on each other with very little friction. As the cartilage does not show up on x-rays, the hip joint usually shows a "space" between the ball and the socket on x-rays of approximately 1/4 inch wide and fairly even in outline (Figure 6.5). The

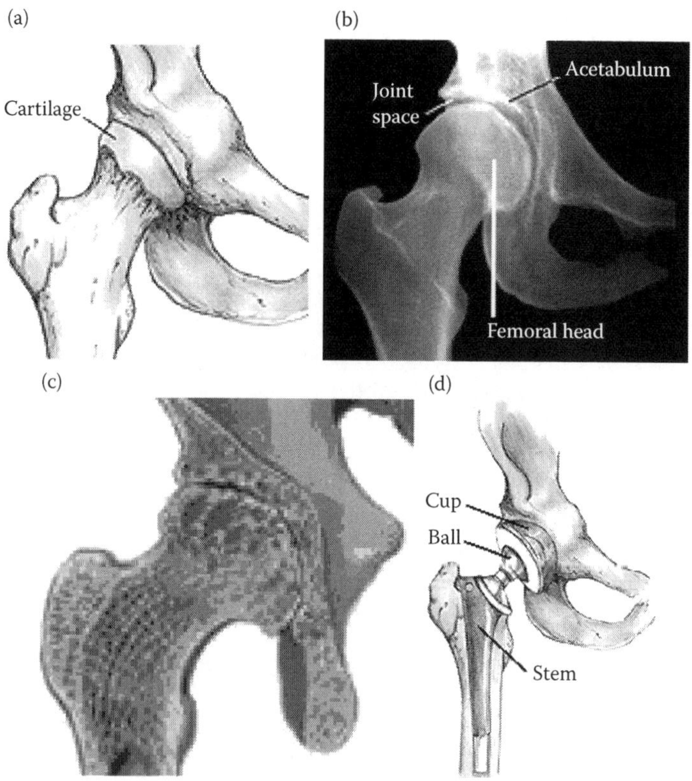

FIGURE 6.5
Schematic diagram (a) and x-ray image of the normal hip joint (b), diseased hip joint (c), and components of THR (d). (From http://www.hipsandknees.com/hip/hipanatomy.htm.)

hip joint is susceptible to fracture and diseases, such as osteoarthritis and rheumatoid arthritis, which eventually lead to irreparable damage of the hip. In osteoarthritis, due to "wear and tear" of the hip, the cartilage is either thinner or absent, leaving bare bone on the head of the femur to grind against the bone of the pelvic socket (Figure 6.5), causing mechanical pain. Rheumatoid arthritis is mainly inflammatory and eventually destroys the cartilage as well as damaging the bone next to the cartilage as it becomes very soft. Diseased and damaged hip joints can be totally replaced by prosthetic joints (Figure 6.5). A case study on the biomaterials employed and the rationale for their use in the artificial THR is discussed in the following section.

In modern THR, also called a hip arthroplasty, the head of the femur is removed and replaced with a metal ball and stem. This stem fits into the shaft of the femur. The surface layer of the pelvis socket is replaced with a plastic or a metal and plastic cup. Thus, the painful parts of the hip joint are completely replaced with synthetic biomaterials, as shown in Figure 6.6.

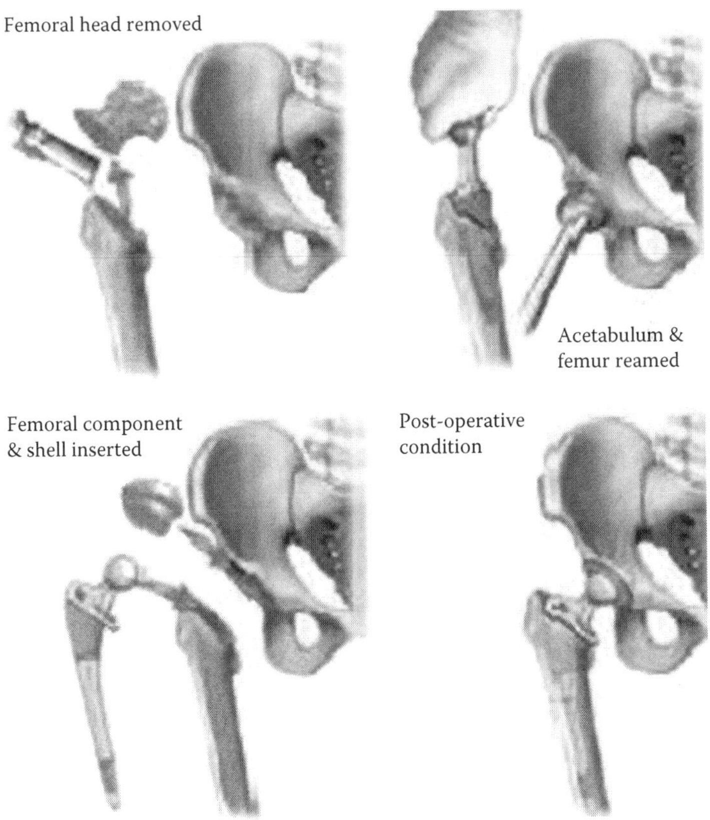

FIGURE 6.6
Schematic diagram of surgical procedures in hip replacement. (From http://www.ehealthmd.com/library/totalhipreplacement/THR_whatis.html.)

Initially, a metal ball and plastic socket was used for the replacement of the hip joint and today, many different shapes, sizes, and designs of artificial components that are stronger, are available for THR.

From materials selection requirements, there are four basic components of the artificial hip: femoral stem, ball that attaches to the stem, acetabular cup that is fixed to the pelvis, and fixation agent that cements the cup and stem to the surrounding bone. The material for the stem should have sufficient strength and fracture toughness. So, metallic biomaterials such as 316L steel, Co-Cr-Mo, and Ti-6Al-4V alloys are the most suitable materials. Early hip designs used both the stem and ball made of steel (Figure 6.7), but its susceptibility to crevice corrosion and pitting and relatively low fatigue strength restricts its use to older and less active persons. The "Charnley" stainless steel hip implant may also cause allergic reaction in some patients because of its nickel content. The "Freeman" hip stem is made up of Co-Cr alloys and has excellent corrosion and fatigue properties. The geometrical shape of the stem is designed to be used without any fixation agent and to encourage bone growth into the (proximal) features of the stem, while the smooth shaft ensures load transfer (Figure 6.7). However, to match the modulus of elasticity of bone with the stem material to avoid stress shielding, titanium alloys were the obvious choice for the femur stem as they have relatively low weight, but with high strength. But due to the poor wear properties of titanium, a two-piece modular femoral component consisting of Ti-6Al-4V alloy stem and ball of different material were used (Figure 6.7). The use of ceramic materials, which are very hard and can be polished to a fine surface finish,

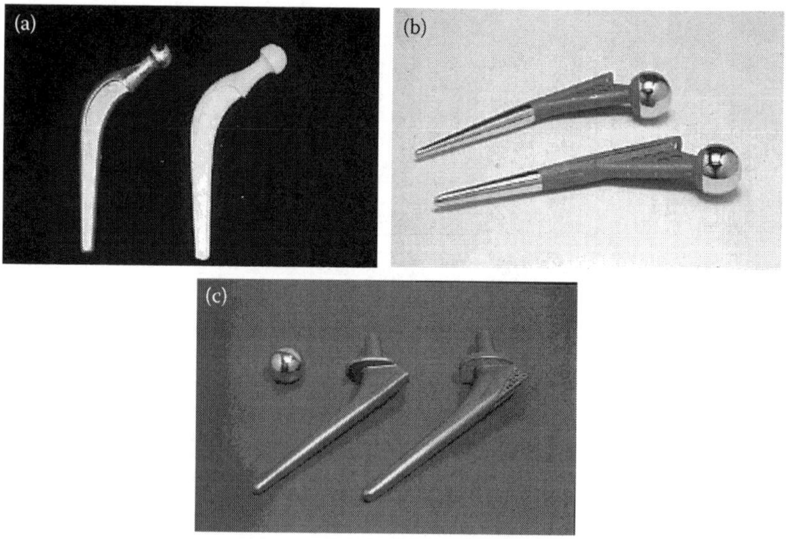

FIGURE 6.7
Pictures of (a) stainless steel, (b) Co-Cr and (c) titanium alloy hip implants. (Extracted from http://www.materials.qmul.ac.uk/casestud/implants/.)

can minimize the wear. Hence, the high purity polycrystalline alumina or zirconia is used for the ball component.

Traditionally, implants were made with a metal femoral head and a plastic acetabulum. The acetabular cups are commonly made of ultrahigh molecular weight polyethylene as it has a very low coefficient of friction. But polyethylene also inevitably wears, especially in young and active patients. So, a ceramic femoral head and articulating it against a ceramic acetabular component can minimize particle debris, which cause early implant failure. The ceramic-on-ceramic surfaces of alumina oxide have been shown to last longer than traditional metal and plastic components.

The commonly used bone cement to hold the femoral and acetabular components in place is an acrylic polymer called polymethylmethacrylate (PMMA). The PMMA polymerizes in situ during surgery and its main disadvantage is the considerable heat generated during the curing process, which causes cell death in the surrounding bone. Also, it has poor resistance to fracture and the cracks (fatigue fractures) that occur over time in the cement can cause the prosthetic stem to loosen and become unstable. Therefore, new implant designs were introduced to attach the stem and the cup directly to bone without the use of cement. Designs for cementless fixation have a surface topography that is conducive to attracting new bone growth. Mostly, they are textured or have a surface coating of hydroxyapatite around much of the implant, so that the new bone actually grows into the surface of the implant. Cementless implants require a longer healing time than cemented replacements, as they depend on new bone growth for stability. There have been many improvements in both the materials and the methods used to hold the femoral and acetabular components in place. In a hybrid hip technique, one component, usually the acetabular socket, was inserted without cement, and the other component, usually the femoral stem, was inserted with cement.

6.5 Summary

Many metallic materials exhibit biocompatibility, appropriate mechanical properties, and are of reasonable cost. Metallic biomaterials are grouped into three major metal groups: iron-based stainless steels, cobalt-based alloys, and pure titanium and titanium alloys. All exhibit corrosion resistance through passivation with the formation of either chromium oxide or titanium oxide. The stainless steels (ASTM F138/139, F1314, F1586, and F2229) are used for temporary implant applications as bone screws and plates, as they also corrode inside the body under highly stressed and oxygen depleted regions. The Co-Cr alloys (ASTM F75, F799, and F562) have superior fatigue and ultimate tensile strength. Therefore, they are the ideal materials for implant applications, which require long service life without failure, such as dental applications and recently for artificial joints. The titanium and its alloys (ASTM F67, F136, 1295, and 2146) provide superior corrosion resistance compared to stainless steel and Co-Cr alloys, but with much lower (approximately half) moduli. The thermal SME and superelasticity of NiTi alloy provides newer possibilities for implant applications, such as to restrict, dilate, push apart, or pull together body components. Nanostructured metallic materials have been shown to directly signal the adsorption of the required matrix proteins, favor the adhesion correct cells, and ensure the early integration with tissues with overall improved biological performance.

Glossary

Age hardening: A process of increasing hardness and strength by the precipitation of particles of a phase from a supersaturated solid solution alloy.

Anodize: A process of coating a metal with an oxide layer.

Arthroplasty: A surgery done to reconstruct or replace a diseased joint.

Corrosion: A destructive chemical reaction of a metal with the environment to one of its compounds. For example, the corrosion of iron by oxygen and water to produce iron oxides (rust).

Forging: A process of working of a metal to some predetermined shape by hammering, upsetting, pressing, or rolling, either hot or cold, or by a combination of several of these processes.

Grain: A solid polyhedral group of atoms bound together in a regular geometric pattern.

Hardness: A property of resistance of metal to plastic deformation by indentation. Most common method of measurements are Rockwell, Brinell, Scleroscope, and Vickers.

Martensite: A hard product that is formed when steel is cooled very rapidly.

Passivation: A combined process of removal of contaminates from the surface of a metal by means of a chemical dissolution, mostly by acid treatment, and spontaneous formation of a protective oxide film.

Pitting corrosion: A localized corrosion occurring at high concentrations of chlorides, moderately high temperatures, and acidic conditions, leading to perforation of the material.

PRE: Pitting resistance equivalent number gives indication of the pitting resistance of stainless steels. The PRE can be calculated as $= \%Cr + 3.3 \times \%Mo + 16 \times \%N$.

Wrought alloys: Products produced by rolling and extrusion as well as forging of a metal that has been cast into a form or shape that is suitable for further processing.

EXERCISES

6.1 What type of metallic systems are mostly widely used as biomaterials?
6.2 Why does 316 stainless steel have a very low carbon content?
6.3 How will you improve the mechanical properties of austenitic stainless steels?
6.4 What is the role of chromium and molybdenum additions to the cobalt-based alloys?
6.5 Why is MP35N alloy expected to have very good mechanical properties?
6.6 How does titanium and its alloys acquire superior corrosion resistance?
6.7 What are the advantages of using titanium-based alloys for implant applications compared to other metallic system?
6.8 Why are shape memory alloys more suitable as orthodontic wires?
6.9 How does a silver–tin mercury amalgam set?
6.10 What type of gold casting alloys are used for dental applications?
6.11 What are the reasons for the failure of metallic implants with conventional grain size?
6.12 Which major properties of metallic materials are anticipated to change on reducing the grain size to nanometer size?
6.13 How can nanostructured metallic implants enhance tissue integration?

References

Angenete, J. 2004. *A TEM investigation of the influence of nitrogen and cold working on the microstructure of solid solution annealed austenitic stainless steel (316L)*, 02-24 Figures 3 and 5, NanoAnalys, SKI Report 29, by Magnus Hansson and SeijiYamamaoto, Goteburg, Sweden.

Black, J. 1999. *Biological performance of materials: Fundamentals of biocompatibility*. New York: Marcel Dekker.

Bordjih, K. et al. 1996. Evaluation of the effect of three surface treatments on the biocompatibility of 316L stainless steel using human differentiated cells. *Biomaterials* 17:491–500.

Brunski, J. B. 2004. Metals. In *Biomaterials science: An introduction to materials in medicine*, ed. B. D. Ratner, A. S. Hoffman, F. J. Schoen, and J. E. Lemons, 137–53. San Diego, CA: Elsevier Academic Press.

Davis, J. R. 2003. *Handbook of materials for medical devices*. Materials Park, OH: ASM International.

Duerig, T. W. et al. 1990. *Engineering aspects of shape memory alloys*. London: Butterworth-Heinemann.

de Oliveria P. T. and A. Nanci. 2004. Nanotexturing of titanium-based surfaces upregulates expression of bone sialoprotein and osteopontin by cultured osteogenic cells. *Biomaterials* 25:403–13.

Gleiter, H. 1989. Nanocrystalline materials. *Prog. Mater. Sci.* 33:223–315.

Gutwein, L. G. and T. J. Webster. 2004. Increased viable osteoblast cell density in the presence of nanophase compared to conventional alumina and titania particles. *Biomaterials* 25:4175–83.

Hahn, H. 1997. Gas phase synthesis of nanocrystalline materials. *Nanostruct. Mater.* 9:3–12.

Horton, R. A. 1988. Investment casting. In *Metals handbook*, Vol. 15, 9th ed., 253–69. Materials Park, OH: ASM International.

Hu, E. and D. Shaw. 1999. Synthesis and assembly. In *Nanostructure science and technology: R&D status and trends in nanoparticles, nanostructured materials, and nanodevices*, ed. R. W. Siegel, E. Hu, and M. C. Roco, 15–33. Washington DC: National Science and Technology Council.

Koch, C. C. 2003. Top-down synthesis of nanostructured materials: Mechanical and thermal processing methods. *Rev. Adv. Mater. Sci.* 5:91–99.

Komarneni, S. et al. 2004. Microwave-polyol process for metal nanophases. *J. Phys.: Condens. Matter* 16:S1305–S12.

Lane, R., B. Craig, and W. Babcock. 2002. Materials ease: Materials engineering with nature's building blocks. *AMPTIAC Q.* 6:31–36.

Long, M. and H. J. Rack. 1998. Titanium alloys in total joint replacement—a materials science perspective. *Biomaterials* 19:1621–39.

Mantovani, D. 2000. Shape memory alloys: Properties and biomedical applications. *JOM* 52:36–44.

McComb, D. 1998. Gallium restorative materials. *J. Can. Dent. Assoc.* 64:645–47.

Medlin, D. J. et al. 2003. Metallurgical characterization of a porous tantalum biomaterial (Trabecular Metal) for orthopaedic implant applications. *Adv. Mater. Proc.* December:31–32.

Park, J. B. and Y. K. Kim. 2003. Metallic biomaterials. In *Biomaterials: Principles and applications*, ed. J. B. Park and J. D. Bronzino, 1–45. Boca Raton, FL: CRC Press.

Pollack, H. W., 1988. *Materials science and metallurgy*, 4th ed. Englewood Cliffs, NJ: Prentice Hall.

Ratner, B. D., A. S. Hoffman, F. J. Schoen, and J. E. Lemons J.E. 2004. In *Biomaterials science : An introduction to materials in medicine*, San Diego: Elsevier Academic Press.

Sato, M. and T. J. Webster. 2004. Nanobiotechnology: Implications for the future of nanotechnology in orthopedic applications. *Expert Rev. Med. Dev.* 1:105–14.

Siegel, R. W. 1991. Cluster-assembled nanophase materials. *Ann. Rev. Mater. Sci.* 21:559–78.

Swihart, M. T. 2003. Vapor-phase synthesis of nanoparticles. *Curr. Opin. Coll. Inter. Sci.* 8:127–33.

Valiev, R. Z. et al. 2003. SPD-processed ultra-fine grained Ti materials for medical applications. *Adv. Mater. Proc. December*:33–34.

Webster, T. J. and J. U. Ejiofor. 2004. Increase osteoblast adhesion on nanophase metals: Ti, Ti6Al4V and CoCrMo. *Biomaterials* 25:4731–39.

Zhu, X. K. et al. 2003. Synthesis of bulk nanostructured Zn by combinations of cryomilling and powder consolidation by room temperature milling: Optimizing mechanical properties. *Scr. Mater*. 49:429–33.

7

Ceramic Biomaterials

7.1 Introduction

Ceramics are polycrystalline inorganic nonmetallic compounds, including metallic oxides, silicates, carbides and various refractory hydrides, sulfides. Humans are also full of natural ceramics, such as bones and teeth. The ceramics used to augment or replace various parts of the body, particularly bone, are called bioceramics and are widely used in many medical applications, such as hip prosthesis, cardiac valves, and dental implants, because of their relative inertness to body fluids, high compressive strength, and aesthetic appearance. Certain type of glasses and glass-ceramics are also used for biomedical applications as bone substitutes. Some carbons have found use as biomedical implants, especially for their blood compatibility in heart valves. The various applications of bioceramics are listed in Table 7.1. This chapter describes the different types of bioceramics, their tissue response, the advantages of nanobioceramics, and some of their processing methods.

7.2 Bioceramics

Among the biomaterials available, bioceramics exhibit some of the most interesting properties. Biomaterials, when implanted into the body, cause some reaction with the host tissues and bioceramics exhibit all the possible tissue/implant interactions. There are four types of interactions: toxic—tissue dies due to chemical leaching from the ceramic; biologically inert—tissue forms a nonadherent fibrous capsule around the implant surface; bioactive—tissue chemically bonds with the implant surface; dissolution of implant—the implant surface dissolves, allowing tissues to refill the space previously occupied by the implant. Based on the tissue response, the bioceramics can be classified as inert, porous, bioactive, and resorbable ceramics (Table 7.2). This is a more appropriate classification than that based on the composition of the materials, as done in the case of metals, polymers, etc. The different type of attachments

TABLE 7.1

Uses of Bioceramics as Implant Materials

Ceramic	Applications
Alumina	Femoral heads, dental implants, otolaryngological applications, maxillofacial reconstruction, coatings for tissue ingrowth, drug delivery devices, middle ear ossicles
Bioglass	Alveolar ridge augmentations, dental implants, coatings for bonding with tissues, otolaryngological applications, periodontal pocket obliteration, maxillofacial reconstruction
Carbon	Cardiac valves, coatings on vascular implants, hand joints
Hydroxyapatite	Coatings for bonding with tissues, dental implants, alveolar ridge augmentations, otolaryngological applications, periodontal pocket obliteration, maxillofacial reconstruction, ocular implants
Tricalcium phosphate	Bone restoration, drug delivery devices, bone spacers
Zirconia	Femoral heads

Source: Compiled from Park, J. B. and Kim Y. K., *Biomaterials – Principles and applications*, Boca Raton, FL: CRC Press, 1–20, 2003; Davis, J. R., *Handbook of materials for medical devices*, ASM International, Materials Park, OH, 2003. With permission from Taylor & Francis Group.

TABLE 7.2

Various Types of Bioceramic-Tissue Attachments

Type of Attachment	Fixation; Examples
Dense, nonporous, nearly inert ceramics attach by bone growth into surface irregularities by cementing the material into the tissues or by press fitting into a bone defect	Morphological; alumina (single crystal and polycrystalline)
Porous inert ceramics allow bone ingrowth to occur, which results in mechanical attachment of the bone to the ceramic material	Biological; porous alumina and hydroxyapatite coatings
Dense, nonporous, surface-reactive ceramics, glasses, and glass–ceramics attach directly by forming a chemical bond with the bone	Bioactive; bioactive glasses, bioactive glass-ceramics, hydroxyapatite
Dense, nonporous or porous, resorbable ceramics are resorbed due to enhanced dissolution rates *in vivo* and so ultimately are replaced by bone	Resorbable; calcium sulfate, tricalcium phosphate

Source: Compiled from Hench, L. L., *J. Am. Ceram. Soc.*, 81, 1705–28, 2005; Davis, J. R., *Handbook of materials for medical devices*, ASM International, Materials Park, OH, 2003. With permission.

between the host tissue and an implant, along with examples of bioceramics used are

1. Nearly inert: This type of implant exhibits minimal interaction with the host tissues and the implant is covered with a nonadherent fibrous tissue as the host tries to isolate itself from the foreign body. The fixation of the implant and the tissue is by pure

mechanical interaction and is known as morphological fixation (alumina and zirconia femoral heads).
2. Porous: The fixation of porous implant is by biological ingrowth of the host tissues into the implant pores. This is also known as biological fixation (hydroxyapatite (HA) and HA-coated porous metals used for femoral stems).
3. Bioactive: The fixation is by chemical bonding between the implant and the host tissues (bioactive glasses, HA, and bioactive glass–ceramics used for dental and orthopedic devices).
4. Resorbable: This type of implant chemically dissolves or is removed from the body by cells. So, there is no fixation of the implant, only replacement of implant with biological tissues (tricalcium phosphates; TCP).

The comparison of the relative reactivity of the bioceramics, which correlates very closely with the rate of formation of an interfacial bond of the various ceramics, is shown in Figure 7.1. The response of the bioactive material is in between that of resorbable and inert materials. Every material elicits some type of response and the concern is trying to find something that is minimal, so that it is as close to being inert as possible. Any biomaterial must display qualities of biocompatibility, meaning that it does not elicit a negative response, and must also display biodurability, meaning that it resists wear or corrosion. These characteristics of durability and compatibility have long been associated with biomaterials, but recently, attention is also focused on a third property: bioactivity. Materials that integrate bioactivity, work in some means to increase the healing process.

Most of the biomaterials are found to have some bioactive attachment with different rates of bonding and thickness of bonding. So, the more appropriate definition is "A bioactive material is one that elicits a specific biological response at the interface of the material which results in the formation of bond between tissues and the material." The comparison of the interfacial layer thickness of the various bioactive materials is shown in Figure 7.2. More detailed discussion on bioactivity is presented in a later section on bioactive ceramics.

7.2.1 Nearly Inert Bioceramics

Bioinert ceramics resist corrosion and wear, but maintain good biocompatibility while in the human body. Examples of bioinert ceramics are aluminum oxide, zirconium oxide, and single-phase calcium aluminum silicates. Due to their high strength, they are typically used in load-bearing applications, such as femoral heads in hip prostheses and dental implants. Some nonstructural support uses of alumina are as ventilation tubes, sterilization devices, and drug delivery systems. The high-purity alumina (aluminum oxide, Al_2O_3) is

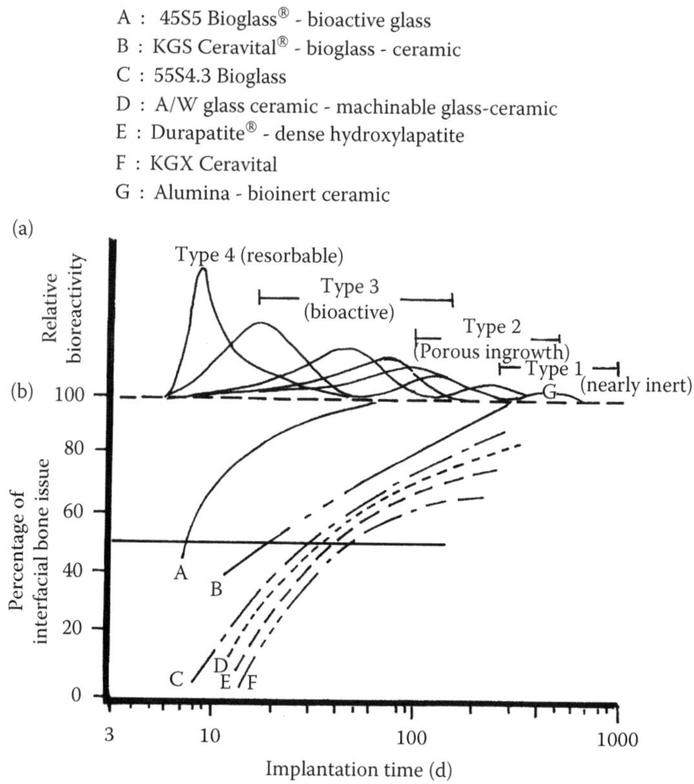

FIGURE 7.1
Bioactivity spectrum of various bioceramics: relative rate of bioreactivity (a) and time dependence of formation of bone bonding at an implant interface (b). (From http://www.bg.ic.ac.uk/Lectures/Hench/BioGlass/cal3.htm.)

obtained from bauxite ore and medical grade alumina contains more than 99.5% Al_2O_3 with silica and alkali oxide impurities less than 0.1% (ASTM F603-78). The naturally occurring single crystal of alumina is known as sapphire or ruby, depending on the impurity that give rise to its color. Single crystal alumina or sapphire has been used in dental implants, although its use in this application is declining with the advent of more advanced materials, such as resin-based composites.

Most of the alumina implants are made with polycrystalline alumina and the strength of alumina depends on its grain size and porosity. As smaller the grain size, lower the porosity and higher the strength; very fine-grained alumina with grain size < 4 μm and with elastic modulus of 380 GPa is used. The alumina implants are usually produced by sintering at 1600°C–1700°C and a small amount of magnesia (MgO, < 0.5%) is used as a sintering aid and to limit the grain growth during sintering (Davis 2003). Sintering is a process of bonding ceramic powder by cold pressing it into a desired shape and then heating

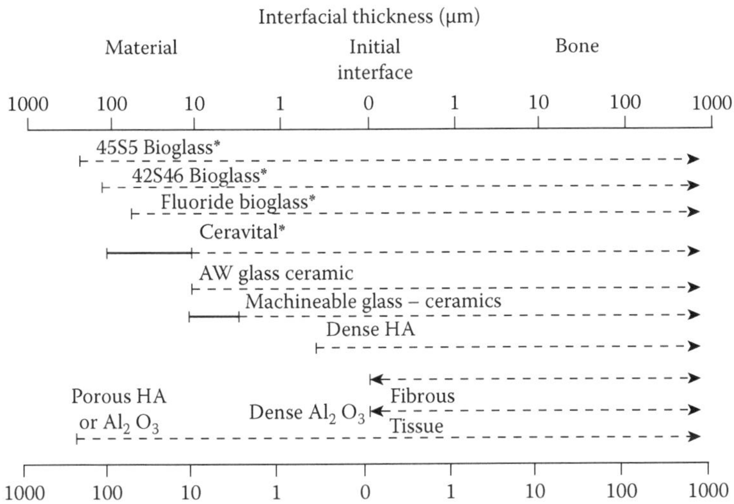

FIGURE 7.2
Comparison of interfacial thickness of reaction layer of bioactive implants or fibrous tissue of inactive bioceramics in bone. (From http://www.bg.ic.ac.uk/Lectures/Hench/BioGlass/cal3.htm.) * registered trademark.

at a temperature below the melting point of the main constituent to form a strong cohesive body. The physical and mechanical properties of alumina are summarized in Table 7.3. For more than 25 years, the high hardness and superb tribiological properties of alumina have permitted its use on load bearing and wearing surfaces, such as total hip prostheses (Hench 1991). However, the stress shielding due to the high elastic modulus of alumina may cause bone atrophy and loosening of the acetabular cup in older patients with osteoporosis or rheumatoid arthritis. Also, an increase in grain size can drastically decrease the mechanical properties. So, the highest quality control during the implant production, and knowledge about the age, joint disease nature, and the biomechanics of the repair, are the key to success for alumina prostheses.

Zirconia (ZrO_2) also has excellent biocompatibility and good tribiological properties. It is used in hip prostheses as the articulating ball. As zirconia undergoes a large volumetric change during phase transformation at high temperatures, partially stabilized zirconia (PSZ) is used for implant applications. The PSZ contains a dopant oxide, such as ytteria (Y_2O_3, around 6 mol.%), used to stabilize the high-temperature phase (Billotte 2003). The lower elastic modulus and higher strength (Table 7.3) are the potential advantages of zirconia in load-bearing applications.

Carbon exhibits excellent compatibility with tissue and is used as a bioinert material. Three different classes of carbon materials can be distinguished: pyrolytic carbon (low-temperature isotropic carbon, LTI), vapor-deposited carbon (ultralow-temperature isotropic carbon, ULTI) and glassy-carbon (vitreous carbon). Pyrolytic carbon is commonly used in artificial heart valves

TABLE 7.3

Physical and Mechanical Characteristics of Bioceramics

Properties	**Alumina ISO 6474**	**Alumina ASTM F603**	**Yttria-Stabilized Zirconia ASTM F1873**	**Pyrolytic (LTI) Carbon**	**HA**	**Bioglass 45S5**
Content (%)	≥ 99.5%	≥ 99.5%	≥ 93.2% + yttria	0% Si	…	…
Density (g/cm^3)	> 3.90	> 3.94	> 6.0	1.5–2.2	3.16	2.66
Average grain size (μm)	< 7	≤ 4.5	≤ 0.6	3–4 nm		
Vickers hardness (GPa)	> 2000 (10^6 psi)	18	1200	150–250	600	450–460
Compressive strength (MPa)	…	4000	1200	517	500–1000	…
Flexural strength (MPa)	400	45,000	800	…		…
Elastic modulus (GPa)	380	380	200	18–28	80–110	35
Fracture toughness (K_{1c}) MPa	5–6	…	15	4.8	1.0	…
Weibull modulus	…	8	10	…	12	…

Source: Compiled from Park, J. B. and Kim Y. K., *Biomaterials – Principles and applications*, Boca Raton, FL: CRC Press, 1–20, 2003; Davis, J. R., *Handbook of materials for medical devices*, ASM International, Materials Park, OH, 2003; Hench, L. L., *J. Am. Ceram. Soc.*, 81, 1705–28, 2005. With permission from Taylor & Francis Group.

and has been the most popular material for this application for the last 30 years. It is obtained by the thermal decomposition (pyrolysis) of hydrocarbon such as propane and methane in the absence of oxygen. Properties that make this material suitable for biomaterials applications include good strength (Table 7.3), wear, resistance, and durability, and most importantly, thromboresistance, or the ability to resist blood clotting. Pyrolytic carbon is also used for small orthopedic joints, such as fingers and spinal inserts (Davis 2003).

7.2.2 Porous Bioceramics

The porous bioceramics have the advantage of bioinertness combined with mechanical stability when bone grows into the pores of the ceramic implant. The porous prostheses act as a scaffold for bone growth. Typically, a pore size > 100 μm is necessary for bone growth to maintain its vascularity and long-term viability. But the interconnectivity of pores may be more critical than the pore size.

Some marine corals have a high degree of uniform pore size and interconnectivity. The coral genus, *Porites*, has pores in the range of 140–160 μm and the coral genus, *Goniopora*, has a larger pore size of 200–1000 μm, with all the pores interconnected in both the corals. They are used as investment materials for casting materials with a highly controlled pore size and interconnected microstructure. This process of duplicating the porous microstructure of corals is called replamineform process and consists of firing the machined required shape coral to drive of carbon dioxide of the calcium carbonate ($CaCO_3$) skeleton to form calcia (CaO) while maintaining the original coral microstructure. The desired material such as calcium phosphate is then cast into the porous CaO structure and finally the negative cast of the original coral structure is retained by removing the CaO by ageing in a dilute acid (Davis 2003). The calcia is easily removed by dissolving in dilute hydrochloric acid. Porous materials of cobalt alloys, alumina, titania, calcium phosphates, polymethyl methacrylate, polyurethane, and silicone rubber have been formed by the replamineform process. Foaming agents, such as calcium carbonate, which evolve gases during heating, or soluble metals and salts are mixed with the ceramic materials to form a porous structure. The size and shape of the soluble particles determine the pore size and structure, which are subsequently removed with a suitable etchant (Hench 1982).

As the porosity increases, the strength of the ceramic material decreases drastically. Much surface area is also exposed and environmental effects become more important. So, the use of low-strength porous ceramics is severely restricted to non load-bearing applications. If load bearing is not a primary requirement, porous ceramics can provide a functional implant. Porous alumina has also been used as a bone spacer, where sections of bone have to be removed due to disease.

TABLE 7.4

Composition of Bioactive Bioceramics

Bioceramic	I_b value	SiO_2 wt.%	Na_2O wt.%	CaO wt.%	P_2O_5 wt.%	MgO wt.%	CaF_2 wt.%
45S5 Bioglass®	12.5	45.0	24.5	24.5	6.0	...	
KGS Ceravital®	5.6	40–50	5–10	30–35	10–50	2.5–5.0	
A/W glass–ceramic	3.2	34.0	...	44.7	16.2	4.6	0.5
Durapatite®	3.1	18	1200 HV	150–250			

Source: Compiled from Park, J. B. and Kim Y. K., *Biomaterials – Principles and applications*, Boca Raton, FL: CRC Press, 1–20, 2003; Davis, J. R., *Handbook of materials for medical devices*, ASM International, Materials Park, OH, 2003; Hench, L. L., *J. Am. Ceram. Soc.*, 81, 1705–28, 2005. With permission from Taylor & Francis Group.

7.2.3 Bioactive Bioceramics

Some special compositions of glasses, ceramics, and glass–ceramics are found to develop a mechanically strong bond to bone (Hench 1982). These materials are termed "bioactive ceramics." The common feature of bioactive ceramics is a time-dependent, kinetic modification of the surface that occurs upon implantation. A hydroxylcarbonate apatite (HCA) layer is formed on its surface, which provides the bonding interface with tissues. The HCA phase is chemically and structurally equivalent to the mineral phase in bone. This biological similarity of the HCA layer that has formed on the bioactive implant surface is responsible for interfacial bonding. A few more specific compositions of bioactive glasses have been found to bond to soft tissues as well.

The bioactive properties of the HA and bioactive glasses are found to be remarkably different. So, a simple way of grading the bioactivity of a material is based on the "Index of bioactivity" (I_b), which is the time ($t_{0.5bb}$) taken for more than 50% of the interface between bone and an implant to chemically bond together. The I_b values ($= 100/t_{0.5bb}$) can be calculated from the curves as shown in Figure 7.1, and some typical I_b values are listed in Table 7.4. Based on the I_b values, bioactive ceramics can be further grouped as "Class A" and "Class B" bioactive materials.

Class A bioactivity: Materials with I_b values greater than 8 and consist of bioactive materials, such as bioactive glasses, that not only act as a matrix for bone cell growth (osteoconductive process), but also increase the rate of bone cell proliferation. An extra and intracellular response is elicited by a Class A bioactive material at the interface. Such materials are said to be osteoproductive.

Class B bioactivity: Materials with an I_b value less than 8, but greater than 0 and include bioactive materials such as synthetic HA that are only osteoconductive. Thus, the material only exhibits an extracellular response at the interface.

Also Class A bioactive materials show faster rates of *in vitro* hydroxylcarbonate-apatite layer precipitation (within 20 h) and higher rates of bond to bone formation in contrast to Class B bioactive materials. Class A bioactive materials also have the capability of bonding to soft tissues, while Class B can only bond to bone. But, these materials are not osteoinductive (induce new bone formation), as this requires the presence of growth factors such as bone morphogenic proteins (BMP) and other factors, which are only present in natural bone. The BMP activates precursor cells to differentiate into osteogenic cells, thereby causing bone cells to multiply and increase the rate of bone matrix formation. The osteoproductive materials cause the existing bone cells to produce a matrix at an increased rate and enhance the rate of proliferation of existing osteoprogenitor cells, but does not cause precursor cells to become osteogenic.

7.2.3.1 Bioactive Glasses

Ceramics in various forms and compositions are presently in use. Most silicate ceramics (SiO_2–Na_2O–CaO) have a SiO_2 content of 65 wt.% or more. These silicate ceramics are more commonly called glass. The 65 wt.% silica glasses are extremely bioinert. The bioactivity was first demonstrated for a certain compositional range of bioactive glasses that contained SiO_2, Na_2O, CaO, and P_2O_5 in specific proportions, as listed in Table 7.4. The three key compositional features of these glasses that differentiate them from traditional soda-lime–silica glasses are

1. Less than 60 mol.% SiO_2
2. High Na_2O and CaO content
3. High CaO/P_2O_5 ratio

Under this compositional range of relatively low silicon and high alkaline content, the glass surface becomes highly reactive on exposure to an aqueous medium, which leads to a rapid ion exchange with the environment. The sodium ion is released rapidly followed by slower release of calcium and silica ions. Under certain conditions in the solution, these ions precipitate to form the calcium-phosphate mineral layer, which is involved in bonding with the bone. Most of the bioactive silica glasses are based on the formula "45S5," signifying 45 wt.% SiO_2 (S = the network former) and 5:1 molar ratio of Ca to P. As the addition of P_2O_5 to the SiO_2–Na_2O–CaO matrix makes the glass extremely bioactive, glasses with substantially lower molar ratios of Ca to P do not bond with bone. Also, the addition of as little as 3 wt.% Al_2O_3 to the 45S5 formula prevents bonding. However, substitutions of 5–15 wt.% B_2O_3 for SiO_2 or 12.5 wt.% CaF_2 for CaO has no significant effect on the ability of the material to form a bone bond.

The approximate regions of bone bonding and soft-tissue bonding for the Na_2O–CaO–P_2O_5–SiO_2 glass system, for a constant 6 wt.% of P_2O_5, are shown in Figure 7.3. The best region for bone bonding is shown in the middle of the diagram (Region A) and corresponds to the composition of the 45S5 glass. Thus, region A is termed as the bioactive-bone-bonding boundary. The conventional silicate glasses such as glassware or microscope slides, with composition within region B, have a very low reactivity and behave as nearly inert bioceramics.

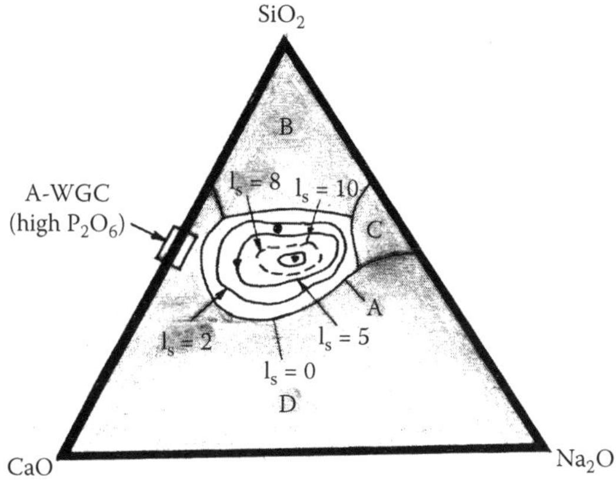

FIGURE 7.3
Compositional regions for bone bonding and soft-tissue bonding of bioactive glasses and glass–ceramics. (From http://www.bg.ic.ac.uk/Lectures/Hench/BioGlass/cal3.htm.)

They are nonbonding and elicit a fibrous capsule at the implant–tissue interface. The glasses within region C have a very high reactivity and are nonbonding. In fact, they are resorbable and disappear within 10–30 days of implantation. Compositions within region D do not form glass and so have not been tested as implants. The bioactive glasses that lie within the compositional range in region E (dashed line region) can strongly adhere to the soft tissues.

Glass–ceramics are polycrystalline ceramics formed by controlled crystallization of glasses (Davis 2003). The nucleation and growth of small crystals (< 1 micron) as well as their distribution influence the formation class ceramics. A range of low-alkali (0–5 wt.%) bioactive silica glass–ceramics called "Ceravital" were found bonded to bone. The addition of small amounts of Al_2O_3, Ta_2O_5, TiO_2, Sb_2O_3, or ZrO_2 for nucleation and growth to Ceravital, inhibits bone bonding. A two-phase glass–ceramic consisting of fluorinated apatite [$Ca_{10}(PO_4)_6(OH_1F_2)$] and calcium silicate [β-wollastonite, $CaSiO_3$] crystals in a residual silica glassy matrix, called "A/W glass–ceramic," also bonds with bone and is found to have a very high interfacial bond strength (Kokubo 1992). The addition of Al_2O_3 or TiO_2 to the A/W glass–ceramic also inhibits bone bonding, but incorporation of a second phosphate phase [β-whitlockite, $Ca_9Mg_{0.7}Fe^{2+}{}_{0.5}(PO_4)_6(PO_3OH)$] does not alter the bioactivity. So, alumina containing a machinable, multiphase, bioactive glass-ceramic composed of phlogopite [(Na,K) $Mg_3[AlSi_3O_{10}]F_2$, mica, and apatite crystals have also been developed to bond to bone. However, the aluminum ions are well incorporated in the crystal lattice, as shown in the formula, and are not involved in the surface reaction kinetics (Davis 2003). The disadvantages of multiphase glass–ceramic are its brittleness and the limitation of composition to improve the mechanical strength. So, they are used as fillers in bone cement, dental restorative composites, and coating materials.

The sequence of interfacial reactions involved in forming a bond between bone and single-phase bioglass has been well studied. It involves 11 sequential

Reaction stages		
	5	Crystallization of the amorphous $CaO-P_2O_5$ layer by incorporation of OH^- and CO_3^{2-} ions from solution to form hydroxylcarbonate apatite layer
	4	Migration of Ca^{2+} and PO_4^{3-} ions and formation of amorphous $CaO-P_2O_5$-rich layer on SiO_2 layer
	3	Condensation and repolymerization of a SiO_2-rich layer on the surface
	2	Breaking of Si–O–Si bonds and formation of Si–OH (silanols)
	1	Rapid exchange of Na^+ or K^+ with H^+ or H_3O^+ from solution
		Bioactive glass

FIGURE 7.4
Surface reaction stages of a bioactive glass. (From Hench, L. L., *J. Am. Ceram. Soc.*, 81, 1705–28, 2005; Davis, J. R., *Handbook of materials for medical devices*, ASM International, Materials Park, OH, 2003. With permission.)

stages of complete bonding of bioglass to bone of which 1–5 are the chemical stages and 6–11 are the biological stages (Hench 2002). The chemical stages are related to the stimulated formation of silica-rich film and a calcium phosphate film on the surface of the material, as schematically shown in Figure 7.4. For multiphase materials, such as Ceravital or A/W glass–ceramic, the time-dependent surface changes for each phase and each interface between the phases has to be considered.

7.2.3.2 Calcium Phosphate Ceramics

Calcium phosphate ceramics, such as HA ($Ca_{10}(PO_4)_6(OH)_2$), TCP ($Ca_3(PO_4)_2$), and tetracalcium phosphate (TTCP, $Ca_4P_2O_9$), are the most widely used bioceramics. This is because the mineral phase of human bone and teeth consists primarily of calcium and phosphate ions. The calcium-to-phosphorus (Ca/P) ratio is a very useful parameter to understand the solubility and acidity of calcium phosphates. The Ca/P ratio of all calcium phosphates varies from 0.5 to 2.0, but for Ca/P ratios below 1, both acidity and solubility rates are very high, therefore, these compounds are not suitable as biomaterials. The list of calcium phosphate biomaterials arranged according to their Ca/P ratio is shown with their abbreviations and chemical formula in Table 7.5. The crystal structure and morphology of HA, octacalcium phosphate, and amorphous calcium phosphate are shown in Figure 7.5.

Among the various calcium phosphates, HA is the thermodynamically stable phase at physiological pH and has a Ca/P ratio of 1.66. HA belongs to the apatite mineral family [$A_{10}(BO_4)_6X_2$] and crystallizes in a hexagonal structure with unit cell dimensions $a = 0.943$ nm and $c = 0.688$ nm, respectively (Hench 2005). Ions such as carbonate, hydroxyl, fluoride, chloride, and traces of magnesium may be incorporated into the HA structure. The substitution of hydroxyl ion with fluoride improves the chemical stability of HA

TABLE 7.5

Ca/P Ratio of Calcium Phosphates Used as Biomaterials

Name	Abbreviation	Chemical Formula	Ca/P Ratio
Amorphous calcium phosphate	ACP	$Ca_{10-x}H_{2x}(PO_4)_6(OH)_2$	1.5
Octacalcium phosphate	OCP	$Ca_3H_2(PO_4)_6.5H_2O$	1.33
Tricalcium phosphate	TCP	$Ca_3(PO_4)_2$	1.50
Hydroxyapatite	HA	$Ca_{10}(PO_4)_6(OH)_2$	1.67
Tetracalcium phosphate	TetCP	$Ca_4O(PO_4)_2$	2.0

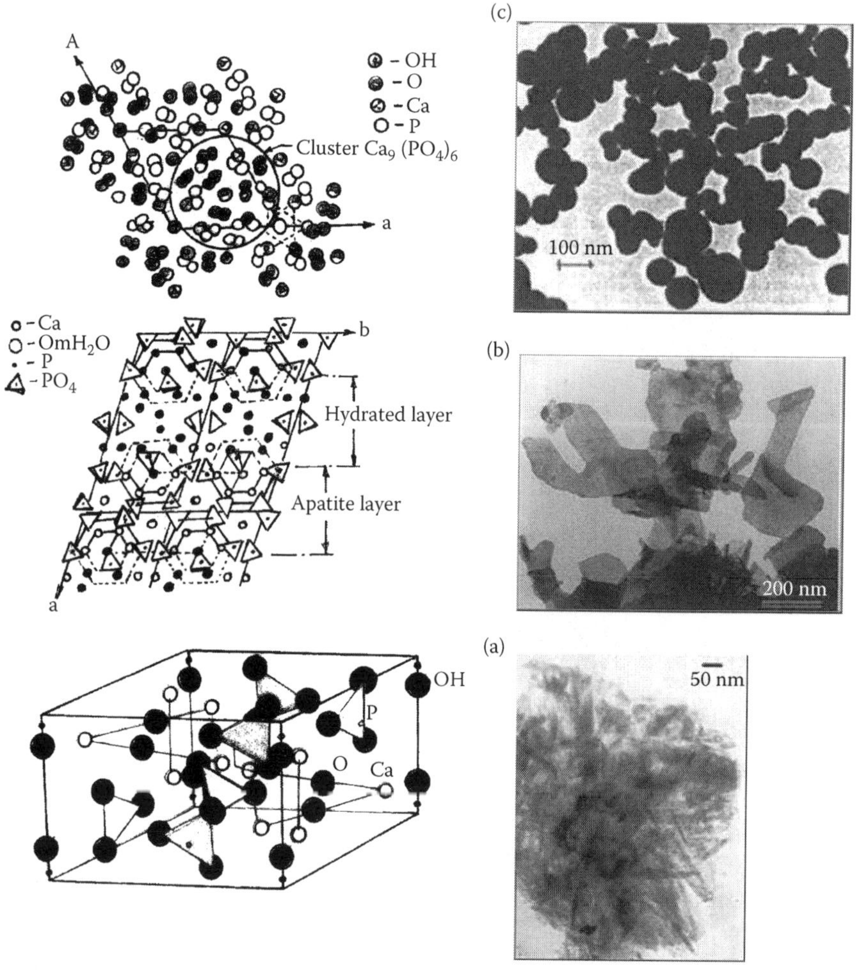

FIGURE 7.5

Crystal structure and morphology of calcium phosphates: hydroxyapatite (a), octacalcium phosphate (b), and amorphous calcium phosphate (c).

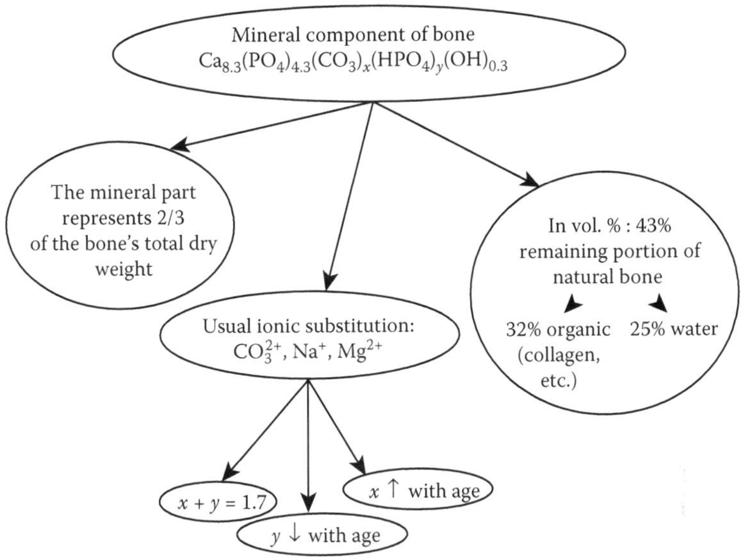

FIGURE 7.6
Schematic representation of the composition of mineral phase of bone. (Reproduced from Vallet-Regí, M., *J. Chem. Soc. Dalton Trans.*, 100, 97–108, 2001. With permission from The Royal Society of Chemistry.)

due to the symmetrical shape of fluoride ion as compared to the asymmetric coordination of hydroxyl ion with two atoms. The mineral phase of bone is a calcium-deficient carbonate HA with a Ca/P ratio of about 1.5, which strictly speaking is chemically and compositionally similar to TCP, while being structurally similar to stoichiometric HA (Ca/P = 1.67), as schematically shown in Figure 7.6. Apatites with Ca/P ratios ranging from 1.67 to 1.33 originate from the loss of Ca^{2+} ions from the unit cell; hence the name calcium-deficient HA with the formula Ca_{10-x} $(HPO_4)_x$ $(PO_4)_{6-x}$ $(OH)_{2-x}$ (Siddharthan 2004).

HA forms a direct chemical bond with hard tissues and the bonding mechanism of dense HA has been found to be very different from that for bioactive glasses with a very ultrathin bonding zone of 0.05–0.2 μm thick. Moreover, the crystallites of the bone mineral are found to be in perfect epitaxial alignment with the apatite crystals of the implant material. Many methods have been developed to produce synthetic HA directly or by conversion from other calcium compounds. The aqueous precipitation of HA is the most frequently prepared chemical route. The porous structure of certain marine coral is similar to bone and is composed of calcium carbonate. So, the coral has been converted into HA by a hydrothermal exchange process (Sivakumar 1996). Both coral and coralline HA are used to repair, replace, and correct bone disorders. The polycrystalline HA has a high elastic modulus of 40–117 GPa compared to enamel, the stiffest hard tissue with an elastic modulus of 74 GPa. Poisson's ratio of HA and bone are similar (≈ 0.3). The typical physical properties of HA are shown in Table 7.3. The wide variations in the properties of polycrystalline HA are due to the variations in the method and processing conditions affecting the phase purity, density, and grain size.

7.2.4 Bioresorbable Bioceramics

Resorption or biodegradation is the ability of the body to degrade the bioceramic and it is found to depend on chemical composition, physical form (porous/dense, particulate/block), and crystallinity. It occurs by

- Physiochemical dissolution depending on the local pH and solubility product
- Physical disintegration due to chemical attack of grain boundaries into small particles
- Biological factors such as phagocytosis, which causes a decrease in local pH

The rate of degradation varies for different bioceramics. Nearly all calcium phosphate ceramics are resorbable when exposed to physiological environments and the rate of resorption increases with decreasing Ca/P ratio. Thus, TCP is resorbed more rapidly than HA. TCP undergoes polymorphic transformation from β-TCP to α-TCP at temperatures between 1120°C and 1290°C and the solubility of α-TCP is higher than β-TCP. So, the rate of biodegradation increases as

- With α-TCP > β-TCP > HA phases
- Surface area increases
- Crystal and grain size decreases
- Substitution of CO_3^{2-}, Mg^{2+} and Sr^{2+} ions in HA increases

The rate of biodegradation decreases with the substitution of F^- and Mg^{2+} ions in HA and TCP phases, respectively (Davis 2003).

The resorbed bioceramic has to be replaced by the formation of new tissues, but if the bioceramic is resorbed too fast, then pores may occur. Hence, the relationship between resorption rate of bioceramic and growth rate of bone tissue should be considered in selecting the resorbable ceramics. A combination of HA and TCP phases, called biphasic calcium phosphates (BCP) ceramics, has been attempted for faster bone formation and better bone bonding (Kumar 2000). The BCP is soluble and gradually dissolves in the body, seeding new bone formation as it releases calcium and phosphate ions into the biological medium. Additionally, BCP has been proposed as a potential matrix for a bioactive drug delivery system in which the *in situ* release of a therapeutic agent is favored by the bioresorption of the TCP ceramics besides biocompatibility and osteoconductivity.

7.3 Nanostructured Bioceramics

The ceramics, per se, are very hard, brittle, and difficult to machine. These properties of ceramics have discouraged the exploiting of their beneficial properties for potential applications. Nanostructured ceramics exhibit promising properties when their grain size is reduced below 100 nm, and the fabrication of nanostructured ceramics is an exciting prospect in materials research. With a reduction in grain size, these ceramics exhibit superplastic behavior, i.e., they can be deformed to great lengths (up to 300% of its original length). Zirconia, a hard, brittle ceramic, has even been rendered superplastic. In fact, nanocrystalline ceramics possess good formability and machinability combined with excellent physical, chemical, and mechanical properties. Nanocrystalline ceramics can be pressed and sintered into various shapes at significantly lower temperatures, whereas it would be very difficult, if not impossible, to press and sinter conventional ceramics even at high temperatures.

Nanophase ceramics can be designed to possess the chemical composition, surface properties (specifically, topography), mechanical properties (namely, ductility), and grain size distribution similar to those of physiological bone (which contains 70 wt.% HA with grain sizes less than 100 nm). Conventional materials, such as titanium and titanium alloys, do not simulate the chemical, surface, mechanical, or grain size distribution found in physiological bone.

The *in vitro* cell culture study on the *efficacy* of nanophase alumina, titania, and HA provided the first evidence of enhanced adhesion of osteoblasts (bone-forming cells), decreased adhesion of fibroblasts (cells that contribute to fibrous encapsulation and callus formation, which may lead to implant loosening and failure), and decreased adhesion of endothelial cells (cells that line the vasculature of the body) on the nanophase bioceramics (Webster 2000). Furthermore, evidence of enhanced osteoblast proliferation, alkaline phosphate activity, and concentration of calcium in the extracellular matrix on nanophase bioceramics compared to respective conventional larger grain size materials were found (Webster 2001). The nanophase bioceramics established enhanced functions of osteoblasts and osteoclasts, which may result in the active formation and maintenance of healthy juxtaposed bone *in vivo* to improve orthopedic/dental implant efficacy. The synthesis, characterization, and *in vitro* and *in vivo* results of various nanostructured bioceramics are highlighted in the subsequent sections.

7.4 Synthesis and Characterization of Nano Bioceramics

Bioceramic nanoparticles can be viewed as the fundamental building blocks of nanotechnology and they are the starting point for many "bottom-up" approaches for preparing nanostructured biomaterials and biomedical

TABLE 7.6

Comparison of Ceramic Powder Production Methods

	Composition		Particle	
Properties/Method	**Purity**	**Distribution**	**Size**	**Distribution**
Coprecipitation	High	Homo	Fine	Narrow
Solid state reaction	Medium	Hetero	Coarse	Broad
Gas phase reaction	High	Homo	Ultrafine	Narrow
Hydrothermal	High	Homo	Fine	Narrow

devices. Their synthesis is an important component of rapidly growing research efforts in nanotechnology and a wide range of nanoparticles of bioceramics can be prepared by a variety of methods. The properties of the ceramic powder depend on the methods of production and a comparison of some powder characteristics produced by the various conventional methods is listed in Table 7.6. The high-purity ultrafine powders are obtained by using the gas phase reactions. Coprecipitation and hydrothermal methods involve the synthesis in liquid phase and are suitable for the production of the fine structure homogeneous powder. However, washing, drying, and calcining process stages and use of high liquid volumes and surfactants are necessary to produce high purity materials at high yields. The solid state reactions are the most widely used for commercial production of cost-efficient powders, because the raw materials are simply calcined to obtain the products. But the powders are coarse and heterogeneous in both size and purity. The various methods available for the production of nanophasic bioceramics are listed in Table 7.7, along with a brief description of the process involved. The advantages and disadvantages of the methods are also indicated. Some are specific, sophisticated production procedures developed for high performance nano-bioceramic powders and some are currently used for commercial production.

7.4.1 Synthesis and Characterization of Nano Alumina

Alumina, considered a bioactive bioceramic, has been used for both dental and orthopedic applications in the treatment of hand and elbow fractures, edentations, and arthoplasty. However, nanophase alumina has shown evidence for the first time of its ability to stimulate material characteristics (such as surface roughness, grain size, etc.) of bone that enhances protein interaction, subsequent osteoblast adhesion, and other cell functions, similar to bioactive materials. The nanophase alumina powder was obtained by physical vapor synthesis (PVS) process (NanophaseTechnologies, Inc., USA). In the PVS method, the solid is vaporized by jets of thermal energy, as shown in Figure 7.7. By also using a reactive gas, such as oxygen, in the cold gas stream, molecular clusters of oxides or other compounds of the evaporated material are formed. Then, the vapor and the gas are cooled to reduce the temperature to form nanometric

TABLE 7.7

Methods Available for Nanoceramic Synthesis

Method	Process Description	Advantages	Disadvantages
Precipitation under low temperature, microwaves, ultrasonics	Salt precursor is dissolved. On addition of base, compound hydroxide precipitates in water. Salts are washed and dried	Simple approach, low production cost, stoichiometry control	Agglomeration of particles and residual surface contamination
Sol-gel synthesis	Hydrolysis of reactive organic-metal precursors results in hydroxide compound gels that are heated to get the ceramic oxides	Grow nanosized particles in different matrices	Properties depend on the rate of hydrolysis and drying
Reverse micelles/ microemulsions: oil in water; water in oil; bicontinuous	Surfactant dissolved in organic solvent creates micelles (spherical aggregate) wherein synthesis occurs by alkoxide hydrolysis or metal salt precipitation	Size control by reactive precursor concentration in micelle	High amount of surfactant. Sensitive to temperatures
Mechanical deformation. Milling or shock deformation	Coarse-grained precursor material undergoes severe mechanical deformation by ball milling or friction/sliding wear	Nanomaterials of immiscible systems can be produced	Contamination from the milling media
Vapor condensation by thermal evaporation, sputtering, laser	Supersaturated vapors of the materials are condensed under inert gas and/or in oxydizer	Extremely low contamination levels, control of size, high density, directional, and high-speed vapor	High costs with low yields
Spray pyrolysis	Salt solutions are sprayed in atomizer to form aerosols that flow in inert gas stream to transform into particles	High purity and homogeneity	Large volume of solvent used. Difficulties of increasing the yield
Flame decomposition	Metal-organic precursors vaporized by combustion, oxidize and rapidly condense in inert gas stream and flame reactor	Production of commercial quantities	Control of size and morphology difficult

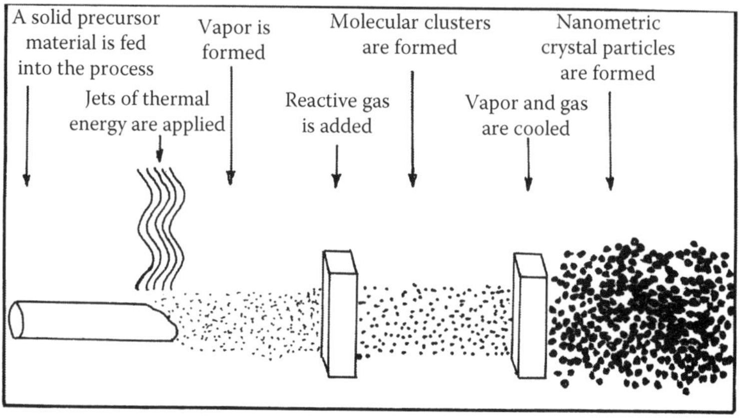

FIGURE 7.7
Schematic diagram of physical vapor synthesis method. (From Nanophase Technologies Corporation Home Page.)

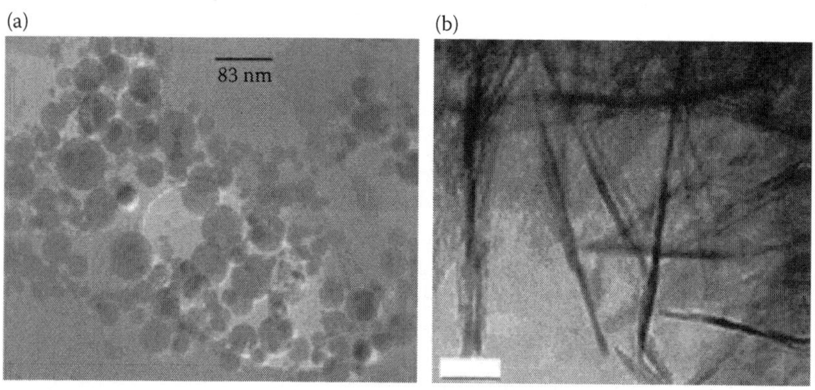

FIGURE 7.8
TEM micrographs of alumina nanoparticle (a) and nanofibers (b) (bar = 20 nm). (From Nanophase Technologies Corporation Home Page; Tepper, F., Lerner, M., and Ginley, D., *Am. Ceram. Soc. Bull.*, 80, 57–60, 2001. With permission.)

particles. The morphology of the nanophase alumina powder prepared by this method is shown in Figure 7.8. The *in vitro* osteoblast and osteoclast functions on nanophase alumina of varying particulate size, chemistry, and phase were studied in detail to find out what formulation might be most beneficial for bone regeneration and the results are summarized in Table 7.8. These studies (Webster 1999, 2001) clearly established that nanophase (23 nm grain size) alumina in comparison to conventional (177 nm grain size) alumina has

- Greater surface roughness (35–50%), number of grain boundaries, and larger surface area
- Greater porosities with pores of smaller diameter (four times)

TABLE 7.8

Summary of the Properties and Cellular Response on Nanophase and Conventional Phase Alumina

	Alumina		
Properties	**Conventional**	**Nanophase**	
Sintering temperature (°C) and time (2 h)	1200	1100	1000
Grain size (nm)	> 100 (177–167)	49–45	24
Porosity (%)	2.4	3.4	4.5
Pore diameter (Å)	29.4	11.1	6.9
Composition (anatase and rutile wt.%)	90 and 10	90 and 10	
Contact angle (deg)	18.6	10.8	6.4
Surface roughness (nm)	17	19	20
Surface area (μm²/μm)	1.15	…	1.73
Osteoblast cell density after 4 h for seeding of 3500 cells/cm²	2300	3125 and 2050 (67 nm)	3340
Cell morphology	Well spread		Rounded
TRAP[a] activity by osteoclast after 10 and 13 days	Nil	…	≈ 6
	Nil	…	≈ 5
Resorption pits by osteoclast after 10 and 13 days (no/cm²)	Nil	…	≈ 3
	≈ 3	…	≈ 6

Source: Reprinted from Webster, T. J., Siegel, R. W., and Bizios, R., *Biomaterials*, 20, 1221–27, 1999. With permission from Elsevier; Reprinted from Webster, T. J. et al., *Biomaterials*, 22, 1327–33, 2001. With permission from Elsevier; Reproduced from Sato, M. and Webster, T. J., *Expert Rev. Med. Dev.*, 1, 105–14, 2004. With permission from Expert Reviews Ltd.

[a] nmol of p-nitrophenyl phosphate-cleaved/min/g protein.

- Lower contact angle (three times lower) corresponding to an increased wettability and thus an increase in hydrophilicity and surface reactivity
- Greater concentration of protein adsorption (17%) and of select proteins like vitronectin and denatured collagen (due to smaller pore structure)
- Enhanced (46%) osteoblast adhesion and the presence of a critical grain size for increased osteoblast adhesion between 49 and 67 nm after 4 h
- Enhanced synthesis of tartrate-resistant acid phosphatase (TRAP) by osteoclast-like cells after 10 days
- Enhanced formation of resorption pits (33%) by osteoclast-like cells after 13 days

Collectively, nanophase alumina has optimal surface properties (higher surface area and lower contact angle) and surface features (large nanoscale pores close to protein size) to selectively adsorb proteins that mediate specific osteoblast adhesion (such as fibronectin and vitornectin) more effectively (Sato 2004). The adsorbed protein was also unfolded to a larger extent to expose a larger number of osteoblast adhesive epitopes. This together with nanometer surface roughness improved both osteoblastic and osteoclastic responses, while simultaneously inhibiting fibroblast functions on nanophase alumina.

Nanophase alumina was further modified to closely simulate the physical geometry of the inorganic component of bone. So, to match the aspect ratio of the HA in bone, alumina nanofibers with dimensions approximately 2 nm in diameter and 50 nm in length (Figure 7.8) were synthesized by a proprietary sol-gel method. In a sol-gel method, a homogeneous solution of reactant precursors (a sol) through hydrolysis reaction followed by condensation is irreversibly converted into a three-dimensional polymer (a gel), forming an elastic solid. The gel formed is surrounded by interconnected pores, and this can be dried to form a rigid solid with interconnected nanoscale porosity and hence a high surface area. Alternately, fibers can also be drawn from the gel. The advantages and disadvantages of the sol-gel process for the synthesis of nanomaterials are listed in Table 7.7. The nanofibrous alumina was formed by drying and heating at 400°C and has a high surface area of around 450–600 m^2/g. Increased osteoblast adhesion, proliferation, and deposition of calcium-containing mineral was observed on nanofibrous alumina-compacted substrates in comparison with similar substrates of nanospherical particulate alumina, which has also shown enhanced osteoblast and osteoclast function than the conventional micron grain size alumina. The similarity of the nanofiber shape with aspect ratio to that of the mineral phase of the bone could influence the conformation of adhesive proteins, which could influence osteoblast behavior. The alumina nanofiber heated and sintered at 400°C closely matches the stoichiometry of boehmite (AlOOH), which differs in chemical composition to the nanophase and conventional spherical alumina sintered compacts. Therefore, osteoblast functions on various phases of alumina nanofiber were also studied. The boehmite nanofiber alumina changed to gamma, gamma + delta, theta + delta, and alpha phases of alumina when sintered at 600°C, 800°C, 1000°C, and 1200°C. Increased osteoblast functions were observed on theta + delta compared to boehmite nanofiber alumina. The nanometer surface features, chemistry, and crystallinity were different for both the alumina nanofibers (Webster 2005).

The nanoscale architecture of alumina was investigated for tissue engineering applications. The impact of the nanoscale pores on osteoblast response was studied on nanoporous alumina. The nanoporous alumina was fabricated by a single or a two-step anodization process, which is an electrochemical process of growing oxide on the surface of a biased conductive solid (anode, aluminium) by passing a current through a solution. It is a cheap and easy method to produce highly controlled porous alumina with pores in the nanometer scale 30–80 nm in diameter and by a two-step anodization, regular distribution of the pores due to a self-organization

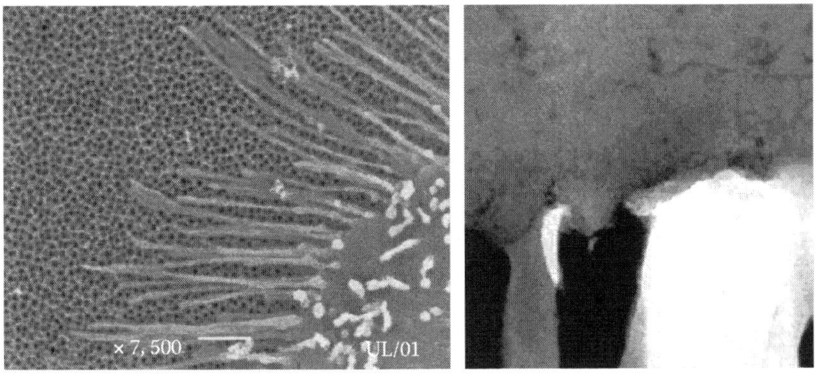

FIGURE 7.9
SEM micrograph of HOB cells cultured for 24 h (a) and TEM micrograph of cross section of HOB cells cultured for 21 days (b) on nanoporous alumina. (Reprinted from Karlsson, M. et al., *Biomaterials*, 24, 3039–46, 2003. With permission from Elsevier.)

process can be formed. The SEM characterization of osteoblast adhesion and morphology on the surface showed that the cells had extended their processes into the pores and were indeed able to respond to the nanoscale features with the cell protrusions (filopodia) attaching to the pores of the alumina (Figure 7.9). Evidence for the adsorption of fibronectin with the right conformation of the exposure of the cell-binding receptors has also been shown on porous alumina substrate. This glycoprotein is known to play a major role in the differentiation of osteoblasts and thus in mineral formation (Karlsson 2003).

Collectively, the various forms of nanophase alumina ceramics clearly indicates significant biointegration and cell growth with decreased grain size, which may lead to improved osseointegrative potentials compared to conventional grain size alumina. Also, a sharp increase in osteoblast function has been observed for spherical grain sizes less than 60 nm and for nanofibrous alumina (diameter 2; length > 50 nm).

Similar to alumina, titania (TiO_2), the native oxide of titanium, is also known to be a bioinert bioceramic. So, nanophase titania has also been studied for osteoblast functions. The nanophase titania with 32-nm grain size was prepared by the PVS process (Nanophase Technologies, Inc., USA) as described earlier. The nanophase titania of various grain sizes was prepared by sintering the 32-nm grain size titania compacts at 600 or 800°C and conventional alumina (large grain sizes greater than 100 nm) at a temperature of 1200°C. Compared to conventional grain size titania, enhanced osteoblast proliferation, alkaline phosphate activity, and concentration of calcium in the extracellular matrix on nanophase titania have been observed. By contrast, evidence for decreased adhesion of fibroblasts and adhesion of endothelial cells (cells that line the vasculature of the body) has been provided by the nanophase titania compared to conventional titania (Webster 2003).

Both nanophase alumina and titania have clearly demonstrated evidence for enhanced functions of osteoblasts and osteoclasts. The nanophase alumina implied relatively more osteoblast adhesion relative to the nanophase titania. However, the grain sizes and ceramic type were different. Similarly, theta + delta nanofiber alumina has shown increased osteoblast functions compared to boehmite nanofiber alumina. The nanometer surface features, chemistry, and crystallinity were different for both the alumina nanofibers. Hence, it may be observed that the enhanced cellular response to nanophase ceramics was independent of surface chemistry and material phase, but dependent on the surface topography (surface roughness in nanometer dimension) of the nanophase ceramics (Sato 2004).

7.4.2 Synthesis and Characterization of Nano Calcium Phosphate Ceramics

HA is sensitive to nonstoichiometry and impurities because of its complex composition ($Ca_{10}(PO4)_6(OH)_2$) and crystal structure ($P6_{3/m}$). The densification of HA to form solid products at high temperatures results in grain growth and decomposition into undesired phases with poor mechanical and chemical stability. So, HA is mostly used as powder, coatings, porous bodies, and non load-bearing implants. The application of nanostructured HA can lead to superior chemical homogeneity and microstructural uniformity, and also high-quality dense apatite can be formed at low sintering temperatures. The fabrication of nanostructured HA is also a challenge to replicate the precise structure of natural bone. In addition, nanostructured HA is expected to have superior mechanical properties in comparison with conventional micron-size HA.

Many novel methods are available for the synthesis of nanocrystalline calcium phosphate ceramics, including coprecipitation process, precipitation using emulsion, microemulsion, and templates, synthesis using microwaves and ultrasonics, refined solid reaction method, mechanochemical method, hydrothermal reaction, and sol-gel techniques (Rameshbabu 2005). Depending upon the technique, nanoceramics with various morphology, stoichiometry, and level of crystallinity have been obtained.

The wet chemical route has been shown to generate the desired stoichiometry, crystalline phase, and grain size at low temperatures. The high-resolution TEM micrograph, as shown in Figure 7.10, indicates uniform morphology of nanocrystalline HA (Ahn 2001). The nanocrystalline HA was thermally stable up to 1300°C and fully dense and transparent HA was formed in 30 min at a low temperature of 900°C with pressure-assisted sintering (load 100 MPa). The sintered compact possessed a uniform and ultrafine microstructure with an average grain size of 100 nm with no glassy or amorphous interfaces along the grain boundaries (Figure 7.11). The ultrafine microstructure results

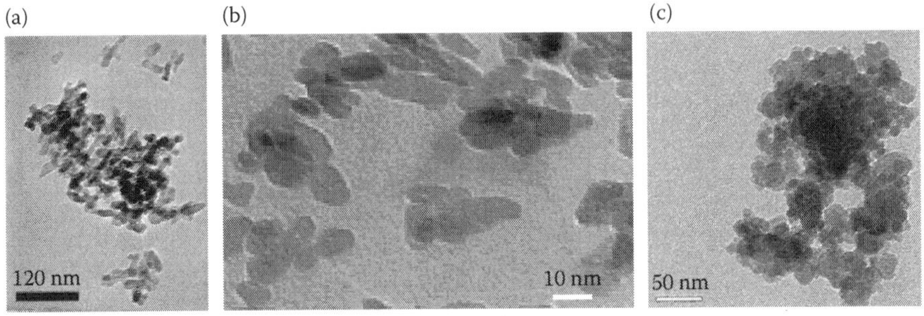

FIGURE 7.10
TEM micrographs of nanocrystalline HA powder synthesized by precipitation (a), sol-gel method (b), and mechanochemical method (c). (Reprinted from Ahn, E. S. et al., *Nano Lett.*, 1, 149–53, 2001. With permission from The American Chemical Society.)

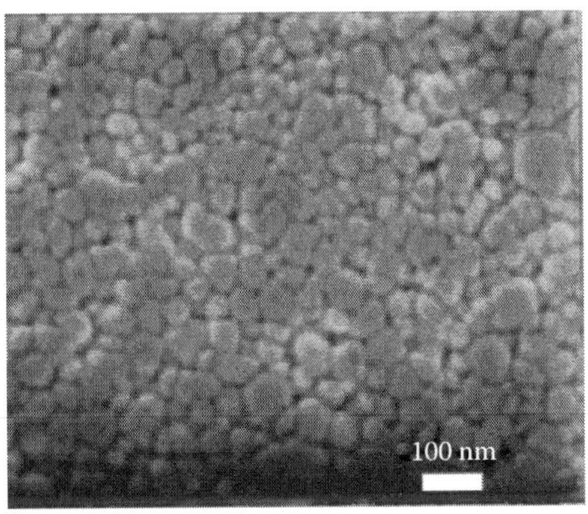

FIGURE 7.11
SEM micrographs of polished cross-sections of dense nanocrystalline HA. (Reprinted from Ahn, E. S. et al., *Nano Lett.*, 1, 149–53, 2001. With permission from The American Chemical Society.)

in a 70% improvement in bending strength (193 MPa) over the conventional coarse-grained HA (38–113 MPa).

In the precipitation method of preparation, nano-HA properties are influenced by the temperature, reagents concentration, addition rate, stirring, maturation, and presence of impurities. It is reported that HA precipitated at 22°C has an average width of 11 nm and a length of 110 nm, and at 95°C, the width is 33–110 nm and the length is 55–220 nm. The reaction temperature affects the crystallinity, reaction rate, and morphology of HA (Lazić et al. 2001). Microwave plays an important role in reactions in aqueous media and has been used for precipitation of nanosized HA (Rameshbabu 2005). It is found that the pH value and the complex reagent such as EDTA in microwave synthesis of HA play an important role in the final HA nanostructures with different shapes. Sol-gel techniques have been used to form HA nanoparticles in the shape of an ellipsoid, with an average size of crystals in the long

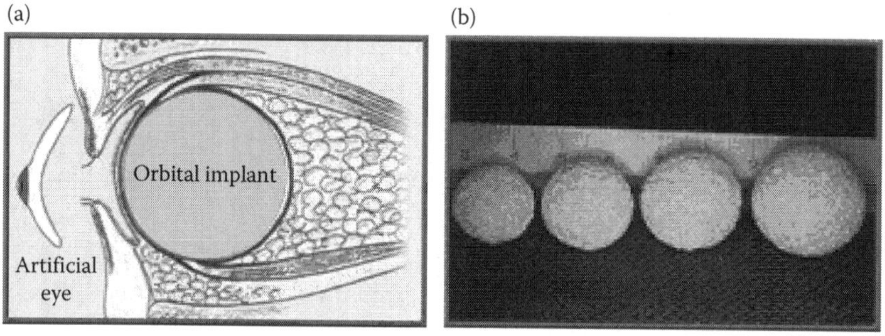

FIGURE 7.12
Schematic diagram of an orbital implant with artificial eye (shown removed) (a) and coral HA-based orbital implants (b). (From Bio-Eye® Hydroxyapatite Orbital Implant, Integrated Orbital Implants, Inc., San Diego; http://www.ioi.com/default2.htm.)

axis in the range of 20–30 nm, as shown in Figure 7.10. The mechanochemical processing seems to be advantageous in producing nanocrystalline HA with uniform morphology in a simple way under normal temperature and pressure, as shown in Figure 7.10. These selected examples clearly indicate that the morphology of nanophase HA can be optimized to form implants to enhance its integration with tissues.

The spark plasma sintering (SPS) is a recent process that enables sintering of materials in short periods by charging the spaces between the powder particles with electrical energy and using a high sintering pressure. It has many advantages, such as rapid and uniform sintering, sintering with fewer additives, and easy operation, compared to that of conventional systems using hot press (HP) sintering or hot isostatic pressing. The SPS process has the potential to fabricate dense nanostructured HA-sintered compacts.

The osteoblast and osteoclast functions on nanophase HA were studied in detail in comparison to conventional grain size HA. The HA was prepared by precipitation method, and by changing the temperature and time of precipitation, the grain size of HA was controlled. For nanophase grain size (< 100 nm) and conventional grain size (> 100 nm), the reaction conditions were 24 h stirring at room temperature and 1–3 h at 90°C, respectively. Sintering was done at 1100°C for 1 h to fabricate compacts for cell culture study. The average surface grain size of the nanophase compact was 67 nm and the conventional grain size phase compact was 132–179 nm. Similar to nanophase alumina and titania, enhanced osteoblast proliferation, alkaline phosphate activity, and concentration of calcium in the extracellular matrix have also been observed on nanophase HA compared to conventional HA (Webster 2001). Also, evidence for enhanced synthesis of TRAP and enhanced formation of resorption pits by osteoclast-like cells has been provided by nanophase HA similar to devitalized bone used as reference. Interestingly, 12 times more synthesis of TRAP and 25% greater resorption pits were obtained when osteoclast-like cells were cultured for 13 days on nanophase HA compared to nanophase alumina (Webster 2001). The increased surface roughness and wettability of nanophase HA seem to mediate the enhanced functions of osseous cells, as also observed earlier. The nanometer-sized grains and high-volume fraction of grain boundaries in nanostructured HA coatings have also been found to increase osteoblast adhesion, proliferation, and mineralization (Catledge 2002).

Numerous techniques for the synthesis, fabrication, and consolidation of nanophase materials are reported in the literature. Further, processing methods to create nanoscaled features on materials are also being intensively developed due to the tremendous need in various applications. Hence, it is possible that these techniques can be transferred to biomaterial applications, both for enhancing the material–cell functions and for inexpensive fabrication. But, resultant properties vary widely with the processing methods and the starting material used. So, further analysis and additional processing steps are essential for biomaterial applications. Also, this requires innovative techniques for processing nanostructured biomaterials. However, this is a much easier and promising route to pursue than developing new materials for biomedical applications.

7.5 Case Study

When an eye is removed due to injury or disease, an artificial eye replaces the volume in the orbit (bony cavity surrounding the eye) that was occupied by the eye. This small, spherical implant maintains the natural structure of the orbit and provides support for the artificial eye (Figure 7.12). The orbital implant is used to restore the natural appearance of the eye and surrounding tissues. Ocular prosthesis is usually made of plastic or glass and some custom artificial eyes are handcrafted by highly skilled ocularists (eye makers) to precisely match the look of the natural eye. However, until 1989, lack of movement of the artificial eye was a major obstacle to restoring a natural appearance. They also tended to drift (migrate) in the orbit and were often rejected by the body, making further surgery necessary. These problems motivated the search for a better orbital implant. A case study on the use of HA in achieving the natural appearance is discussed in the next section.

The key design features for the relative success of an orbital implant are very light weight (< 2 g) to prevent damage to the delicate muscles of the lower lids over time; natural lid shape to be completely buried within the sclera to eliminate chances of infection; porosity to allow vascular orbital tissues to grow into its structure to lock it into place to prevent migration, to allow it to fight infections from within the implant via the vascular bed infiltrating the implant, and support "healing from within" of any defect in the conjunctival-Tenon's closure; and natural biocompatibility to be readily accepted by the tissues of the orbit. HA meets almost all of these requirements. As discussed earlier, the microarchitecture of certain species of marine coral is almost identical to that of human cancellous bone and the calcium content of these species also allows them to be converted to HA. So, naturally derived HA is virtually identical to the mineral portion of cancellous bone in terms of both porosity and chemical make-up. Consequently, soft tissues readily infiltrate the material, muscles can be attached to it, and the natural "bio-eye orbital implant" thus has the ability to greatly increase artificial eye movement (Shields 1993). Additionally, the natural HA orbital implant can successfully accommodate a motility/support peg, which directly connects the artificial eye to the implant. This is possible due to complete interconnected porosity being filled with fibrovascular ingrowth and the motility/support peg supports the weight of the prosthesis while simultaneously ensuring transfer of any socket movement directly to the prosthesis. The objective of a more natural appearance was thus finally achieved with the help of a natural material using ocean coral. However, the rough surface of coral-derived HA has occasionally led to chronic inflammation, resulting in breakdown of the sclera and conjunctiva. The other disadvantages of the porous HA derived from coral are their source-dependent nonreliable properties. So, synthetic HA-based orbital implants are also being considered as a better and effective alternative (Biswanath 2005).

7.6 Summary

Certain types of ceramics, glasses, and glass–ceramics used as biomaterials are called bioceramics and they can be classified as inert, porous, bioactive, and resorbable ceramics, depending on their cellular response. Inert ceramics, such as aluminum oxide (Al_2O_3) and zirconium oxide (ZrO_2), are used in load-bearing applications in hip prostheses and dental implants. Porous alumina with a pore size typically > 100 μm maintains its vascularity and is used as a scaffold for bone growth. Bioactive ceramics develop a mechanically strong bond to bone or soft tissues through a time-dependent, kinetic modification of the surface upon implantation. Some regions of the Na_2O–CaO–P_2O_5–SiO_2 glass system (45S5) and calcium phosphate ceramics, such as HA ($Ca_{10}(PO_4)_6(OH)_2$), are the most widely used bioactive bioceramics. But, TCP ($Ca_3(PO_4)_2$) is resorbed or biodegraded when exposed to physiological environments and induces the formation of new tissues. Bioceramics exhibit optimal surface properties and surface features when their grain size is reduced below 100 nm to selectively adsorb proteins that mediate specific cell adhesion more effectively. The enhanced functions of osteoblasts and osteoclasts by the nanostructured bioceramics, results in the active formation and maintenance of healthy juxtaposed bone *in vivo* to improve orthopedic/dental implant efficacy.

Glossary

Alumina: Aluminum oxide is a chemical compound of aluminium and oxygen with the chemical formula Al2O3. It is often referred to as alumina.

Bioglass: A glass that can form a bond with live tissue at its surface because of a chemical reaction. It is often referred to as bioactive glass.

Calcium phosphate: A group of compounds of calcium ions (Ca^{2+}) with orthophosphates (PO_4^{3-}), metaphosphates, or pyrophosphates ($P_2O_7^{4-}$) and, occasionally, hydrogen or hydroxide ions.

Fibroblast: A flat, elongated cell associated with fibrous tissues in the body.

Fibronectin: A high molecular weight adhesive glycoprotein (a protein with a sugar attached) involved in many cellular processes, including cell migration/adhesion and serves as a general cell adhesion molecule by anchoring cells to collagen or proteoglycan substrates.

Glass–ceramics: Polycrystalline ceramics formed by controlled crystallization of glass.

Hydroxyapatite: A calcium phosphate compound with calcium and phosphorous in the ratio: 1.67 and with the chemical formula $Ca_{10}(PO_4)_6(OH)_2$.

Osteoblast: A cell associated with the production of bone.

Osteoclast: A large multinuclear cell associated with the absorption and removal of bone.

Polyol: An alcohol with many hydroxyl radicals, like polyethers, glycols, polyesters, and castor oil. It is also known as polyhydric alcohol.

Pyrolytic carbon: A carbon material produced by low-temperature pyrolysis of gaseous hydrocarbon compounds at temperatures ranging from 1000 to 2500 K and deposited on suitable substrates. It has disordered layers compared to graphitic carbon.

Tricalcium phosphate: A calcium phosphate compound with calcium and phosphorous in the ratio: 1.50 and with the chemical formula $Ca_3(PO_4)_2$.

Vitronectin: A multifunctional adhesive glycoprotein that promotes adhesion, spreading, and migration of cells.

Weibull modulus: A dimensionless number used to measure the variability of failure under loading.

Zirconia: Zirconium oxide is a chemical compound of zirconium and oxygen with the chemical formula ZrO_2. It is also referred to as zirconia, but is different from zircon, which is a zirconium silicate ($ZrSiO_4$).

EXERCISES

7.1 What types of ceramics are termed bioceramics and what are their advantages as biomaterials?
7.2 How will you classify bioceramics based on their tissue interactions?
7.3 What are the requirements of medical grade alumina and how it is achieved?
7.4 Why is ytteria added to zirconia for implant applications?
7.5 How is pyrolytic carbon formed and why can it be used in artificial heart valves?
7.6 What are the disadvantages of porous bioceramics?
7.7 How can bioactivity be defined and classified?
7.8 What compositional features of bioactive glass are crucial for bone bonding?
7.9 Why does hydroxyapatite bond with bone?
7.10 How can the biodegradation of bioceramics be modified?
7.11 What are the advantages of nanostructured bioceramics?
7.12 Why do you expect nanophase alumina to have enhanced osteoblast functions?

References

Ahn, E. S. et al. 2001. Nanostructure processing of hydroxyapatite-based bioceramics. *Nano Lett.* 1:149–53.

Billotte W. G. 2003. Ceramic biomaterials. In *Biomaterials: Principles and applications*, ed. J. B. Park and J. D. Bronzino, 21–52. Boca Raton: CRC Press.

Biswanath, K. et al. 2005. Synthetic hydroxyapatite-based integrated orbital implants: A human pilot trial. *Indian J. Ophthalmol.* 53:235–41.

Davis, J. R. 2003. *Handbook of materials for medical devices*. Materials Park, OH: ASM International.

Hench, L. L. 1991. Bioceramics: From concept to clinic. *J. Am. Ceram. Soc.* 74:1487–1510.

Hench, L. L. 2005. Bioceramics. *J. Am. Ceram. Soc.* 81:1705–28.

Hench, L. L. and S. Best. 2004. Ceramics, glasses, and glass-ceramics. In *Biomaterials science: An introduction to materials in medicine*, ed. B. D. Ratner, A. S. Hoffman, F. J. Schoen, and J. E. Lemons, 153–70. San Diego, CA: Elsevier Academic Press.

Hench, L. L. and E. C. Ethridge. 1982. *Biomaterials: An interfacial approach*. New York: Academic Press.

Hench, L. L. and J. M. Polak. 2002. Third-generation biomedical materials. *Science* 295:1014–17.

Hench, L. L. and J. W. Wilson. 1984. Surface-active biomaterials. *Science* 226:630.

Karlsson, M. et al. 2003. Initial in vitro interaction of osteoblasts with nano-porous alumina. *Biomaterials* 24:3039–46.

Kokubo, T. et al. 1992. Chemical reaction of bioactive glass and glass-ceramics with a stimulated body fluid. *J. Mater. Sci.: Mater. Med.* 3:79.

Kumar, T. S. S., I. Manjubala, and J. Gunasekaran. 2000. Synthesis of carbonated calcium phosphate ceramics using microwave irradiation. *Biomaterials* 21:1623–29.

Lazić, S. et al. 2001. The effect of temperature on the properties of hydroxyapatite precipitates from calcium hydroxide and phosphoric oxide. *Thermochim. Acta* 374:13–22.

Park, J. B. and Y. K. Kim. 2003. Metallic biomaterials. In *Biomaterials: Principles and applications*, ed. J. B. Park and J. D. Bronzino, 1–20. Boca Raton, FL: CRC Press.

Rameshbabu, N., K. R. Rao, and T. S. S. K. Kumar. 2005. Accelerated microwave processing of nanocrystalline hydroxyapatite. *J. Mater. Sci.* 40:6319–23.

Sato, M. and T. J. Webster. 2004. Nanobiotechnology: Implications for the future of nanotechnology in orthopedic applications. *Expert Rev. Med. Dev.* 1:105–14.

Shields, J. A., C. L. Shields, and P. DePotter. 1993. Hydroxyapatite orbital implant after enucleation experience with 200 cases. *Mayo Clin. Proc.* 68:1191–95.

Siddharthan, A., S. K. Seshadri, and T. S. Sampath Kumar. 2004. Microwave accelerated synthesis of nanosized calcium deficient hydroxyapatite. *J. Mater. Sci.: Mater. Med.* 15:1279–84.

Sivakumar, M. et al. 1996. Development of hydroxyapatite derived from Indian coral. *Biomaterials* 17:1709–14.

Tepper, F., M. Lerner, and D. Ginley. 2001. Nanosized alumina fibers. *Am. Ceram. Soc. Bull.* 80:57–60.

Vallet-Regí, M. 2001. Ceramics for medical applications. *J. Chem. Soc. Dalton Trans.* 100:97–108.

Webster, T. J., Siegel, R. W., and Bizios, R. 1999. Osteoblast adhesion on nanophase ceramics, *Biomater.* 20:1221–27.

Webster, T. J. 2003. Improved bone tissue engineering materials. *Am. Ceram. Soc. Bull.* 82:23–28.

Webster, T. J. et al. 2000. Enhanced functions of osteoblasts on nanophase ceramics. *Biomaterials* 21:1803–10.

———. 2001. Enhanced osteoclast-like cell functions on nanophase ceramics. *Biomaterials* 22:1327–33.

Webster, T. J., E. L. Hellenmeyer, and R. L. Price. 2005. Increased osteoblast functions on theta + delta nanofiber alumina. *Biomaterials* 26:953–60.

8

Polymeric Biomaterials

8.1 Introduction

A polymer is a substance made up of repeated, small and simple chemical units called monomers. A typical polymer may include tens of thousands of monomers. Because of their large size, polymers are classified as macromolecules. The terms "polymer" and "monomer" are derived from Greek words; poly meaning many, mono meaning one, and meros meaning units. The name of the polymer is often based on its repeating units. Some of the repeat structures of widely used biomedical polymers are listed in Table 8.1.

8.1.1 Polymerization Process

The process of synthesizing polymer from monomer is called polymerization. Polymers can be synthesized by multiple methods, which are broadly divided into two groups: (i) addition polymerization and (ii) condensation polymerization.

8.1.1.1 Addition Polymerization

In addition polymerization, polymers are synthesized by a reaction between two molecules, either the same (to form homopolymer) or dissimilar (to form heteropolymer). The process of addition polymerization to produce polymers involves four steps: (i) activation, (ii) initiation, (iii) propagation, and (iv) termination. Polyethylene, for example, is produced by this method, from the monomer called ethylene when it is exposed to a free radical (•) (see Figure 8.1).

Activation is a process of producing free radicals. Free radicals are very reactive chemical species that have an unpaired electron. Formation of free radicals is achieved, for instance, by the decomposition of a molecule such as benzoyl peroxide. Under optimal conditions, a molecule of benzoyl peroxide can yield two peroxide free radicals. Initiation is a process by which free radicals can react with a monomer (ethylene, in this case) and initiate the polymerization process. Propagation is a rapid reaction of this radicalized

TABLE 8.1
Repeat Structure of Polymers

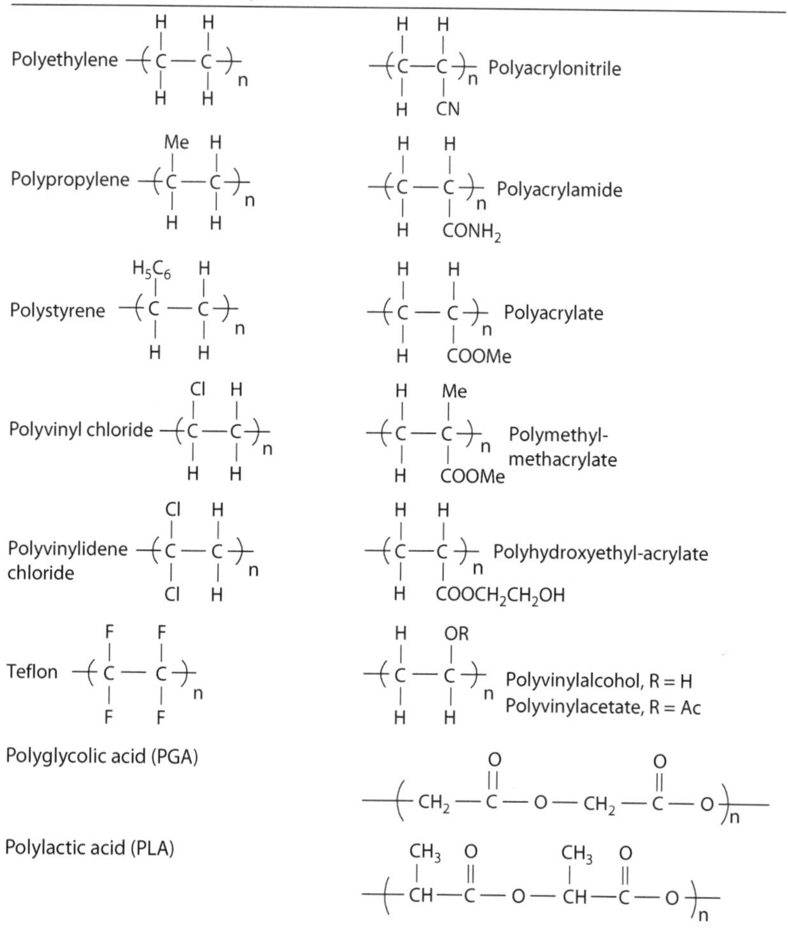

ethylene molecule with another ethylene monomer, which creates a chain that propagates until the growing chain collides or all of the free radicals have reacted. Termination is an end process, which takes place when reacting the free radicals to form a stable molecule. The most common method of termination is by coupling, wherein two radical species react with each other, forming a single stable molecule.

8.1.1.2 Condensation Polymerization

In condensation polymerization, polymers are synthesized when monomers bond together through condensation reaction. Condensation reaction is a chemical reaction in which two molecules react and become covalently

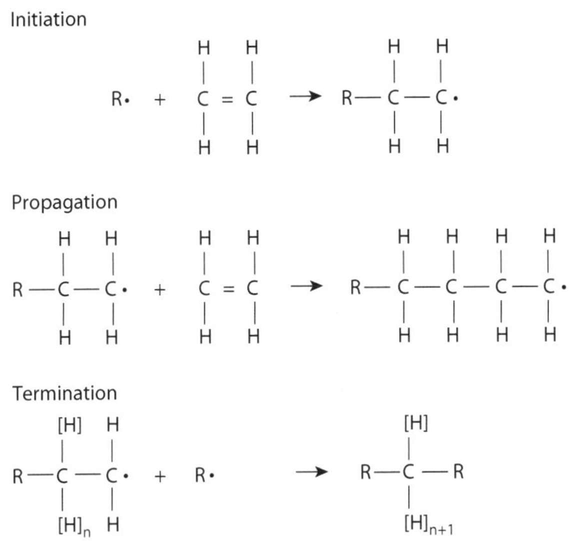

FIGURE 8.1
An example of addition polymerization.

bonded to one another by the concurrent loss of a small molecule (often, but not always, water), with the formation of a polymer chain. Typically, this type of reaction can be achieved through reacting molecules incorporating the functional groups of alcohol, amine, or carboxylic acid. An example of condensation polymerization is the reaction of dimethyl terephthalate and ethylene glycol in the presence of heat to form poly(ethylene terephthalate) (PET) (see Figure 8.2). The condensation polymers are generally characterized by a broad range of polymer chain molecular weights because the condensation reaction is just as likely to occur with another monomer as with a growing polymer chain.

8.1.2 Types of Polymers

Polymers can be classified into two types with respect to the monomer repeating units by which they are synthesized; homopolymer and copolymer. When the polymer is made up of a single repeating unit, it is called a homopolymer (see Figure 8.3a). In a homopolymer, the same monomer units are evenly distributed in the polymer chain. On the other hand, a polymer made from two different monomers is called a copolymer. In this respect, depending on the arrangement of the types of monomers in the polymer chain, it can be further classified into four types (see Figure 8.3a through c): (i) random copolymer, (ii) alternating copolymer, (iii) block copolymer, and (iv) graft copolymer. In a random copolymer, two or more different monomer units are distributed randomly and sometimes unevenly in the polymer chain. In an alternating copolymer, the monomer units are distributed

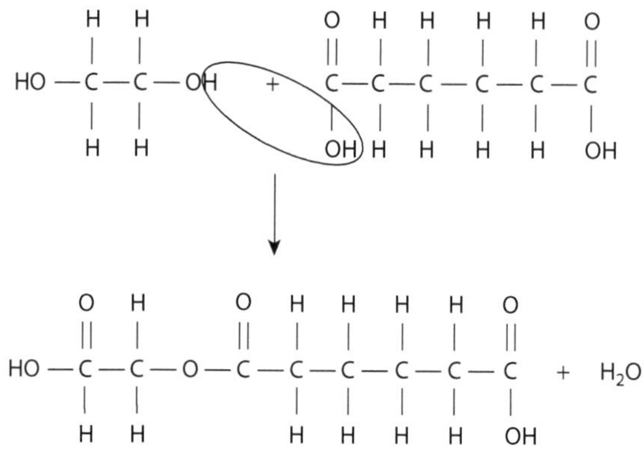

FIGURE 8.2
An example of condensation polymerization.

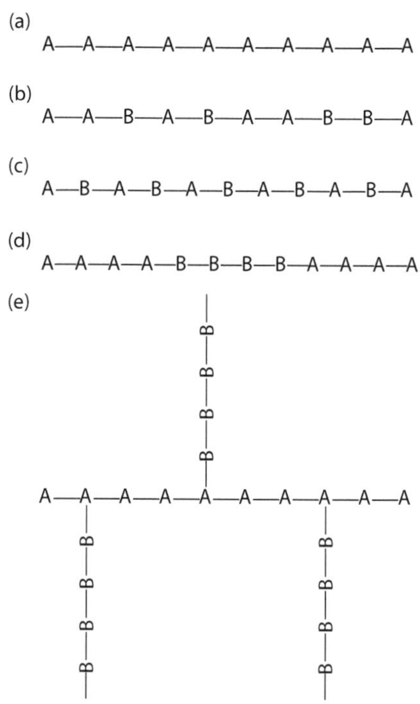

FIGURE 8.3
Molecular structure of (a) homopolymer, (b) random copolymer, (c) block copolymer, and (d) graft copolymer.

in a regular alternating fashion with nearly equimolar amounts of each in the polymer chain. In a block copolymer, instead of a mixed distribution of monomer units, a block of one monomer is attached to a block of another monomer. In a graft copolymer, as the name suggests, side chains of a given monomer are attached to the main chain of another monomer. It should be noted that copolymers always have different properties from those of a homopolymer made from either monomer. The bulk properties of a copolymer depend on the percentage of monomer A to monomer B, the properties of each, and how they are arranged along the chain.

8.1.3 Factors Influencing the Properties of Polymers

The physical and chemical properties of a polymer are largely influenced by molecular weight, regularity of the molecular structure, intermolecular forces, and crystallinity.

8.1.3.1 *Molecular Weight*

Polymer molecular weight is important because it determines many physical properties, including transition temperature, strength, stiffness, toughness, and viscosity. The molecular weight of a polymer is equal to the number of repeating units (i.e., degree of polymerization) multiplied by the molecular weight of the repeating units. In both addition and condensation polymerizations, the length of the chain is determined by purely random events, not all of the chains will be of the same length and, in general, many different chain lengths will be present, thus the molecular weight can only be represented by an average value. There are a number of ways in which the molecular weight can be determined for a polymer. Two main ways are the number average molecular weight (M_n) and the weight average molecular weight (M_w). The number average molecular weight (M_n) is obtained by counting the number of molecules in a given weight of sample. The general expression can be written as: $M_n = \Sigma n_i M_i / \Sigma n_i$, where n_i is the mole fraction of chains with molecular weight M_i. Weight average molecular weight (M_w) is obtained by measurement of the weight of the molecules in the total sample weight. The general expression can be written as: $M_w = \Sigma w_i M_i / \Sigma w_i$, where w_i is the weight fraction of chains with molecular weight M_i.

8.1.3.2 *Molecular Structures*

A schematic of a simple polymer structure is shown in Figure 8.4. This chain-like molecular structure is responsible for its functional properties, in particular physicochemical and mechanical, and these properties may vary from polymer to polymer corresponding to their molecular structures. Three typical types of molecular structures exist, namely, linear, branched, and cross-linked structures (see Figure 8.5). A linear polymer consists of a long chain

A—A—A—A—A—A—A—A

FIGURE 8.4
Schematic of a simple polymer structure. A represents a monomer unit. — represents a covalent bond.

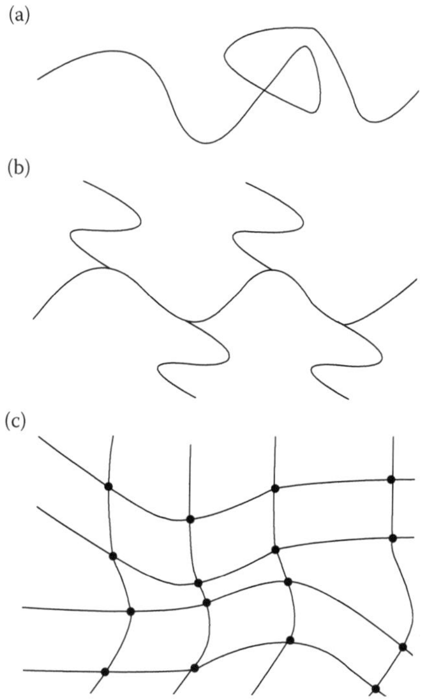

FIGURE 8.5
Types of molecular configuration: (a) linear structure, (b) branched structure, and (c) cross-linked structure.

of monomer repeated units. A branched polymer consists of many branches that are covalently attached to the main chain. A cross-linked polymer has monomers of one chain covalently bonded with monomers of another chain, resulting in a 3D molecular structure. Apart from the molecular structures, other factors such as morphology, composition, molecular weight, and crystallinity also influence the properties of a polymer.

8.1.3.3 Intermolecular Forces

All molecules, both small ones and polymers, interact with each other, attracting each other through electrostatics. Like small molecules, intermolecular forces greatly affect polymers. The intermolecular forces between polymer chains play a large part in determining polymer properties. The intermolecular forces are those forces that are exerted on one molecule of a substance by those of another, and that, in general, affect the macroscopic properties of the polymers. Such forces may be either attractive or repulsive in nature. They are conveniently divided into two types: short-range forces and long-range forces. Short-range forces operate when the centers of the molecules are separated by 3 Å or less. On the other hand, long-range forces operate at greater distances. Generally, if molecules do not tend to interact chemically, the short-range forces between them are repulsive. These forces arise from interactions of the electrons associated with the molecules and are also known as exchange forces. Molecules that interact chemically have attractive exchange forces; these are also known as valence forces. Mechanical rigidity of molecules and effects such as limited compressibility of matter arise from repulsive exchange forces. Long-range forces, or van der Waals forces as they are also called, are attractive and account for a wide range of physical phenomena, such as friction, surface tension, adhesion, and cohesion of liquids and solids, and viscosity. van der Waals forces arise in a number of ways, one being the tendency of electrically polarized molecules to become aligned. Quantum theory also indicates that in some cases the electrostatic fields associated with electrons in neighboring molecules constrain the electrons to move more or less in phase.

The intermolecular forces in polymers are determined by dipoles in the monomer repeating units. Polymers containing amide groups can form hydrogen bonds between adjacent chains; the positive hydrogen atoms in N–H groups of one chain are strongly attracted to the oxygen atoms in C = O groups on another chain. These strong hydrogen bonds result in, for example, the high tensile strength and melting point of kevlar. Polyesters have dipole–dipole bonding between the oxygen atoms in C = O groups and the hydrogen atoms in H–C groups. Dipole bonding is not as strong as hydrogen bonding; therefore, melting point and strength of ethane are lower than kevlar, but polyesters have greater flexibility. Ethane, however, has no permanent dipole. The attractive forces between polyethylene chains arise from weak van der Waals forces. Molecules can be thought of as being surrounded by a cloud of negative electrons. As two polymer chains approach, their electron clouds repel one another. This has the effect of lowering the electron density on one side of a polymer chain, creating a slight positive dipole on this side. This charge is enough to actually attract the second polymer chain.

8.1.3.4 Polymer Crystallinity

According to the arrangement of molecules, polymers can be classified into three types: amorphous, crystalline, and semicrystalline. Amorphous refers to the random alignment of the polymer chains. Amorphous polymers, on the other hand, gradually soften as they are heated, but they do not flow as easily (in a molding process) as crystalline materials. Examples of amorphous polymers are polystyrene, polycarbonate, and polysulfone. Crystalline refers to a structured alignment of the polymer chains in a polymer matrix.

Examples of crystalline polymers are polyethylene, polypropylene, and polyetheretherketone. A semicrystalline polymer is one that contains both crystalline and amorphous regions. It is neither all crystalline nor all amorphous in nature. High-density polyethylene and PET are notable examples of semicrystalline polymers.

Generally, the degree of crystallinity can be obtained from the measurement of density. This is because crystalline polymers are denser than amorphous polymers because of the strong intermolecular bonds between the polymer chains. In polymers, the degree of crystallinity ranges from 0 (amorphous) to >90% (crystalline) and is greatly affected by molecular structure, molecular weight, and processing conditions.

8.1.4 Polymer Characterization

A variety of analytical techniques are used to determine the properties of polymers, including spectroscopic (e.g., nuclear magnetic resonance, Raman, and infrared), mechanical (e.g., tensile, dynamic mechanical, and rheological), microscopic (e.g., electron and optical microscopy), physicochemical (e.g., intrinsic viscosity, differential scanning, calorimetry, and gel permeation chromatography), and scattering (e.g., light and x-rays). By using these techniques, both surface and bulk properties of polymers can be easily determined.

8.2 Polymers as Biomaterials

Polymers are one of the primary classes of biomaterials and are currently widely used in a variety of biomedical applications, owing to their functional properties (because they are most similar to that of soft tissues), surface modifiability, sterilizability, and design flexibility (because the polymer composition and structure can be tailor made to a specific need). The use of polymers in biomedical applications dates back almost to the birth of polymer science, and since then, they have been used for the design of medical prostheses or implants and for the delivery of therapeutic or other biomolecules. Polymers intended for use in biomedical applications must meet certain criteria and regulatory requirements. Biocompatibility is one of the most important requirements. As mentioned previously, biocompatibility is a descriptive term, indicating the ability of a material to perform with appropriate host responses upon implantation within the human body. Polymers that are biocompatible to living cells or tissues or other body parts are generally called polymeric biomaterials. Polymers for biomedical applications should have adequate mechanical properties to match the specific applications, should not induce inflammation or other toxic response, should be fully metabolized once it biodegrades, and should be sterilizable and easily processable into a desired size and shape.

A range of polymers have been developed, in which poly(lactic acid) (PLA), poly(glycolic acid) (PGA), and poly(lactic-co-glycolic acid) (PLGA) are the most widely used synthetic polymers, and collagen, gelatin, and chitosan are the most widely used naturally derived polymers in biomedical applications; in particular, tissue engineering of skin, cartilage, bone, vascular, and nerve. In addition to tissue engineering, polymeric biomaterials are also used in several other biomedical applications, including poly(methyl methacrylate) (PMMA) as bone cement and intraocular lenses, PE as hip implants, PET as cardiovascular implants, poly(vinyl alcohol) (PVA) as cartilage implants, polyurethane (PU) as wound dressing and vascular implants, PGA as degradable sutures, PLGA as bone screws, poly(vinyl siloxane) (PVS) as dental impression materials, poly(ethylene glycol) (PEG) as a drug delivery system, and poly(hydroxyethyl methacrylate) (PHEMA) as soft contact lenses. In the following sections, classification and properties of some of the widely used polymers in biomedical applications are described.

8.3 Classification of Polymeric Biomaterials

Polymeric biomaterials can be classified in several different ways according to their structures, the types of reactions by which they are synthesized, their functional properties, or their applications. Polymeric biomaterials are broadly grouped into two types: naturally derived and synthetic. They can also be classified with respect to their degradation behavior. The degradation property of the polymers is one of the key determinant factors for the selection of polymers for use in a specific human application. Some of the widely used polymers in biomedical applications are listed in Table 8.2 with respect to their biodegradability. The naturally derived polymers are often called biopolymers, which are usually biodegradable, but the rate of degradation corresponds to the molecular configuration and other factors (such as composition, molecular weight, crystallinity, etc.) of the respective polymers. Collagen, gelatin, and chitosan are a few notable examples of biopolymers. Synthetic polymers can be either biodegradable or nonbiodegradable. PLA, PGA, and PLGA are notable examples of biodegradable synthetic polymers, and PMMA, PE, and PET are notable examples of nonbiodegradable synthetic polymers. In the following sections, the structure and key properties of some of the widely used polymers, both naturally derived and synthetic, in biomedical applications are discussed.

TABLE 8.2
Biomedical Applications of Polymers

Polymers	Applications
Nonbiodegradable polymers	
Polymethylmethacrylate (PMMA)	Bone and dental cement, intraocular lens
Polyethylene (PE)	Load-bearing orthopedics, cochlear implants
Polyethylene terephthalate (PET)	Cardiovascular, surgical mesh, and artificial blood vessels
Polyhydroxyethylmethacrylate (PHEMA)	Drug delivery
Polybutylmethacrylate (PBMA)	Bone and dental filling, controlled release
Polyacrylic acid (PAA)	Bone plates, tissue engineering
Polypropylene (PP)	Heart valves, skin patches, sutures
Polytetrafluroethylene (PTFE)	Vascular grafts, reconstructive surgery
Polyamides	Drug delivery, catheters, syringe
Polycarbonate (PC)	Contact lens, syringe, skull implants
Biodegradable polymers	
Polylactic acid (PLA)	Sutures, bone plates, screws, scaffolds
Polyglycolic acid (PGA)	Sutures, bone plates, screws, scaffolds
Polylactic-co-glycolic acid (PLGA)	Tissue engineering, drug delivery, cartilage screws, sutures, wound dressing
Polycaprolactone (PCL)	Drug delivery, bone plates, fixation device
Polyhydroxybutyrates (PHB)	Drug delivery, bone plates
Polydioxanone (PD)	Sutures
Collagen	Prosthetic heart valves, membranes, wound dressing, tissue engineering
Gelatin	Binding agent, tissue engineering, membranes
Chitosan	Drug delivery, tissue engineering, surgical sutures, bone grafting, wound healing

8.4 Naturally Derived Polymers

Naturally derived or biopolymers are polymers that are produced from natural or biological systems (i.e., microorganisms, plants, and animals), or chemically synthesized from biological starting materials (e.g., starch, natural fats, oils, sugars, etc.). These polymers are often biodegradable and the rate of biodegradation may vary from a few weeks to several months, corresponding to their molecular structure. By changing the structure, it is possible to tailor make some of their functional properties. These polymers are beneficial for a number of reasons, such as biocompatibility, biodegradability, nontoxicity, etc. These factors lead to the concept of using biopolymers for a variety of biomedical applications. The most widely used naturally derived polymers in biomedical applications are briefly discussed below.

8.4.1 Collagen

Collagen is the most widely used naturally derived polymer in a variety of biomedical applications, in particular tissue engineering, owing to its biocompatibility and biodegradability. It is a primary structural protein of the natural extracellular matrix (ECM), therefore collagen naturally has a variety of functional characteristics favorable for cells and tissue growth. Although many types of collagen exist in a living organism, the most abundant form of collagen in the native tissue is type I and type III. Type I collagen is composed of two α_1 (I) chains and one α_2 (I) chain with a fiber diameter of about 50 nm. Type III collagen is composed of three α_1 (III) chains with fibers ranging from 30 to 130 nm in diameter. From the structural point of view, collagen is composed of three polypeptides (α-chains) that are each coiled into a left-handed helical pattern, and then these three chains are wrapped around each other into a right-handed helical pattern, resulting in well-organized rope-like fibers of great structural strength. The triple-helix structure of collagen is shown in Figure 8.6. The triple-helical domain has a characteristic primary structure, where glycine in every third amino acid generates repeating (Gly X–Y) *n* units, where X is alanine or proline, and Y is hydroxyproline. In general, collagen extracted from natural tissues is capable of eliciting

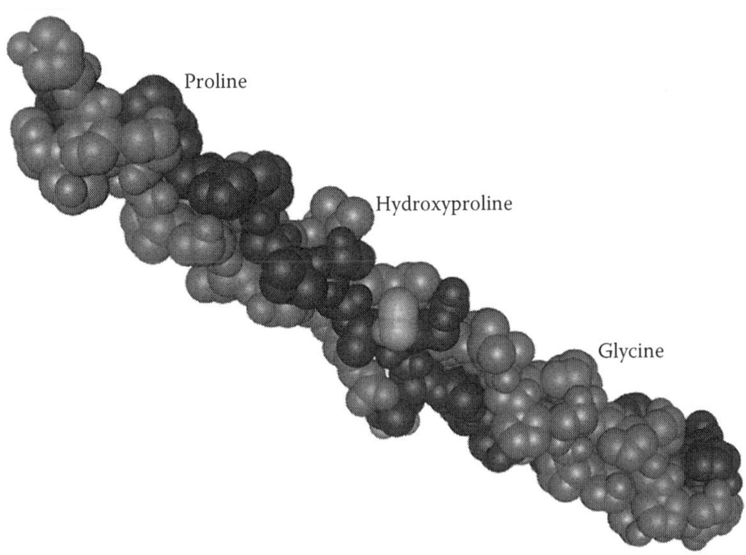

FIGURE 8.6
Triple-helical structure of collagen. (Adapted with courtesy from http://commons.wikimedia.org.)

an immunogenic response upon implantation; therefore, direct use of this type of collagen is limited. Nowadays, a purified form of collagen, known as reconstituted collagen, which has a relatively less immunogenic response, is produced by various biochemical methods and is commercially available for a variety of biomedical applications.

8.4.2 Gelatin

Gelatin is a denatured form of collagen, obtained by acidic and alkaline process. There are two types of gelatin, namely, gelatin A and gelatin B, which are identified by the method of processing from the native collagen. Gelatin A can be obtained by the extraction of collagen using acidic treatment, and gelatin B can be obtained by the extraction of collagen using alkaline treatment. Gelatin B has a higher content of carboxylic groups than gelatin A, owing to their biochemical processing. Although gelatin is a denatured form of collagen, it has its own functional properties. Gelatin is a highly biocompatible, bioresorbable, nontoxic, and nonimmunogenic natural polymer. It does not elicit any noticeable antigenic response and has a low coagulation activity toward platelets. Based on these characteristics, gelatin has some individual importance as a biomaterial for a variety of human health-care applications.

8.4.3 Chitosan

Chitosan is also a naturally derived polymer (polysaccharide), and is obtained by alkaline decetylation of chitin. The chitin is extracted from the exoskeleton of shellfish. Basically, this process consists of two steps: (i) deproteination of the shells with a dilute sodium hydroxide solution and (ii) decalcification with a dilute hydrochloric acid solution. The chitin thus obtained is subjected to N-deacetylation by treatment with a 40–45% sodium hydroxide solution followed by purification procedures, resulting in chitosan. Chemically, it is a copolymer of β(1-4) linked 2-acetamido-2-deoxy-D-glucopyranose and 2-amino-2-deoxy-D-glucopyranose. Its chemical structure is quite similar to the glycosaminoglycans found in native tissue. It is a weak base and thus it is insoluble in water and in a few organic solvents, but it is soluble in dilute aqueous acidic solution with $pH < 6.5$. Chitosan is relatively biocompatible, biodegradable, does not evoke a strong immune response, and is cost effective due to its abundance and diverse processing methods. It shows good antimicrobial and antifungal activities. Further, its plasticity and adhesiveness make chitosan a suitable binder for a number of applications. Chitosan is also readily modified by the covalent attachment of molecules with free carboxylic acids using carbodiimide chemistry. Due to its natural abundance and specific physicochemical and biological properties, chitosan is widely used in a variety of biomedical applications.

8.5 Synthetic Polymers

Synthetic polymers play an increasingly pivotal role in various biomedical applications. These polymers offer many advantages over naturally derived polymers in that they can be easily tailored to provide a wide range of functional properties, particularly, free from concerns of immunogenicity. Further, they are easily processable, surface modifiable, and sterilizable. Synthetic polymers involved in tissue engineering or other biomedical applications fall into two major categories: nonbiodegradable and biodegradable. The choice of which category to use is purely dependent on the specific site of application. Each material has its own characteristics that closely match the physical and/or chemical properties of the specific tissue to be repaired or, on the other hand, to simply support the cell activity and subsequent tissue formation. It is worth mentioning that not all polymers are widely used in biomedical applications, in particular tissue engineering, but there are a few biodegradable polymers that are often used for such applications. The prime reason is that nonbiodegradable polymers almost always elicit a chronic inflammation, called a foreign body response, whereas biodegradable polymers can form a temporary scaffolding to provide sufficient mechanical and biochemical support until new tissue grows. Once the new tissue begins to form, the polymer scaffolding material will then gradually degrade and leave behind a regenerated tissue; therefore, in most cases, there is no chance of a foreign body reaction occurring. The most widely used synthetic polymers, both nondegradable and degradable, in biomedical applications are briefly discussed below.

8.5.1 Nonbiodegradable Synthetic Polymers

8.5.1.1 Poly(methyl methacrylate)

PMMA is a vinyl polymer, synthesized by free radical polymerization from the monomer methyl methacrylate. It is biocompatible, nondegradable, bioinert, and one of the hardest polymers, thus it is mostly used in orthopedic and dental applications. The mechanical properties of PMMA: hardness is 60–97, tensile strength is 55–85 MPa, tensile modulus is 2.2–3.8 GPa, and compressive strength is 100–117 MPa. The thermal properties of PMMA: melting temperature is 130°C and glass transition temperature is 105°C. It has good processability and mechinability. It can be processed by injection molding, extrusion, thermo forming, bending and joining, and casting. PMMA has a long history as a biomaterial and is used clinically as bone cement for fixation of joint replacements and a filler for bone cavities and skull defects. It is also used in hard contact lens and in drug delivery.

8.5.1.2 Poly(ethylene)

PE is also a vinyl polymer, synthesized by free radical polymerization from the monomer ethylene. It is biocompatible, nondegradable, bioinert, and high strength polymer. The mechanical properties of PE: hardness is 50–66, tensile strength is 16–31 MPa, tensile modulus is 0.18–1.6 GPa, and compressive strength is 4–25 MPa. The thermal properties of PE: melting temperature is 110°C and glass transition temperature is –78°C. These properties may vary depending on the density of PE. There are three types of PE with different densities, which can be made by controlling their molecular structure, namely, low-density PE (LDPE), high-density PE (HDPE), and ultra high molecular weight PE (UHMWPE). Among them, UHMWPE is extensively used in biomedical applications, followed by HDPE. UHMWPE has a greater toughness and wear resistance than other PE polymers, therefore it is primarily used in load-bearing orthopedic implants and cochlear (inner ear) implants.

8.5.1.3 Poly(ethylene terephthalate)

PET is a thermoplastic polymer, synthesized by polycondensation reaction of ethylene glycol with either terephthalic acid or dimethyl terephthalate. It is one of the most important polymers used in biomedical applications. It is biocompatible, biostable, hydrophophic, and high strength polymer. It has excellent mechanical properties: hardness is 110, tensile strength is 50–60 MPa, tensile modulus is 2.8–3.1 GPa, and compressive strength is 90 MPa. The thermal properties of PET: melting temperature is 250°C and glass transition temperature is 76°C. It was first commercially manufactured by DuPont in the late 1940s under the trade name Dacron®. Depending on its processing conditions (thermal), it may exist in various forms: amorphous, semicrystalline, and crystalline. PET was first introduced to biomedical applications in the 1950s in the form of sutures, since then it is extensively used in many current medical practices, including cardiovascular implants, surgical mesh, and artificial blood vessels.

8.5.2 Biodegradable Synthetic Polymers

8.5.2.1 Poly(lactic acid)

PLA is one of the most frequently used biodegradable synthetic polymers in biomedical applications, in particular in designing scaffolds for tissue engineering, owing to its functional characteristics that favor cell and tissue growth. Due to its chiral structure, PLA has two enantiomeric forms: (i) the left-handed (L-PLA) and (ii) the right-handed (D-PLA). These two enantiomers have different degradation rates. Hydrolysis is the principal mode of degradation and it is greatly affected by the hydrophilicity and crystallinity of the polymer. The degradation products of PLA are nontoxic and thus they are safe for biomedical applications. The L-PLA is widely used for tissue engineering applications, owing to its superior biocompatibility and prolonged biodegradation compared to D-PLA. Furthermore, it possesses high strength and modulus. By contrast, the D-PLA possesses low strength and modulus, and rapid biodegradation. The racemic mixture D,L-PLA has amorphous characteristics, whereas a pure polymer of either of the stereoisomers has a highly crystalline nature.

8.5.2.2 Poly(glycolic acid)

PGA is the simplest form of linear aliphatic polyester, and is used in various biomedical applications. It is also a biocompatible and a biodegradable polymer. It can be synthesized by ring-opening polymerization of glycolic acid, but does not form any enantiomers like PLA. It is highly crystalline and is a hydrophilic polymer. The percent crystallinity ranges from 45 to 55. Owing to its hydrophilic nature, it is completely absorbed within a few weeks upon implantation, whereas PLA can remain stable for over one year due to its hydrophophic nature and, of course, the presence of an additional methyl group. It exhibits a high tensile strength, modulus, and is too stiff that makes it suitable for a variety of biomedical applications.

8.5.2.3 Poly(lactic-co-glycolic acid)

PLGA is a copolymer that consists of PLA and PGA macromolecular units. By changing the composition of these copolymeric units, the rate of biodegradation and mechanical strength of PLGA can be manipulated. This kind of copolymer has less crystallinity and has a faster degradation rate than that of homopolymers. For example, a copolymer of 50% PGA and 50% L-PLA degrades much faster than each homopolymer. The composition of a copolymer also significantly affects its percent crystallinity. For example, a copolymer of 90% PGA and 10% L-PLA has high crystallinity, whereas a PGA to L-PLA ratio from 25/75 to 75/25 is relatively amorphous. Owing to its biocompatibility and tunable biodegradability, PLGA is nowadays widely used in a variety of tissue engineering applications.

8.6 Polymeric Nanobiomaterials

For the past few years, there has been great interest in the processing of novel polymeric materials in the order of nanometer length scale. Polymers in the form of nanofibers are considered a unique class of material and are in demand for a variety of biomedical applications, in particular tissue engineering and regeneration, compared to other types of nanobiomaterials

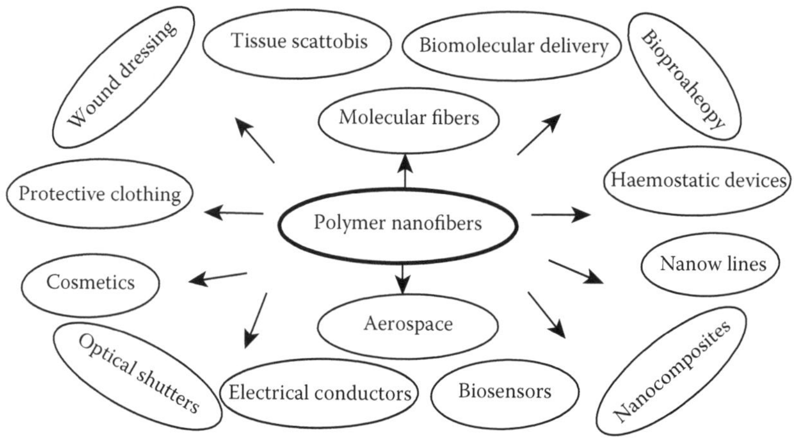

FIGURE 8.7
Applications of polymer nanofibers. (From Murugan, R. and Ramakrishna, S., *Tissue Eng.*, 12, 435, 2006. With permission from Mary Ann Liebert, Inc., publishers.)

(metallic and ceramic nanobiomaterials), owing to their functional properties, design flexibility, and surface modifiability. The polymer nanofibers used for this purpose are often called polymeric nanobiomaterials.

A nanofiber generally refers to a fiber having a diameter size in the range of 1–100 nm. The reduction in the diameter of the fibers to the order of nanometers results in a number of favorable properties, such as large surface area per unit mass, small pore size, flexibility in surface functionalization such as enhancement of solubility, biocompatibility and biorecognition, improved mechanical properties (stiffness and tensile), etc. These specific characteristics make the polymer nanofibers a unique class of nanobiomaterials for a variety of applications, such as scaffolds for tissue engineering, medical and dental implants, and therapeutic and biomolecular delivery. In addition to biomedical applications, polymer nanofibers are also found in other industrial applications (see Figure 8.7). Although some of these applications are in the development stage, a few have been commercially exploited (e.g., nanofilters and nanosensors). In the following sections, we focus our attention toward design strategies of such polymer nanofibers suitable for biomedical applications.

8.7 Processing of Polymer Nanofibers: Current Scenarios

Polymer nanofibers can be processed by multiple methods, including (i) drawing, (ii) template synthesis, (iii) self-assembly, (iv) phase separation, and (v) electrospinning. Comparative merits and demerits of these methods are depicted in Table 8.3 and some of the key aspects are described in the following sections.

8.7.1 Drawing

Drawing is a simple method that is being explored to process polymeric nanofibers because it needs minimum equipment. The drawing process can be better considered as dry spinning at a molecular level. A schematic representation of the drawing method is shown in Figure 8.8, whereby nanofibers are produced when the tip of a micropipette is dipped into the test droplet near the contact line using a micromanipulator and subsequently withdrawn from the liquid at a speed of about 1×10^{-4} ms^{-1}. When the end of the micropipette touches the surface of the droplet, the drawn nanofiber is then deposited. In order to draw fibers, a viscoelastic material is required so that it can endure the strong deformation and at the same time it has to be cohesive enough to support the stress that builds up in the pulling process. Using this method, nanofibers have been fabricated with sodium citrate molecules (Ondarcuhu and Joachim 1998). The droplet of solution is deposited on a surface to allow evaporation to take place. After a few minutes of evaporation, due to the capillary flow, the edge of the droplet is more concentrated and the drawing process can begin. By this drawing process, it is possible to create nanofibers with diameters less than 100 nm. The disadvantage of this process is that it produces fibers one after another; thus it is a time-consuming process. Furthermore, this process can only be applied to viscoelastic materials.

8.7.2 Template Synthesis

Template synthesis is a method that uses a nanoporous membrane as a template during the nanofiber formation. The highlight of this method is the fabrication of various sizes of solid as well as hollow-shaped fibers by optimizing the experimental conditions. A schematic representation of the nanofibers processing method by template synthesis is shown in Figure 8.9. Using this method, aligned polyacrylonitrile nanofibers were processed using aluminum oxide membrane as a template (Feng et al. 2002). In this particular process, when the pressure of the water is increased, it forces the polymer solution through the cylindrical nanopores of the membrane. Once the extruded polymer comes into contact with the solidification solution, it solidifies and forms nanofibers. It was found that the surface of the nanofibers was extremely hydrophobic without any modification by components of low surface energy. Further, it has been suggested that fiber orientation with different diameters can be obtained by using templates with different pore diameters. This method has been widely used to obtain nanotubules and nanofibrils of polymers. However, this method is limited to a few polymers only, which may be a disadvantage of the template synthesis.

TABLE 8.3

Various Methods of Processing Polymer Nanofibers

Methods	General Descriptions	Level of Processability	Level of Productivity	Merits	Demerits
Drawing	A dry spinning process, which typically requires a viscoelastic material so that it can endure the strong deformation and at the same time it has to be cohesive enough to support the stress that builds up in the pulling process	Easy	Lab scale	Simple process, requires minimum equipment	Produces fibers one after another, time-consuming, applicable only to viscoelastic materials
Template	A process that uses nanoporous membrane as a template to extrude nanofibers	Moderate	Lab scale	Feasibility of producing various sizes of hallow and sold fibers	Limited to a few polymers
Self-assembly	A process in which atoms, molecules, and supramolecular aggregates organize and arrange themselves into an ordered structure through weak and noncovalent bonds; typically involves a bottom-up approach	Difficulty	Lab scale	Mimic the biological process in certain circumstances	Complex process, limited to a few polymers, unable to produce long and continuous fibers with control over fiber orientation

Phase separation	A process that involves various steps, typically raw material dissolution, gelation, solvent extraction, freezing and drying, leading to the formation of nanofibrous foam-like structure	Easy	Lab scale	Simple process, tailorable mechanical properties	Limited to a few polymers, longer processing time, unable to produce long and continuous fibers with control over fiber orientation
Electro-spinning	A process that essentially employs electrostatic forces for the production of polymer nanofibrous scaffolds; typically involves a top-down approach	Relatively easy	Lab and industrial scales	Simple and cost effective process, capable of producing long and continuous fibers with control over fiber orientation, versatile to many polymers	Use of high-voltage apparatus

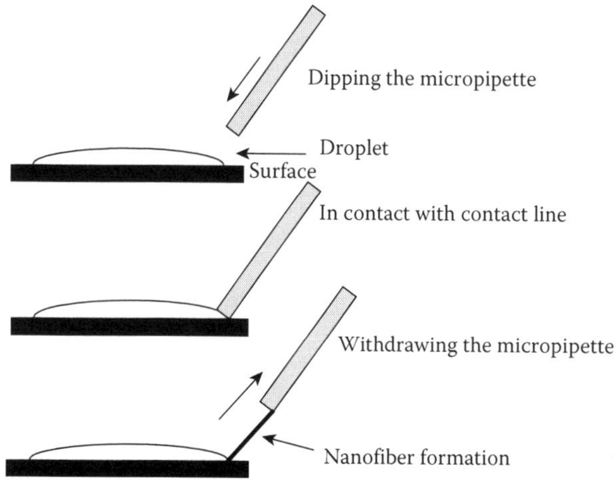

FIGURE 8.8
Schematic of polymer nanofiber processing by drawing method.

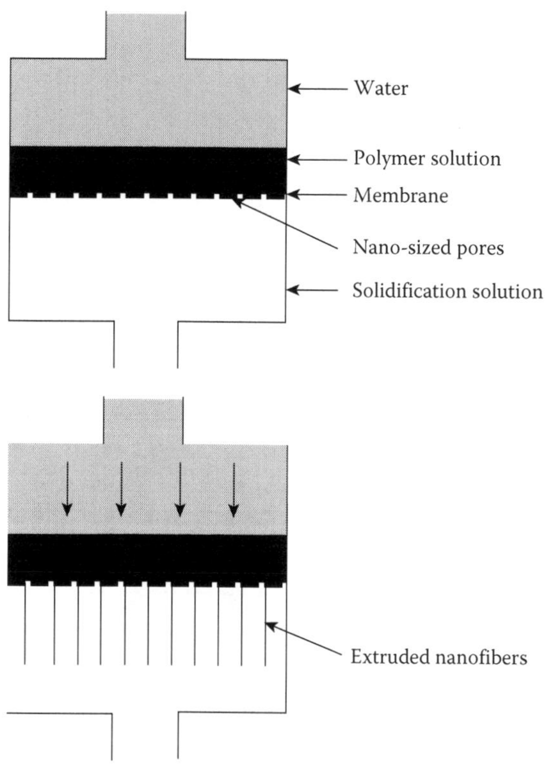

FIGURE 8.9
Schematic of polymer nanofiber processing by template method.

8.7.3 Self-Assembly

Over the past few years, much interest has focused on self-assembling for producing polymer nanofibers. Self-assembly is nothing more than a process in which individual, preexisting components organize themselves into an ordered structure required for specific functions without human intervention. The self-assembly takes place by noncovalent bonding, which typically include hydrogen bonding, ionic bonding, hydrophilic and van der Waals interactions. Although each of these forces is rather weak, their collective interactions could produce a very stable structure that could match the structural features of biological systems. The key challenge in self-assembly is to design molecular building blocks that can undergo spontaneous organization into a well-defined pattern that mimics complex biological systems. There are two experimental examples given below for the processing of nanofibers by self-assembly method.

Peptide-amphiphile (PA) nanofibers were developed by the self-assembling process for cell transplantation (Beniash et al. 2005) and to direct biomineralization of HA (Hartgerink et al. 2001). Beniash et al. (2005) demonstrated the feasibility of PA molecules to self-assemble into 3D nanofibrous scaffold under physiological conditions and their efficacy in cell entrapment was studied. The results indicated that cells entrapped in the nanofibrous network can survive and proliferate well, which suggests that the self-assembled PA system could be used for cell transplantation or other related tissue engineering applications. Hartgerink et al. (2001) further revealed the potential of self-assembled PA nanofibrous scaffold to direct self-biomineralization. The authors reported a PA molecule that self-assembles into a nanostructural gel and mimics some of the key features of the natural ECM of bone tissue. They processed the PA nanofibers with negatively charged surfaces because it is believed that this promotes biomineralization by establishing local ion supersaturation. A schematic representation of self-assembly of PA molecules into a cylindrical micelle is shown in Figure 8.10. The experimental results confirmed that the PA fibers are capable of nucleating HA on their surfaces. It was also noticed that the *c*-axes of HA crystals are coaligned with the long axes of PA fiber that nucleates the structural orientation between collagen and HA observed in the natural bone tissues; therefore, this type of self-assembled system could be promising for mineralized tissue repair. Overall, self-assembly is very popular in the field of biomimetic tissue engineering.

8.7.4 Phase Separation

Phase separation is an interesting method used generally for manufacturing scaffolds for tissue engineering. Phase separation involves various processing steps, typically raw material dissolution, gelation, solvent extraction, freezing, and drying. Of course, these steps to convert the polymer into a nanofibrous structure would take a prolonged time. The unique advantage of this

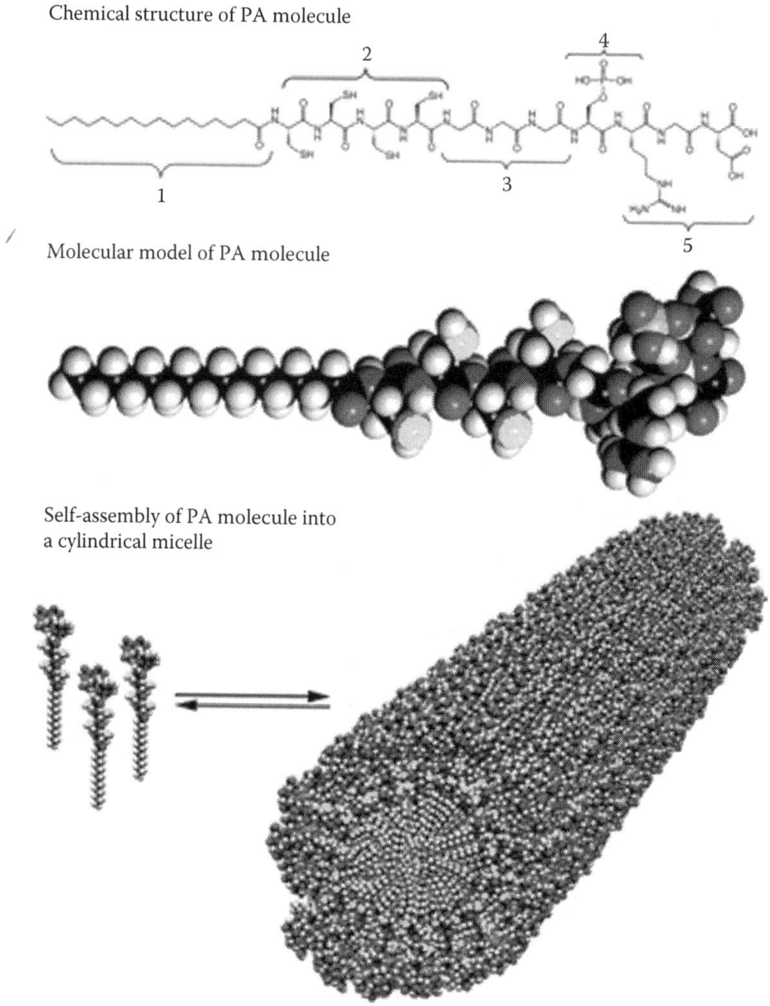

FIGURE 8.10
Schematic representation of self-assembly of PA molecules. (Reprinted from Hartgerink, J. D. et al., *Science*, 294, 1684, 2001. With permission from American Association for the Advancement of Science (AAAS)).

method lies in the possibility of designing 3D nanostructures without using any special equipment. Furthermore, the porosity and mechanical properties of the scaffold can be controlled to some extent, but it is very difficult and perhaps not feasible to maintain the fiber orientation. Tissue scaffolds using poly(L-lactic acid) (PLLA) were fabricated by the authors' group using this phase separation method (Yang et al. 2004). A schematic representation of phase separation involved in the processing of polymer nanofibers is shown in Figure 8.11. The authors processed the scaffolds with a highly porous and

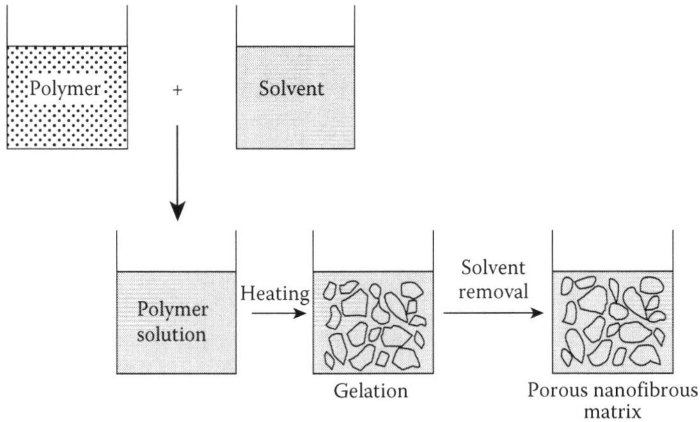

FIGURE 8.11
Schematic of polymer nanofiber processing by phase separation method.

fibrous structure close to natural ECM. The fiber diameters ranged from 50 to 300 nm with an average of 150–250 nm with respect to the polymer concentration used in the experimental process. The scaffolds were further evaluated with neural stem cells under *in vitro* cell culture conditions. The results indicated that the cells differentiated well on the nanofibrous scaffolds and the scaffolds served as a positive cue in supporting neurite outgrowth. This study, therefore, suggests that PLLA nanofibrous scaffolds made by phase separation would be promising for neural tissue engineering. Overall, the phase separation method has gained considerable interest in processing scaffolds for tissue engineering and other biomedical applications.

8.7.5 Electrospinning: A New Approach

Although the above methods have been employed to produce polymer nanofibers, they often encountered some difficulties, especially in controlling the fiber orientation. For many applications, in particular tissue engineering, it is desirable to control not only the fiber diameter, but also the fiber orientation because alignment of the fibers predominantly influences the cell growth. Therefore, importance is given to a method that facilitates a well-defined fiber orientation and control over fiber thickness. In recent years, considerable efforts have been undertaken around the world for the processing of polymer nanofibers with fiber orientation by so-called electrospinning.

Electrospinning is a straightforward, cost-effective, and versatile technique that essentially employs electrostatic forces to produce polymer fibers, ranging in diameter from a few microns down to tens of nanometers. This technique was first introduced by Zelency in 1914. Later, Formhals contributed much to the development of electrospinning and prolifically obtained several patents in the 1930s and 1940s. In those days, it was called electrostatic spray or electrostatic spinning and was renamed electrospinning in the 1990s. However, this technique was not adopted for tissue engineering as a tool for manufacturing tissue scaffolds at the time of invention, but it was used in other industrial applications. Recently, it has been revitalized and is successfully applied in the processing of polymer nanofibers suitable for tissue engineering and other industrial applications, such as molecular filters, chemical sensors, and biosensors. Some of the polymers that have been spun into nanofibers by electrospinning are listed in Table 8.4. The precise merit of this technique is that it could produce scaffolds with most of the structural features required for tissue engineering. It also offers many advantages over conventional scaffold methodologies, for example, it is capable of producing ultrafine fibers with spatial orientation, high aspect ratio, high surface area, and it has control over pore geometry. These are some of the favorable characteristics to be considered for better cell growth because they directly influence the cell adhesion, cell expression, and transportation of oxygen and nutrients. In this light, electrospun polymer nanofibers could serve as a good tissue scaffold and could provide a spatial environment for the growth of new tissue with appropriate functions.

8.7.5.1 Experimental System

The basic configuration of electrospinning, schematically illustrated in Figure 8.12, consists of three major components: (i) a spinneret, (ii) a fiber collector, and (iii) a high-voltage power system. As illustrated in the figure, the spinneret is directly connected to a syringe, which acts as a reservoir for the polymer solution to be electrospun. This polymer solution can be fed through the spinneret with the help of a syringe pump at a steady and controllable feed rate. The feeding rate can be controlled corresponding to the concentration of polymer solution. It is worth pointing out that the material to be spun by this technique must be viscous, but the viscosity may vary depending on the type of materials used. The fiber-collecting device is positioned directly below the spinneret with an appropriate gap. A high-voltage/low-current power system is required for the conversion of polymer solution into a charged polymer jet. The electric power (usually up to 30 kV) is applied across the spinneret and the grounded metallic counter electrode (fiber collector), to facilitate the charged jet to eject from the spinneret tip toward the surface of the fiber collector. The electrospun fibers are collected at the surface of the collector.

8.7.5.2 Spinning Mechanism

Although the experimental design and functional components of electrospinning seem to be extremely simple, the mechanism involved in the spinning of polymer nanofibers is rather complicated. Upon applying an optimized

TABLE 8.4

List of a Few Electrospun Polymers

No.	Polymer	Solvent	Concentration	Perspective Applications
1	Nylon 6,6, PA-6.6	Formic acid	10 wt.%	Protective clothing
2	Polyurethanes, PU	Dimethylformamide	10 wt.%	Protective clothing
		Dimethylformamide	10 wt.%	Electret filter
3	Polybenzimidazole, PBI	Dimethylaccetamide	10 wt.%	Protective clothing
				Nanofiber reinforced composites
4	Polycarboate, PC	Dimethylformamide: tetrahydrofuran (1:1)	10 wt.%	Protective clothing
		Dichlormethane	15 wt.%	Sensor, filter
		Chloroform, tetrahydrofuran		
		Dimethylformamide: tetrahydrofuran (1:1)	15 wt.%	
		Dimethylformamide: tetrahydrofuran (1:1)	20 wt.%	Electret filter
6	Polyacrylonitrile, PAN	Dimethylformamide	600 mg PAN/ 10-5m3	
		Dimethylformamide		
		Dimethylformamide		Carbon nanofiber
		Dimethylformamide		
		Dimethylformamide	15 wt.%	
7	Polyvinyl alcohol, PVA	Distilled water	8–16 wt.%	
		Distilled water	4–10 wt.%	
			1–10 wt.%	

(Continued)

TABLE 8.4

List of a Few Electrospun Polymers (*Continued*)

No.	Polymer	Solvent	Concentration	Perspective Applications
8	Polylactic acid, PLA	Dimethylformamide		Membrane for prevention of surgery-induced adhesion
		Methylene chloride and dimethylformamide		Same as above
		Dichloromethane	5 wt.%	Sensor, filter
			14 wt.%	Drug delivery system
		Dichloromethane		
9	Polyethylene-co-vinyl acetate, PEVA		14 wt.%	Drug delivery system
10	PEVA/PLA		14 wt.%	Drug delivery system
11	Polymethacrylate (PMMA)/ tetrahydroperfluorooctyl acrylate (TAN)	Dimethylformamide: toluene (1:9)		
12	Polyethylene oxide, PEO	Distilled water	7–10 wt.%	
		Distilled water	7–10 wt.%	
		Distilled water	4–10 wt.%	
		Distilled water and ethanol or NaCl	1–4.3 wt.%	
		Distilled water, distilled water and chloroform, distilled water and isopropanol		

		Distilled water: ethanol (3:2)	4 wt.%	Microelectronic wiring, interconnects
		Distilled water, chloroform, acetone		
		Ethanol	4–10%	
			1–10 wt.%	
			1–10 wt.%	
		Isopropyle alcohol + water	10 wt.%	Electret filter
		Isopropanol: water (6:1)		
		Isopropanol: water (6:1)	3–10 wt.%	
		Chloroform	0.5–30 wt.%	
13	Collagen–PEO	Hydrochloric acid	1–2 wt.%	Wound healing, tissue engineering, hemostatic agents
		Hydrochloric acid (pH = 2.0)	1 wt.%	Wound healing, tissue engineering
14	Polyaniline (PANI)/PEO blend	Chloroform		Conductive fiber
		Camphorsulfonic acid	2 wt.%	Conducting fiber
		Chloroform	2–4 wt.%	Conducting fiber

(*Continued*)

TABLE 8.4

List of a Few Electrospun Polymers (*Continued*)

No.	Polymer	Solvent	Concentration	Perspective Applications
15	Polyaniline (PANI)/polystyrene (PS)	Chloroform		Conductive fiber
		Camphorsulfonic acid	2 wt.%	Conductive fiber
16	Silk-like polymer with fibronectin functionality	Formic acid	0.8–16.2 wt.%	Implantable device
17	Polyvinylcarbazole	Dichloromethane	7.5 wt.%	Sensor, filter
18	Polyethylene terephthalate PET	Dichloromethane and trifluoracetic	4 wt.%	
		Dichloromethane: trifluoroacetyl acid (1:1)	2–18 wt.%	
19	Polyacrcylic acid polypyrene methanol, PAA-PM	Dimethylformamide		Optical sensor
20	Polystyrene, PS	Tetrahydrofuran, dimethylformamide, CS2 (carbon disulfide), toluene	18–35 wt.%	
		Methylethylketone	8%	Enzymatic biotransformation
		Chloroform, dimethylformamide	2.5–10.7%	
		Tetrahydrofuran	25 wt.%	
		Dimethylformamide	30 wt.%	(Flat ribbons)
		Tetrahydrofuran	15 wt.%	Catalyst, filter
		Tetrahydrofuran	15 wt.%	Catalyst, filter
		Tetrahydrofuran	15 wt.%	Catalyst, filter

		Tetrahydrofuran	15 wt.%	Catalyst, filter
21	Polymethacrylate, PMMA	Tetrahydrofuran, acetone, chloroform		
22	Polyamide, PA	Dimethylacetamide		Glass fiber filter media
23	Silk/PEO blend	Silk aqueous solutions	4.8–8.8 wt.%	Biomaterial scaffolds
24	Polyvinyl phenol, PVP	Tetrahydrofuran	20, 60% (wt./vol.)	Antimicrobial agent
25	Polyvinylchloride, PVC	Tetrahydrofuran/dimethylformamide 80/20, 60/40, 50/50, 40/60, 20/80, 0/100 (vol. %)	10 wt. 100/0	
26	Cellulose acetate, CA	Acetone, acetic acid, dimethylacetamide	12.5–20%	Membrane
27	Mixture of PAA-PM (polyacrylic acid-poly(pyrene methanol)) and polyurethane	Dimethylformamide	265 wt.%	Optical sensor
28	Polyvinyl alcohol (PVA)/silica	Distilled water		
29	Polyacrylamide, PAAm		1–10 wt.%	
30	PLGA	Tetrahydrofuran:dimethylformamide (1:1)	1–20 mL	Scaffold for tissue engineering
31	Collagen	Hexafluoro-2-propanol		Scaffold for tissue engineering

(*Continued*)

TABLE 8.4

List of a Few Electrospun Polymers (*Continued*)

No.	Polymer	Solvent	Concentration	Perspective Applications
32	Polycaprolactone, PCL	Chloroform:methanol (3:1) toluene:methanol (1:1), and dichloromethane:		
33	Poly(2-hydroxyethyl methacrylate) HEMA	methanol Ethanol: formic acid (1:1), ethanol	12, 20 wt.%/8, 16, 20 wt.%	(Flat ribbons)
34	Poly(vinylidene fluoride) PVDF	Dimethylformamide: dimet-hylacemide ta/(1/1)		(Flat ribbons)
35	Polyether imide, PEI	Hexafluoro-2-propanol	10 wt.%	(Flat ribbons)
36	Polyethylene gricol, PEG	Chloroform	0.5–30 wt.%	
37	Nylon-4,6, PA-4,6	Formic acid	10 wt.%	Transparent composite
38	Poly(ferrocenyldimethylsilane)	Tetrahydrofuran: dimethylf-ormamide	20 wt.%	
39	Nylon 6 (PA-6)/montmoril-lonnite (Mt)	Hexa-fluoro-isopropanol (HFIP), HFIP/ dimethylformamide 95/5 (wt.%)	10 wt.%	
40	Poly(ethylene-co-vinyl alcohol)	Isopropanol/water: 70/30 (%w/v)	2.5–20% w/v	Biomedical
41	Polyacrylnitrile (PAN)/TiO_2			Photovoltaic and conductive polymers
42	Polycaprolactone (PCL)/metal			ZnO: cosmetic use
43	Polyvinyl pyrrolidone, PVP			
44	Polymethaphenylene isophthalamide			

Source: Reprinted from Huang, Z. M. et al., *Comp. Sci. Tech.*, 63, 2223, 2003. With permission from Elsevier.

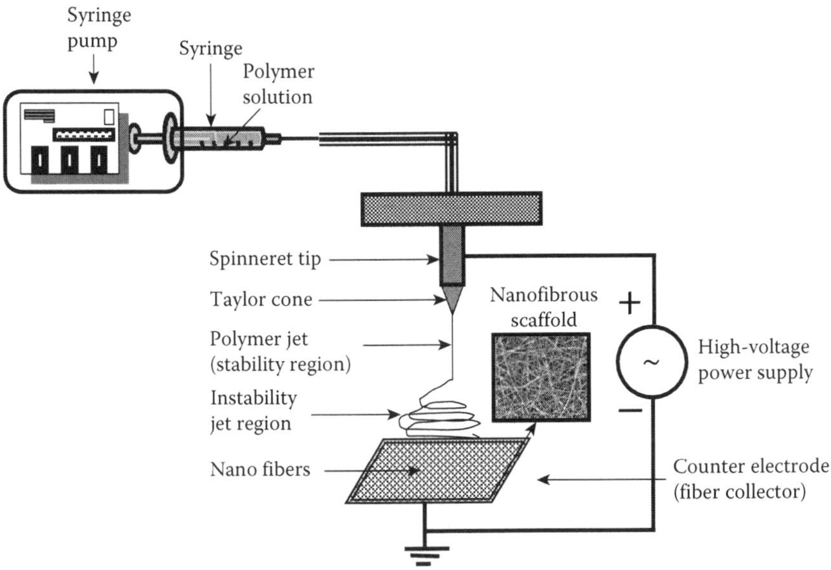

FIGURE 8.12
Schematic of an electrospinning system. (From Murugan, R. and Ramakrishna, S., *Tissue Eng.*, 12, 435, 2006. With permission from Mary Ann Liebert, Inc., publishers.)

electric potential to the spinneret, a pendent droplet of the polymer solution at the tip of the spinneret gets electrified, thereby inducing charge accumulation on the surface of the droplet that subsequently allows the droplet to deform into a cone, known as Taylor's cone. This deformation is commonly caused by two electrostatic forces: (i) electrostatic repulsion between the surface charges of the droplet and (ii) Columbic force exerted by the strong external electric field applied. Once the applied electric field surpasses a critical value (threshold), the electrostatic force tends to exceed the viscoelastic force and the surface tension of the polymer droplet, and a fine charged polymer jet is forced to eject from the tip of the Taylor cone. This polymer jet then moves toward the counter electrode, accompanied by rapid evaporation of the solvent molecules and, while in transit, the different polymer strands in the jet are separated out due to the mutual repulsion, a phenomenon called "splaying," which gives rise to a series of ultrafine dry fibers. These fibers can be collected on a grounded metallic target (fiber collector); typically in the range of a few micrometers to nanometers.

It is worth mentioning that different types of fiber collectors are available corresponding to spatial orientation (see Figure 8.13). For example, rotating-type collectors can be used to obtain aligned nanofibers, whilst static-type collectors can be used to obtain random nanofibers. The alignment of the fibers is rather complicated and numerous parameters influence the fiber orientation, including the rotational speed and shape of the counter electrode,

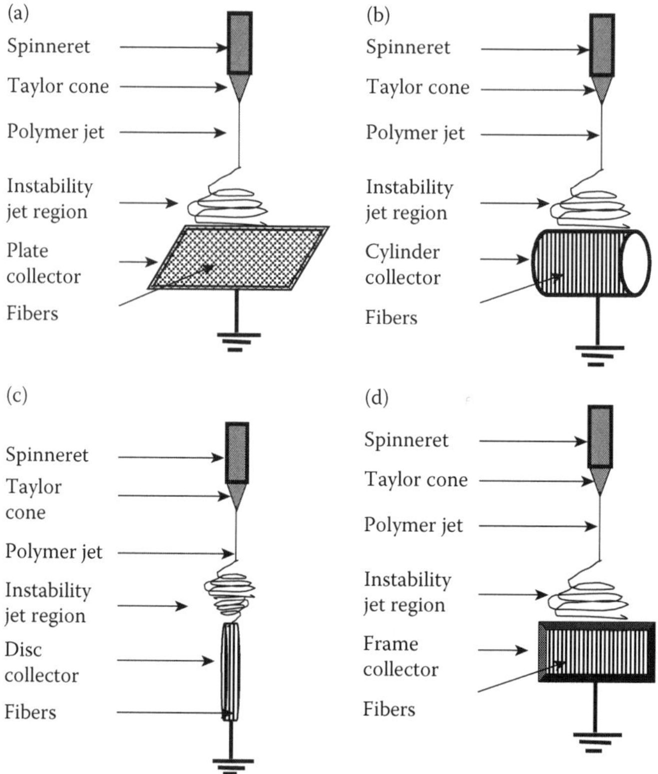

FIGURE 8.13
Different types of fiber collector. (From Murugan, R. and Ramakrishna, S., *Tissue Eng.*, 12, 435, 2006. With permission from Mary Ann Liebert, Inc., publishers.)

the concentration of polymer solution, the dielectric constant of the solvent, the strength and shape of the electric field, and the environmental conditions, such as relative humidity and temperature.

8.8 Electrospun Polymer Nanofibrous Scaffolds

This section explicates how electrospinning can be adopted to produce nanofibrous scaffolds using a few biodegradable polymers for example.

8.8.1 Collagen Nanofibrous Scaffold

As native collagen of the ECM is in the form of a nanofibrous structure, it is highly beneficial if the collagen can be processed into nanofibers for a variety of biomedical applications, in particular tissue engineering. The electrospinning technique has been employed to fabricate this type of collagen into nanofibers (Matthews et al. 2002). The experimental conditions involved in the fabrication are briefly described as follows: collagen (type I) was dissolved in an organic solvent of 1,1,1,3,3,3 hexafluoro-2-propanol (HFP) (8%) and the homogeneous solution was placed in a 1-mL syringe for spinning. A high voltage (25 kV) was applied to the collagen solution. The solution was extruded at a constant flow rate (5.0 mL/h) by keeping the distance between the syringe needle and the collector at 12.5 cm. Once the applied voltage reached threshold, the fibers were forced to eject and accumulate on the fiber collector. The spinning condition can be standardized by varying the experimental parameters, such as solution concentration, flow rate, voltage applied, needle size, and the distance between the syringe needle and the collector.

The morphology of fibers obtained from the above condition was studied by scanning electron microscopy (SEM). Figure 8.14a shows a SEM

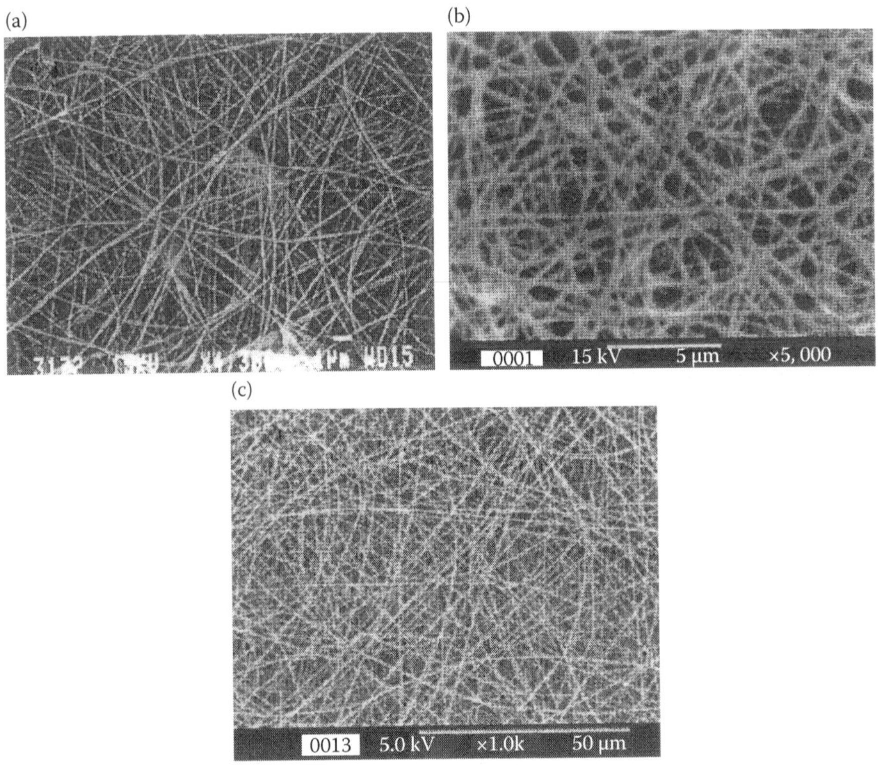

FIGURE 8.14
SEM photographs of polymer nanofibers made of (a) collagen, (b) gelatin, and (c) chitosan. (Reprinted from Matthews, J. A. et al., *Biomacromolecules*, 3, 232, 2002. With permission from American Chemical Society; Reprinted from Huang, Z. M. et al., *Polymer*, 45, 5361, 2004. With permission from Macmillan Publishers Ltd; Reproduced from Ohkawa, K., et al., *Macromol. Rapid Commun.*, 25, 1600, 2004. With permission from Wiley-VCH Verlag GmbH & Co. KGaA.)

micrograph of electrospun collagen. It indicates that the diameters of the collagen fibers are in nanometer scale range, thereby confirming the formation of nanofibers. The average fiber diameter was determined as 100±40 nm. As this morphology is quite analogous to the native ECM, it can be used as a scaffold for tissue engineering to promote cellular growth and other related metabolic functions.

8.8.2 Gelatin Nanofibrous Scaffold

Spinning gelatin macromolecules into a nanofibrous matrix is highly beneficial for a variety of biomedical applications. The electrospinning technique has been employed to fabricate gelatin nanofibers (Huang et al. 2004). The detailed experimental conditions are described as follows: gelatin was first dissolved in 2,2,2-trifluoroethanol (TFE) (7.5%) and the resultant solution was placed in a 5-mL syringe. The distance between the spinneret and the collector was kept at 12 cm. Once a high voltage (10.5 kV) was applied to the gelatin solution, it was extruded at a constant mass flow rate (0.8 mL/h), resulting in a series of ultrafine fibers. These fibers were collected on a grounded metallic target in the form of nonwoven mat. The aforementioned measurements are optimal for spinning, and were standardized by varying the experimental parameters, such as solution concentration, flow rate, voltage applied, and distance between the syringe needle and the collector.

Figure 8.14b shows a SEM micrograph of the electrospun gelatin fibers obtained from the above optimal condition, indicating its surface morphology. The diameters of the fibers are in the order of nanometer scale, ranging from 80 to 300 nm. The average fiber diameter was found to be 140 nm. The gelatin was electrospun from different solution concentrations in the range of 5–15% and it was found that the concentration above 7.5% produced better fibers without any bead formation, whereas a concentration below 7.5% produced fibers with irregular beads. Table 8.5 gives a comparative data on the size of the fiber diameters of the gelatin obtained from the various solution concentrations. These data indicate that the fiber diameter increases with the increase in the solution concentration. Further, fibers formed using the solution of 7.5% concentration have a higher tensile modulus and strength as compared to fibers obtained from the other solution concentrations; thus, fibers formed at this concentration may be used as a good scaffold for tissue engineering applications.

8.8.3 Chitosan Nanofibrous Scaffold

As chitosan is a widely used polysaccharide in biomedical applications, it has been electrospun into nanofibers (Ohkawa et al. 2004). The experimental parameters involved in the processing of a chitosan nanofibrous scaffold are given in Table 8.6, but the spinning mechanism is quite similar to the aforementioned methods. The chitosan was electrospun into nanofibers using

TABLE 8.5

Effect of Polymer Concentration on the Size of Gelatin Fibers

Polymer Concentration (%w/v)	Fiber Diameter Range (nm)	Average Diameter (nm)
5	50–175	100
7.5	80–300	140
10	130–540	240
12.5	200–750	340
15	630–4800	1900

Source: Huang, Z. M. et al., *Polymer*, 45, 5361, 2004.

TABLE 8.6

Processing Condition of Spinning Chitosan Nanofibers

Spinning Factors	Measurements
Solution concentration	8%
Flow rate	–
Distance	15 cm
Voltage	15 kV
Solvent	Trifluoroacetic acid

Source: Reproduced from Ohkawa, K. et al., *Macromol. Rapid Commun.*, 25, 1600, 2004. With permission from Wiley-VCH Verlag GmbH & Co. KGaA.

different solution concentrations and it was found that the concentration less than 7% produced beads on the fibers, while 8% produced an almost uniform fiber network. Here, trifluoroacetic acid (TFA) was chosen as a solvent for chitosan because (i) it forms salts with the amino groups of chitosan macromolecules and this salt then destroys the rigid interaction between the chitosan macromolecules, which makes them ready for spinning, and (ii) the high volatility of TFA is advantageous for the rapid solidification of the electrified polymer jet. A SEM micrograph of an electrospun chitosan scaffold is shown in Figure 8.14c, indicating the formation of fibers at nanometer scale range. The micrograph indicates that the scaffold is composed of randomly oriented fibers with diameters ranging from 390 to 610 nm. The average diameter of the fibers was determined as 490 nm. Further, it shows an interconnected porous architecture throughout the fibrous matrix, which is quite similar to that of natural ECM; thus, it can be suitable for tissue reconstructive applications.

8.8.4 Poly(L-lactic acid) Nanofibrous Scaffold

As PLLA is a highly biocompatible synthetic polymer, there has been great interest in spinning it into nanofibers. Many research groups have successfully electrospun the PLLA nanofibers with spatial orientations, which obviously shows the potential of PLLA. The spinning details, according to the reported data (Yang et al. 2005), are: PLLA solution (1 and 2%) was prepared by dissolving in dichloromethane (DCM) and n,n-dimethyl-formamide (DMF) (70:30). These two polymer concentrations were chosen for spinning fibers with different spatial orientations (aligned and random). The solution was extruded at a constant flow rate (1.0 mL/h) by keeping the distance between the syringe needle and the fiber collector at 10 cm. A high voltage (12 kV) was applied to the syringe needle using a regulated DC power system. Once it reached the threshold, long and ultrafine fibers were forced to eject and deposit on the grounded metallic target in the form of a nonwoven mat.

The electrospun PLLA scaffolds were examined for their (i) fiber size, (ii) fiber shape, and (iii) pores. A SEM was employed to study their morphology. Figure 8.15a through c show SEM micrographs of electrospun PLLA, providing complete details about the size and shape of the fibers and their nature of porous architecture. They can be categorized into two types of fiber patterns: (i) ANF and (ii) RNF, as shown in Figures 8.15a and b, respectively. The micrograph exhibits a high order of alignment on the fiber orientation for ANF, whereas fibers are randomly oriented in the form of a nonwoven mat for RNF. The fiber diameters are on the order of nanoscale (150–500 nm) with an average diameter of 300 nm for ANF. The average fiber diameter was found to be 700 nm for RNF. It was noticed while spinning that the fiber diameter increases with increasing PLLA concentration. The micrographs denote that the average diameter of the ANF is smaller than that of the RNF, which can be attributed to the rotating speed of the fiber collector. Figure 8.15c shows the SEM micrographs of PLLA nanofibers produced by Bognitzki et al. (2001). These fibers have a beautiful porous architecture with nanopores. The average pore size is in the range of 100 nm in width and 250 nm in length. Furthermore, the investigators noticed that elongation of the pores along the fiber axis is the result of a uniaxial extension of the polymer jet in the electric field.

8.8.5 Poly(glycolic acid) Nanofibrous Scaffold

By using electrospinning, Boland et al. (2003) demonstrated the ability of spinning PGA nanofibers. The key factors involved in this spinning process are given in Table 8.7. The SEM micrographs of electrospun PGA indicate the formation of nanofibers with two different spatial orientations, depending on the rotational speed of the mandrel. Figure 8.15d and e represent aligned and randomly orientated fibers, respectively. Due to the different rotational velocity of the collector, it is able to produce fibers with different spatial orientations. It was noticed that the higher speed of the mandrel yielded an aligned form of fibers and the lower speed yielded randomly oriented fibers. The fibers are on the order of nano- and submicron-scale range with an average diameter of 1.19 ± 0.41 μm. Further, elastic moduli of these fibers, fabricated using 1/7 w/v solution concentration, was found to be 104.9 MPa, which is

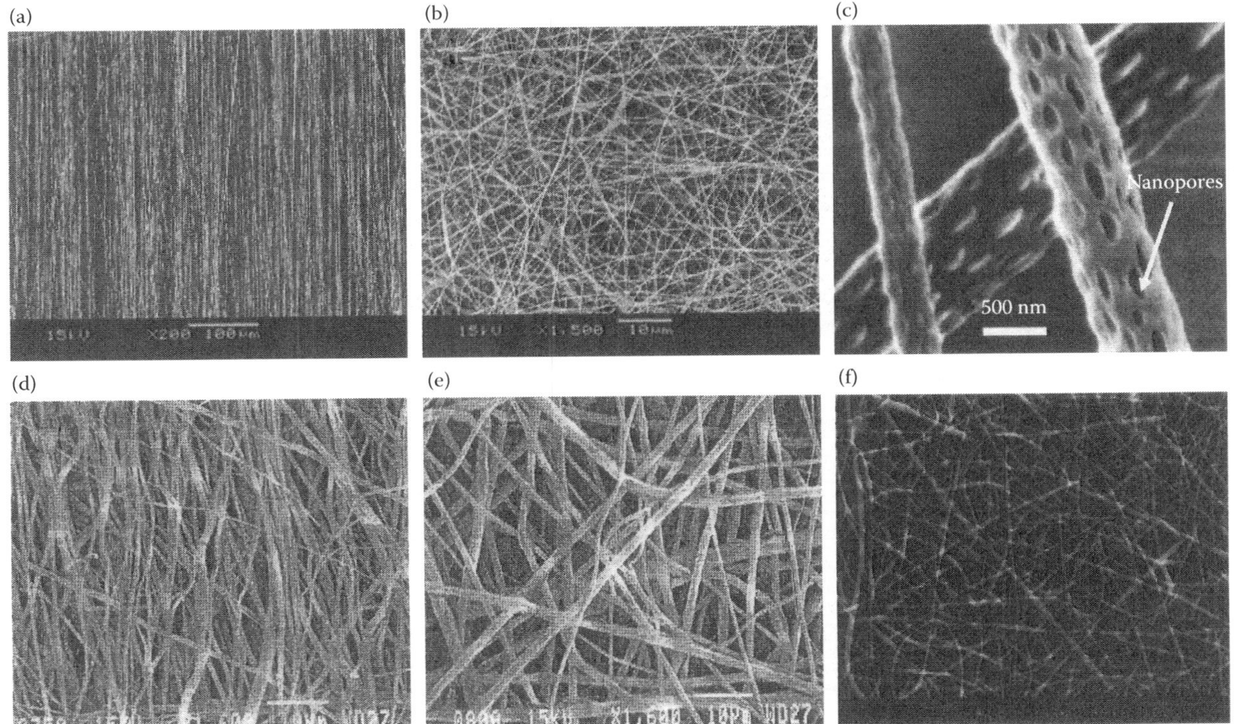

FIGURE 8.15
SEM photographs of polymer nanofibers made of (a) PLLA (aligned fibers), (b) PLLA (random fibers), (c) PLLA (porous fibers), (d) PGA (aligned fibers), (e) PGA (random fibers), and (f) PLGA. (Reprinted from Yang, F. et al., *Biomaterials*, 26, 2603, 2005. With permission from Elsevier; Reproduced from Bognitzki, M. et al., *Adv. Mater.*, 13, 70, 200. With permission from Wiley-VCH Verlag GmbH & Co. KgaA; Boland, E. D. et al., *J. Macromol. Sci. Pure Appl. Chem.*, A38, 1231, 2003; You, Y. et al., *J. Appl. Polym. Sci.*, 99, 1214, 2005. With permission from John Wiley & Sons, Inc.)

TABLE 8.7

Processing Condition of Spinning PGA Nanofibers

Spinning Factors	Measurements
Solution concentration	1/7 w/v
Flow rate	1.0 mL/h
Distance	27.5 cm
Voltage	22 kV
Solvent	Hexafluoro 2 propanol

Source: Reprinted from Boland, E. D. et al., *J. Macromol. Sci. Pure Appl. Chem.*, A38, 1231, 2003. With permission from Taylor & Francis Group.

the highest value among the fibers obtained from the other concentrations. This kind of nanofiber is attractive for tissue engineering applications as a scaffold.

8.8.6 Poly(lactic-co-glycolic acid) Nanofibrous Scaffold

Keeping the merits of the PLGA copolymer, it has been electrospun in the form of nanofibrous structures suitable for tissue engineering applications as a scaffold (You et al. 2005). Although the authors electrospun the PLGA at various solution concentrations, PLGA nonwoven structures were obtained by electrospinning PLGA/chloroform at a concentration of 15%. The spinning conditions are given in Table 8.8. The morphology of electrospun PLGA fibers can be seen from Figure 8.15f. The average fiber diameter of PLGA was found to be 760 nm. The authors noticed that the nature of solvent such as volatility and polarity has a significant influence on the morphology and diameter of the electrospun fibers, similar to conductivity of solution. In order to reduce the fiber diameter, electrospinning of PLGA was carried out with quaternary ammonium salt. The salt is soluble in the electrospinning solvent of PLGA and hence is easily removable from the electrospun fibers. The addition of small amounts of salt to the polymer solution caused a significant decrease in the average fiber diameters to 450 nm and the fibers were amounted in a straight shape. This kind of PLGA nonwoven structure may be used as a biodegradable scaffold in tissue engineering applications.

8.9 Biomedical Applications of Polymer Nanofibers

As previously mentioned, the use of polymer nanofibrous biomaterials for biomedical applications is highly beneficial over conventional microfibrous biomaterials, owing to their functional properties. From a biological

TABLE 8.8

Processing Condition of Spinning PLGA Nanofibers

Spinning Factors	Measurements
Solution concentration	15%
Flow rate	4.0 mL/h
Distance	5–10 cm
Voltage	15–20 kV
Solvent	Chloroform

Source: Reprinted from You, Y. et al., *J. Appl. Polym. Sci.*, 99, 1214, 2005. With permission from John Wiley & Sons, Inc.

viewpoint, almost all human tissues and organs consist of various natural biomaterials in nanofibrous forms or structures. All of them are characterized by well-organized hierarchical structures from macro to nanoscale. For example, bone tissue consists mainly of collagen nanofibrous matrix impregnated with HA nanocrystals, which typically leads to the concept of nanofibrous biomaterials for use in human health-care applications. Furthermore, it is recognized that cells attach and organize well around fibers with diameters smaller than those of the cells. This information clearly indicates the potential of nanobiomaterials in biomedical applications and some of these applications, whose potential has already been demonstrated to certain levels, are discussed in the following sections.

8.9.1 Medical Prostheses

Polymer nanofibers fabricated via electrospinning have been proposed for a number of medical prostheses applications. Since the early 1980s, polymer nanofibers have been proposed for vascular and breast prostheses applications. Polymer nanofibers were deposited as a thin porous film onto a prosthetic device that was designed for implantation into the central nervous system (Buchko et al. 2001). This coating film with a gradient fibrous structure works as an interphase between the prosthetic device and the neural system, and is expected to efficiently reduce the stiffness mismatch at the tissue/device interface and hence prevent device failure after implantation. On the other hand, as abdominal procedure is routinely practiced,adhesion has become a common cause of complication after the operation, which includes small bowel obstruction, female infertility, chronic debilitating pain, and difficulty in future operations. Pertaining to this, Zong et al. (2002) examined the effect of using an electrospun PLGA mat impregnated with antibiotics (Mefoxin®) as an anti-adhesion membrane based on an *in vivo* rat model. They concluded that the membrane was effective in reducing post-surgery adhesion and could act as a physical barrier as well as a local drug delivery vehicle. Therefore, the combined features of composition adjustment, drug-loading capability, and easy-handling ability make these polymeric nanofibrous biomaterials ideal candidates for future clinical evaluations.

8.9.2 Dental Restoration

Polymer nanofibers can be used as reinforcement in dental composites suitable for dental restoration applications. A dental restoration material is generally made of some kind of dental resin, such as bis-GMA and triethylene glycol dimethacrylate (TEGDMA), and a certain amount (up to 70 wt.%) of fillers (e.g., silica or ceramic particles). In practice, it has been found that the fillers, initially used for the purpose of improving mechanical properties, can eventually play a side effect in accelerating the damage of the dental composite due to the stress concentration resulting from the introduction of the fillers. Investigation of the composites used for a longer time period was considerably less optimistic. To overcome this problem, Fong (2003) incorporated the electrospun Nylon 6 nanofibers prepared from 10 wt.% 1,1,1,3,3,3,-hexafluro-2-propanal with a diameter less than one micron and a uniform cylindrical shape was introduced into the bis-GMA/TEGDMA resin. A three-point bending test of this modified dental composite indicated that flexural strength, elastic modulus, and work of fracture were notably increased after embedding into the resin. However, mass fraction of Nylon 6 nanofibers added beyond 5% did not improve the mechanical properties of the dental composite significantly.

The use of polymer nanofibers as reinforcement for engineering composites has so far provided only marginal enhancement in terms of strength and stiffness properties. Nevertheless, limited research work in this direction has indicated that polymer nanofibers are effective in improving fracture toughness of the composites. Fracture toughness is one of the key considerations in developing polymer composite dental devices, such as orthodontic brackets. An additional merit of using nanofibers as reinforcement is that no adverse effect on the transparency of the developed composite dental device can result when the fiber diameter becomes smaller than the wavelength of a visible light. These advantages make polymer nanofibers very promising candidates for the future development of dental prostheses (orthodontic devices) that are lightweight, have optimal mechanical property, and possess desired aesthetic features.

8.9.3 Wound Dressing

Driven by some major factors, such as an increasingly aging population with chronic wounds, unexpected suffering of civilians from terrorist attacks, warfare conflicts, and frequent casualties from traffic accidents, there is an increasing demand for advanced wound care products. In this regard, new technology will dramatically accelerate the development of innovative dressing materials for wound healing. An ideal dressing is one that can provide an environment at the surface of the wound in which healing can take place at the maximum rate consistent with the reproduction of the healing wound with an acceptable cosmetic appearance. Modern dressings are developed to serve the purpose of facilitating wound healing, apart from the basic function of covering wounds from further infection.

Polymer nanofibers can also be used for the treatment of wounds or burns of human skin, as well as designed for hemostatic devices with some unique characteristics. With the aid of electric field, fine fibers of biodegradable polymers can be directly sprayed/spun onto the injured location of skin to form a fibrous mat dressing (see Figure 8.16), which allows wounds to heal by encouraging the formation of normal skin growth and eliminating the formation of scar tissue that would occur in a traditional treatment. Nonwoven nanofibrous membrane mats for wound dressing usually have pore sizes ranging from 500 nm to 1 μm, small enough to protect the wound from bacterial penetration via aerosol particle-capturing mechanisms. High surface area of 5–100 m^2/g is extremely efficient for fluid absorption and dermal delivery. Kenawy et al. (2003) attempted to generate fibrinogen nanofiber mats for potential use as a wound dressing or hemostatic bandage. In

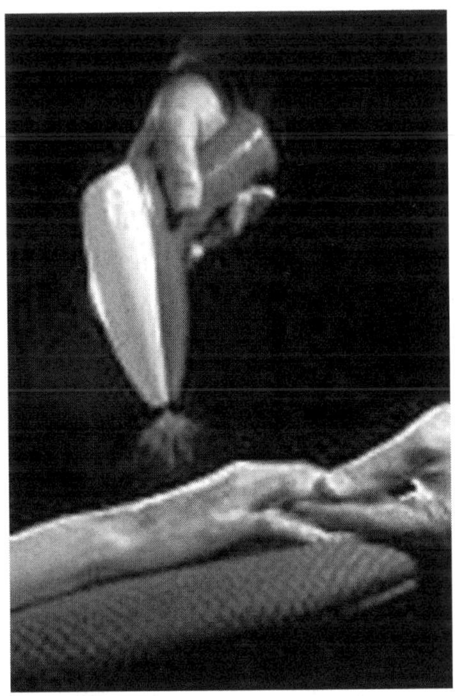

FIGURE 8.16
Photograph showing electrospray of polymer directly onto skin. (Reprinted from Huang, Z. M. et al., *Comp. Sci. Tech.*, 63, 2223, 2003. With permission from Elsevier.)

another report, the performance of PU nanofibrous membranes as dressings was examined *in vivo* using a pig model (Valentine et al. 1984). All these reported data suggest the potential of polymer nanofibers in wound dressing applications.

8.9.4 Drug Delivery

Delivery of drugs to patients in the most physiologically acceptable manner has always been an important concern in drug delivery medicine. In general, the smaller the dimensions of the drug and the coating material required to encapsulate the drug, the better the drug is absorbed by the human being. A wide variety of polymeric materials have been used as delivery matrices, and the choice of the delivery vehicle polymer is determined by the requirements of the specific applications. Drug delivery with polymer nanofibers is based on the principle that the dissolution rate of a particulate drug increases with increasing surface area of both the drug and the corresponding carrier if necessary. For controlled drug delivery, in addition to their larger surface area, polymer nanofibers also have other advantages. For example, unlike common encapsulation involving some complicated preparation process, therapeutic compounds can be conveniently incorporated into the carrier polymers using electrospinning. The resulting nanofibrous membrane containing drugs can be applied topically for skin and wound healing applications, or post-processed for other kinds of drug release. However, thus far, the study on drugs encapsulated by polymer nanofibers is still limited.

Kenawy et al. (2002) studied the delivery of tetracycline hydrochloride based on the fibrous delivery matrices of poly(ethylene-co-vinylacetate), PLA, and their blend (50:50), based on electrospun nanofibrous scaffolds for the delivery of tetracycline hydrochloride. The results demonstrated that the initial rate of release of tetracycline from the scaffold is high during the first 10 to 12 h, probably due to the release of the drug sequestered on the nanofiber surface. Electrospun PEVA showed a higher release rate when compared to the electrospun nanofiber meshes of pure PLA or PLA-PEVA blend. The results indicated that the rate of release of the drug can be controlled by modulating the ratio of PLA and PEVA in the polymeric blend. Therefore, the nanofibrous delivery system showed potential to be employed in the treatment of periodontal diseases. Ignatious and Baldoni (2001) described electrospun polymer nanofibers for pharmaceutical compositions, which can be designed to provide rapid, immediate, delayed, or modified dissolution, such as sustained and/or pulsatile release characteristics. As the drug and carrier materials can be mixed together for electrospinning of nanofibers, the likely modes of the drug in the resulting nanostructure products are: (1) drug as particles attached to the surface of the carrier, which is in the form of nanofibers; (2) both drug and carrier are nanofiber-form, hence the end product will be the two kinds of nanofibers interlaced together; (3) the blend of drug and carrier materials integrated into one kind of fiber containing both components; and (4) the carrier material is electrospun into a tubular form in which the drug particles are encapsulated. Modes (3) and (4) may be preferred. However, as the drug delivery in the form of nanofibers is still in the early stages of exploration, a real delivery mode after production and efficiency has yet to be realized.

8.9.5 Tissue Scaffolds

The emerging field of tissue engineering can be considered as an outgrowth of the advanced polymer nanotechnology. Since human cells can attach and organize well around the fibers with diameters smaller than those of the cells, polymer nanofibers have enormous potential for use in engineering mechanically stable and biologically functional scaffolds suitable for tissue reconstructions. For the treatment of tissues or organs malfunctioning in a human body, one of the challenges to the field of tissue engineering/biomaterials is the design of ideal scaffolds/synthetic matrices that can mimic the structure and biological functions of the natural ECM. In this regard, nanoscale fibrous scaffolds are suitable for replicating the physical structure of the natural ECM and can provide an optimal template for cells to attach, migrate, and grow. The successful regeneration of biological tissues and organs calls for the development of fibrous structures with fiber architectures beneficial for cell deposition and cell proliferation. Of particular interest in tissue engineering is the creation of structurally stable and biologically functional 3D scaffolds.

Biodegradable polymeric nanofibrous scaffolds are generally recognized as one of the key determinant factors for the success of tissue engineering. It is believed that converting polymers into fibers and networks that mimic native structures will ultimately enhance the utility of these materials, as large diameter fibers do not mimic the morphological characteristics of the native fibrils. Polymer nanofibers have been considered for use as scaffolds for engineering tissues, such as skin, cartilage, bone, blood vessel, heart, and nerve. The tissue engineering applications of polymer nanofibers are discussed in detail in Chapter 10.

8.10 Summary

This chapter deals with the structure, property, and applications of polymeric biomaterials with their recent advances. Recently, polymers in the form of nanofibers have been considered for use in various biomedical applications, owing to their functional properties compared to their microscale counterparts. There are multiple methods available for processing polymer nanofibers. Among them, electrospinning is recognized as one of the most practical methods, owing to its mass production rate, cost effectiveness, versatility, and simplicity. The past decade has seen considerable efforts in the use of polymer nanofibers for various biomedical applications, including tissue engineering, drug delivery, wound dressing, medical, and dental implants. The majority of current investigations has made use of the advantage of high surface area to volume and length to diameter ratios of polymer nanofibers, but other features in terms of mechanical, physical, chemical, and biological properties are needed to explore and realize the full potential of polymer nanofibers. Overall, polymers are a versatile class of biomaterials, and polymers in the form of nanofibers are a relatively new generation of biomaterials, the so-called nanobiomaterials.

Glossary

Biodegradable polymer: A polymer that is able to decompose by means of biological activity.

Biodegradation: Decomposition of a material or implant by biological activity.

Collagen: A fibrous protein with a triple-helical structure that functions to hold tissues together.

Decalcification: A process of removal of calcium.

Deproteination: A process of removal of proteins.

Electrospinning: A process that essentially employs electrostatic forces to produce polymer fibers, ranging in diameter from a few microns down to tens of nanometers.

Free radicals: Highly reactive molecules capable of oxidizing other molecules.

Homopolymer: A polymer consisting of only one type of repeat unit.

Implant: Any medical device made from single or multiphase materials intended for human health care.

Molecular weight: The sum of the atomic weights of all atoms in a molecule.

Monomer: A simple molecule entity that combines with others to form a polymer.

Nano: A unit prefix meaning one billionth (1/1,000,000,000).

Nanofiber: A fiber that has nanoscale dimensions.

Polymer: A substance consisting of a long molecule of repeated subunits.

Polymerization: A chemical reaction in which two or more small molecules (monomer) combine to form larger molecules (polymer).

Prosthesis: A medical device that is capable of replacing the organs or tissues of the body.

Scaffold: A temporary supporting structure for growing cells and tissues.

Self-assembly: A process of atoms and molecules adhering in a self-regulating fashion by weak chemical bonds to generate structural organization over many length scales.

van der Waals force: A weak physical force that holds together two molecules or two different parts of the same molecule.

EXERCISES

8.1 Define monomer and polymer and provide some example.
8.2 What is polymerization and what are their types?
8.3 What are the differences between addition and condensation polymerization?
8.4 Classify various types of polymers according to their arrangement of monomer repeated units.
8.5 Name the two types of polymers with respect to their degradation behavior and give some examples.
8.6 What are the key factors influencing the properties of polymers?
8.7 Define nanofiber. What are the methods for the processing of polymer nanofiber?
8.8 Explain the mechanism involved in electrospinning and provide some examples of polymers that have been electro spun.
8.9 What are the major components of electrospinning?
8.10 Name the different types of fiber collectors and describe their purpose.
8.11 What are the biomedical applications of polymer nanofibers?

References

Beniash, E. et al. 2005. Self-assembling peptide amphiphile nanofiber matrices for cell entrapment. *Acta Biomater.* 1:387.

Bognitzki, M. et al. 2001. Nanostructured fibers via electrospinning. *Adv. Mater.* 13:70.

Boland, E. D. et al. 2003. Tailoring tissue engineering scaffolds using electrostatic processing techniques: A study of poly(glycolic acid) electrospinning. *J. Macromol. Sci. Pure Appl. Chem.* A38:1231.

Buchko, C. J., K. M. Kozloff, and D. C. Martin. 2001. Surface characterization of porous, biocompatible protein polymer thin films. *Biomaterials* 22:1289.

Feng, L. et al. 2002. Super-hydrophobic surface of aligned polyacrylonitrile nanofibers. *Angew Chem. Int. Ed.* 41:1221.

Fong, H. 2003. Nylon 6 nanofiber reinforced BIS-GMA/TEGDMA dental restorative composite resins. *Polymer Preprint* 44:100.

Hartgerink, J. D., E. Beniash, and S. I. Stupp. 2001. Self-assembly and mineralization of peptide-amphiphile nanofibers. *Science* 294:1684.

Huang, Z. M. et al. 2003. A review on polymer nanofibers by electrospinning and their applications in nanocomposites. *Comp. Sci. Tech.* 63:2223.

———. 2004. Electrospinning and mechanical characterization of gelatin nanofibers. *Polymer* 45:5361.

Ignatious, F. and J. M. Baldoni. 2001. US Patent No. PCT/US01/02399.

Kenawy, E. R. et al. 2002. Release of tetracycline hydrochloride from electrospun poly(ethylene-co-vinylacetate), poly(lactic acid), and a blend. *J. Control. Rel.* 81:57.

———. 2003. Electrospinning of poly(ethylene-co-vinyl alcohol) fibers. *Biomaterials* 24:907.

Matthews, J. A. et al. 2002. Electrospinning of collagen nanofibers. *Biomacromolecules* 3:232.

Murugan, R. and S. Ramakrishna. 2006. Nano-featured scaffolds for tissue engineering: Spinning methodologies. *Tissue Eng.* 12:435.

Ohkawa, K. et al. 2004. Electrospinning of chitosan. *Macromol. Rapid Commun.* 25:1600.

Ondarcuhu, T. and C. Joachim. 1998. Drawing a single nanofibre over hundreds of microns. *Europhys. Lett.* 42:215.

Valentine, J., S. Blocker, and J. Chang. 1984. Gunshot injuries in children. *J. Trauma* 24:952.

Yang, F. et al. 2004. Fabrication of nano-structured porous PLLA scaffold intended for nerve tissue engineering. *Biomaterials* 25:1891.

———. 2005. Electrospinning of nano/micro scale poly(L-lactic acid) aligned fibers and their potential in neural tissue engineering. *Biomaterials* 26:2603.

You, Y. et al. 2005. Effect of solution properties on nanofibrous structure of electrospun poly(lactic-co-glycolic acid). *J. Appl. Polym. Sci.* 99:1214.

Zong, X. et al. 2002. Structure and process relationship of electrospun bioabsorbable nanofiber membranes. *Polymer* 43:4403.

9

Composite Biomaterials

9.1 Introduction

Single-phase components (also called monolithic) do not always provide all the properties necessary for a given application, which leads to the concept of composites. For better understanding, the relationship between stiffness and strength of some of the widely used biomaterials are shown in Figure 9.1 (Mano et al. 2004). It can be seen from the figure that metals and ceramics are stiffer and possess higher strength than biological hard tissues, whilst polymers mostly possess lower modulus and can have strengths of the same order of magnitude as hard tissues. It should be noted that biological hard tissues exhibit larger spectra of mechanical properties than the monolithic biomaterials. Therefore, there is a need for compounding various monolithic biomaterials in order to obtain composite biomaterials that have mechanical properties quite similar to those of biological hard tissues. It is also noted that the mechanical and biological properties of the hydroxyapatite (HA)/collagen composites are better than their constituents and quite similar to biological hard tissues. Thus composites are a better choice for a variety of biomedical applications than the monolithic biomaterials. In addition, there is a possibility of tailoring their properties better than their each constituent, and to eliminate or minimize the problems associated with the monolithic biomaterials. These facts greatly increase the use of composites in a variety of biomedical applications.

Composite can be defined as a heterogeneous combination of two or more materials, differing in morphology or composition on a microscale, in which one of the materials, called the reinforcing phase, is in the form of fibers or particles, and is embedded in the other material, called the matrix phase (see Figure 9.2). The term "composite biomaterials" refers to those composites that are biocompatible on implantation. The reinforcing material and the matrix material can be metal, ceramic, or polymer. Typically, reinforcing materials are strong with low densities, while the matrix is usually a ductile, or tough, material. The major role of matrix material is (i) to bind the reinforcing materials together, (ii) to transfer stresses between the

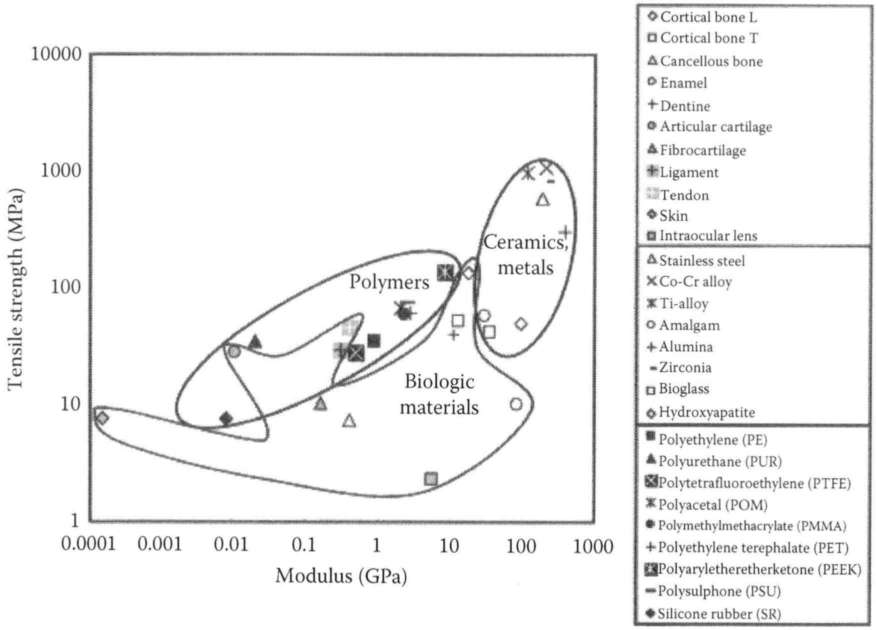

FIGURE 9.1
Tensile strength vs. modulus of biomaterials with relevance for composite design. (Reprinted from Mano, J. F. et al., *Comp. Sci. Tech.*, 64, 789, 2004. With permission from Elsevier.)

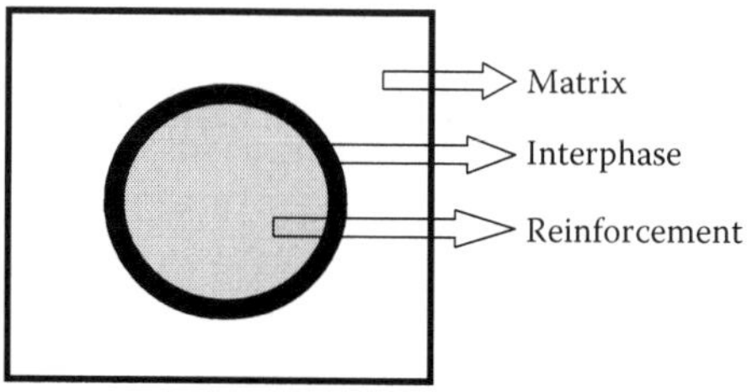

FIGURE 9.2
Schematic representation of constituents of composite biomaterials.

reinforcing materials, and (iii) to protect them against environmental attack and damage due to mechanical abrasion. By selecting the right combination of reinforcing material and matrix material, it is possible to obtain a composite biomaterial with a wide range of mechanical and biological properties, which are not available in monolithic biomaterial; thereby, performance of the composite biomaterials with host tissues can be improved on implantation.

9.2 Classification of Composite Biomaterials

Composite biomaterials are generally classified on the basis of the geometry of the reinforcing materials (see Figure 9.3). The reinforcing materials in the composites may be fibers (called fibrous composites) or particles (called particulate composites). The following sections briefly address the processing aspects of those composite biomaterials.

9.2.1 Fibrous Composite Biomaterials

By the incorporation of fibers in a polymer matrix, it is possible to increase the stiffness, strength, fatigue life, and other mechanical properties of the composites. Fibers are widely used to achieve mechanically strong composite biomaterials. There are four types of fibers used as reinforcing materials: (i) carbon fibers (CF), (ii) ceramic fibers (e.g., alumina), (iii) polymer fibers (e.g., PET), and (iv) metal fibers (e.g., stainless steel wire). Among them, CFs are the most widely used reinforcing material in the development of composite biomaterials because of their biocompatibility, bioinertness, and favorable mechanical properties. Numerous medical devices, such as bone plates and screws, hip replacement stems, dental posts, brackets, and arch wires, are fabricated using CF-reinforced composites, which are also discussed in detail in Section 7.4. It is worth mentioning that CFs are mainly produced from precursors of polyacrylonitrile (PAN), pitch, and rayon. Among them, PAN-based CFs possess superior strength. From a biomaterials points of view; CFs are extensively used as a mechanical enhancer and are used exclusively in combination with polymer matrix material (e.g., high-density polyethylene; HDPE) in the development of mechanically improved composites for load-bearing applications.

The CF-reinforced HDPE composites can be produced by extrusion compounding and injection molding (Sousa et al. 2003). In brief, short CF (25 wt.%)

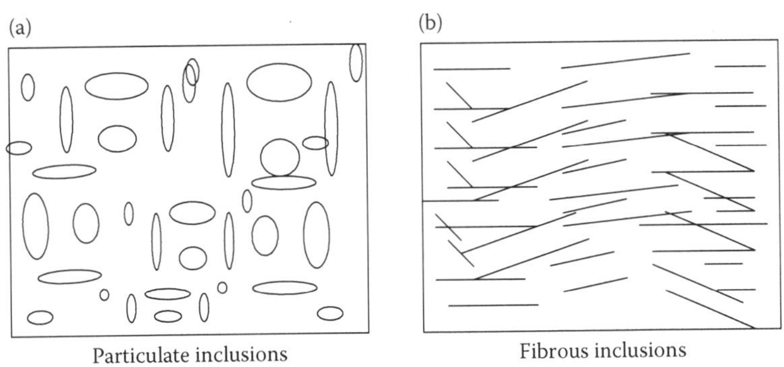

FIGURE 9.3
Types of reinforcing materials.

reinforced composites of HDPE were compounded in twin screw extrusion using a temperature profile between 160°C and 210°C. Separate polymer and fiber feeding ports were used in order to avoid fiber breakage that would eventually occur during the simultaneous conveying of the solid pellets and the CFs before the melting of the polymer phase. The extrude was chopped manually in 60-mm long segments for subsequent injection molding. In order to assess the reinforcement efficiency of CFs, the composites were compounded and molded into dumb-bell tensile test specimens with rectangular cross section (4×9 mm^2) in a single processing stage, using a compounding injection molding. The device combines a corotating twin screw extruder with an injection molding unit machine. It is worth mentioning that the main advantages of compounding injection molding for the processing of thermoplastic polymer-based (e.g., HDPE) composites as compared to the traditional approach are the single heat history, the reduction of molecular degradation, the superior maintenance of fiber morphology, and the reduction of fiber damage due to the elimination of extra handling granulation step. In order to minimize fiber breakage during the compounding step, the feeding of the CFs was performed using a separate port after melting the HDPE. The properties of the composites have been assessed and found that they possess excellent strength, stiffness, and fatigue resistance. The morphological structure of the composite is shown in Figure 9.4. The composite exhibits a shell/core morphology with very distinct orientation patterns at both the shell and core regions, which constrains the mechanical performance exhibited. The experimental results confirmed that mechanically strong polymer composite materials can be manufactured by compounding and injection molding technique.

9.2.2 Particulate Composite Biomaterials

By the incorporation of particulate in a polymer matrix, it is possible to stiffen or harden the composites; thereby, obtaining mechanically strong composite biomaterials. Until recently, only ceramic particles have been used as reinforcing materials. For example, HA particulate-reinforced polymers are widely used in bone and dental restoration because of their excellent mechanical behavior. In the 1980s, Bonfield and group proposed the use of HA particulate-reinforced HDPE composites, introducing the so-called bone analog concept (Bonfield et al. 1981). The research motivation was the development of new generation composite biomaterials having adequate mechanical and biological behavior that allows for their use in hard tissue applications. They found that the mechanical behavior of the composites depends on characteristics of HA particulate. The HA particle size and respective distribution greatly influences the mechanical properties of the composites. For example, stiffness of the HDPE/HA composite is propositional to the HA volume fraction. Nevertheless, although the HA particulates increase the composites stiffness and enhance the creep behavior, the higher the HA content, the higher the number of interfaces between

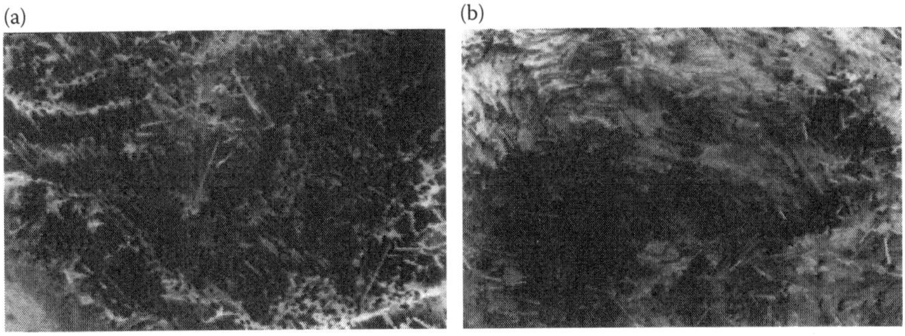

FIGURE 9.4
Scanning electron microscopy micrographs of HDPE/C fibrous composite biomaterials produced by compounding injection molding: (a) shell zone and (b) core region. (Reprinted from Sousa, R. A. et al., *Comp. Sci. Tech.*, 63, 389, 2003. With permission from Elsevier.)

the polymer and the ceramic, which has to be taken into account, since failure can preferentially occur at the interface when the implant is under mechanical loading.

The development of HA particulate-reinforced HDPE composites with high mechanical specification was recently reported (Di Silvio et al. 2002) and their *in vitro* cellular behavior using primary human osteoblasts (HOB) was also studied. The authors developed HDPE/HA composites by incorporation of HA particulate, at 20 and 40 vol.% of HA, into HDPE matrix material through twin screw extrusion and compression molding. The blocks were machined into 13-mm discs with a controlled machining process, in order to reduce topographical differences. The manufacturing conditions and machining process were carefully controlled to give a reproducible material surface roughness with minimal batch variation. A representative scanning electron micrograph (SEM) of the surface of the composite is shown in Figure 9.5, which indicates the distribution of HA throughout the polymer matrix. The effect of surface composition was examined *in vitro* using HOB. The cells were seeded onto the test materials (HDPE/HA), containing 20 and 40 vol.% of HA, at a density of 7×10^5 cells mL^{-1}, followed by incubation at 37°C in humidified air with 5% CO_2 for various time periods. A few representative SEM micrographs of cell-cultured composites are shown in Figure 9.6. SEM observations of cell-cultured test materials showed normal osteoblast morphology, in which most of the cells were in the process of cell division. The results also indicated that there is an increased number of dividing cells found on the material containing 40 vol.% of HA. Further, the results showed that material containing 40 vol.% of HA enhanced cellular activity by increasing proliferation rate and differentiation compared to the material containing 20 vol.% of HA. The overall experimental results obtained have shown that the volume of HA has a significant effect on the bioactivity of the composites. Although both the composites provided a favorable site for cell adhesion, growth, proliferation, and differentiation, the

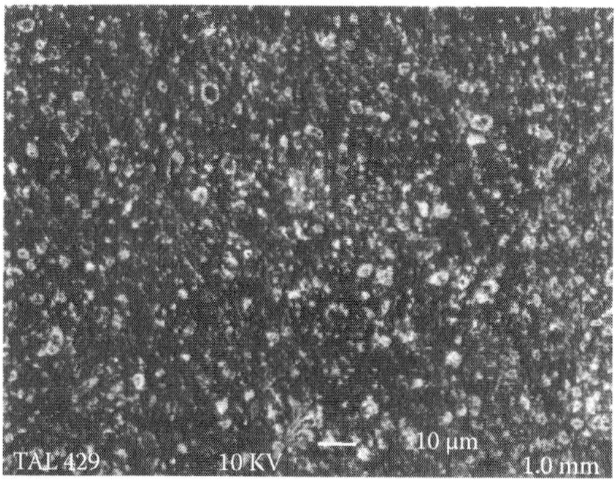

FIGURE 9.5
Scanning electron micrograph of the surface of HDPE/HA, showing the distribution of HA throughout the polymer matrix. (Reprinted from Di Silvio, L., Dalby, M. J., and Bonfield, W., *Biomaterials*, 23, 101, 2002. With permission from Elsevier.)

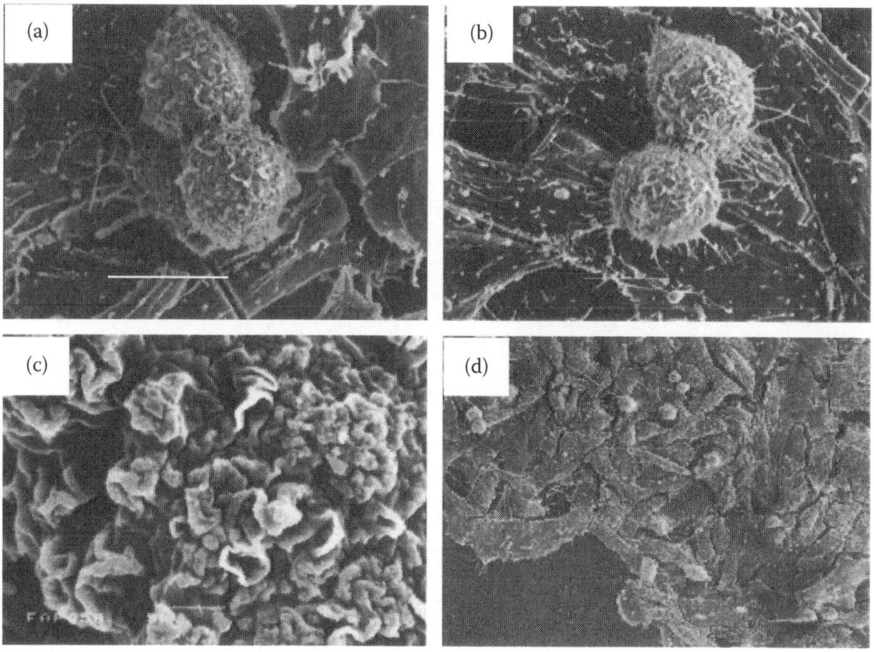

FIGURE 9.6
Scanning electron micrographs of HOB cells cultured onto HDPE/HA containing (a) 20 vol.% of HA, (b) 40 vol.% of HA, (c) magnified view of HOB cell surface morphology during division, and (d) HOB cell layer approaching confluence on composite matrix with many dividing cells. (Reprinted from Di Silvio, L., Dalby, M. J., and Bonfield, W., *Biomaterials*, 23, 101, 2002. With permission from Elsevier.)

composite containing 40 vol.% of HA appeared to produce highly organized collagenous matrix, and high levels of alkaline phosphatase (ALP) activity; thus, this material may be a better choice than the composite containing 20 vol.% of HA for hard tissue applications.

9.3 Biological Responses to Composite Biomaterials

Composite biomaterials implanted at the defective site of the human body tend to elicit a certain response from the host tissue, depending on their characteristics, particularly surface reactivity. According to their interaction with host tissues, the composite biomaterials can be classified into three types: (i) nearly bioinert composites, (ii) bioactive composites, and (iii) bioresorbable composites. The nearly bioinert composite materials refer to any composite that has minimal interaction with their surrounding tissue on implantation. This type of material generally does not cause any response from their host tissues because they neither chemically nor biologically bond to living tissue. This is because this type of biomaterial has already reacted with another reactive substance. As a result, cells can live adjacent to the composites, but do not form a bond with them. Alumina-coated biometals, carbon/carbon, and carbon/polyaryletheretherketone (PEEK) are a few notable examples. The bioactive composite materials refer to any composite that elicits a specific biological response at the interface, which results in the formation of a bond between the host tissues and the implanted material. HA/collagen, HA/PE, and HA/Ti-6Al-4V are a few notable examples of bioactive composites. The bioresorbable composite refers to any composite material that has the ability to undergo resorption over time upon implantation. TCP/collagen, TCP/PLA, and TCP/PCL are a few examples of this kind of bioresorbable composite.

9.4 Biomedical Applications of Composite Biomaterials

Composite biomaterials are mostly used in hard tissue repair or regenerative applications (see Figure 9.7), owing to their mechanical consistency that matches biological hard tissues. A graphical representation of mechanical consistency of various composite materials is given in Figure 9.8 in comparison with a natural bone, which suggests that polymer-based composites possess mechanical consistency quite similar to natural bone. It may also be noted that most of the biological hard tissues, such as bone, cartilage, and tooth are essentially made of composites constituted by several

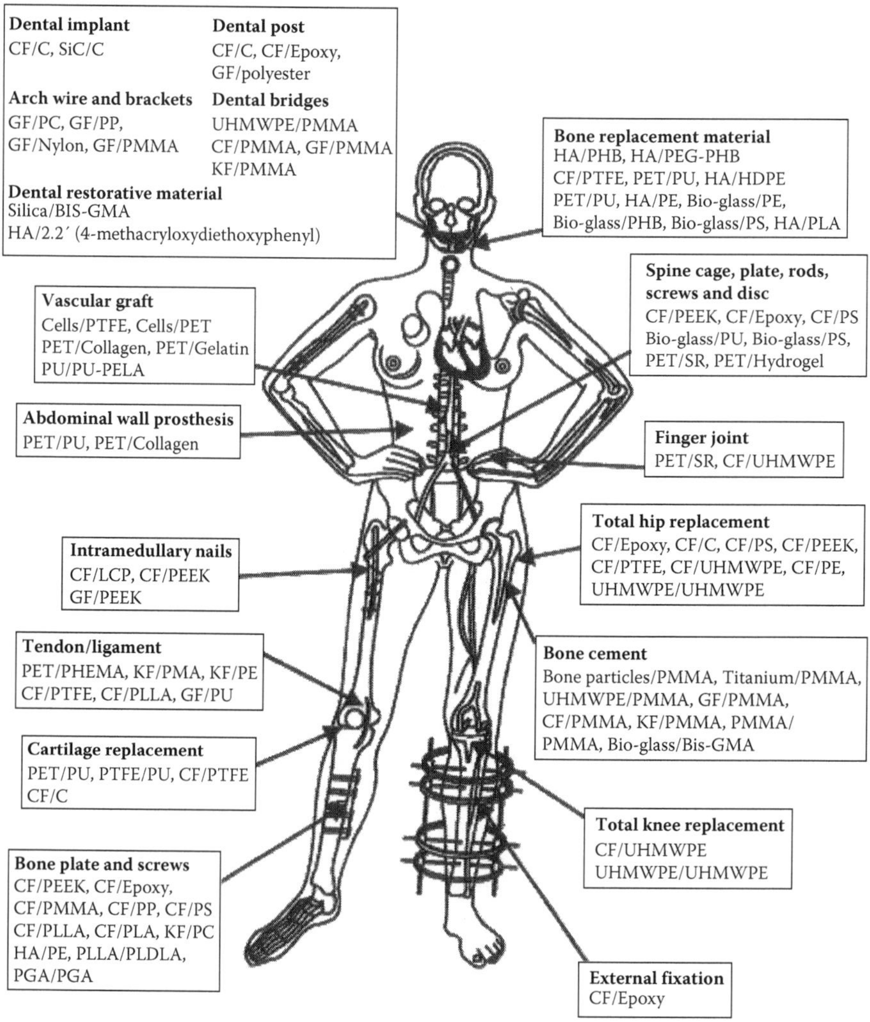

FIGURE 9.7
Clinical uses of composite biomaterials. (Reprinted from Ramakrishna, S. et al., *Comp. Sci. Tech.*, 61, 1189, 2001. With permission from Elsevier.)

organic and inorganic materials, which further stimulate the use of composite biomaterials for hard tissue applications. The composite, therefore, can be treated as the only material that uniquely exhibits a range of properties equivalent to bone, and thus it could be possible to eliminate some of the problems associated with current synthetic bone repair biomaterials. In this section, some of the widely used composite biomaterials in hard tissue applications reported in the literature over the last three decades are presented.

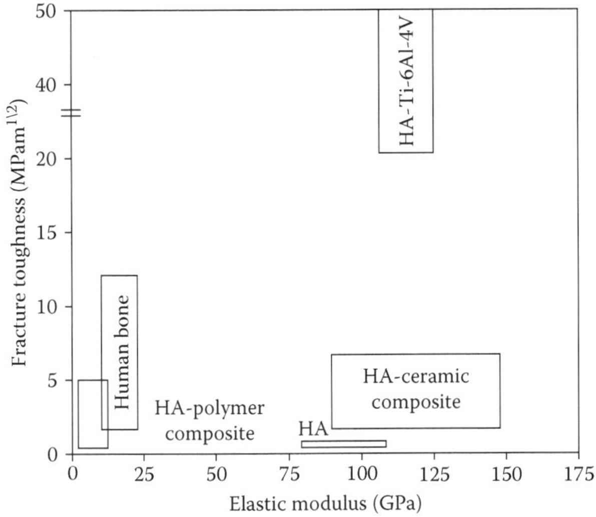

FIGURE 9.8
Mechanical consistency of various HA-based composite biomaterials. (Reprinted from Murugan, R. and Ramakrishna, S., *Comp. Sci. Tech.*, 65, 2385, 2005. With permission from Elsevier.)

9.4.1 Bone Fracture Repair

Bone is a complex and highly specialized form of connective tissue providing the supporting structure for the body. Bone is often called dynamic tissue because it has the capability of self-remodeling according to the applied mechanical environment, which is generally known as Wolff's law. Density of the living bone is influenced by the stress condition applied to the bone. Higher applied stress leads to denser bone. Conversely, if the applied stress is lower than the normal physiological load, the bone mass decreases, leading to bone weakening. Bone is generally weak in tension and shear, particularly along the longitudinal plane.

There are many types of bone fractures depending on the crack size, orientation, morphology, and location. Bone fractures are treated in several ways, depending on the patient's degree of skeletal maturity, the amount of displacement, the type of break, and the presence of associated injuries. Bone fracture repair may be broadly grouped into two types, namely, external fixation and internal fixation. External fixation approach is currently employed in the management of severe soft tissue injuries associated with unstable long bone fractures or significant joint injuries. They are commonly used for multiple fractures in trauma or burns, and for stabilizing pelvis diastasis or fractures. In the external fixation approach, the bone fragments are held in alignment through various means, such as splints, casts, braces, and external fixator systems, in order to maintain the reduction. Most of the external fixation systems are generally made of metals, such as stainless steel and Ti-based alloys. These metallic construct are heavy, which reduces the surgeon's ability to visualize the fracture by x-rays, and limits the ability to fine-tune the limb alignment, which ultimately leads to the search for new materials. Composite materials have unique advantages for use in external fixation of fractures because of their excellent fatigue behavior, high stiffness and strength, low density, radiolucency, and ability to be designed into various shapes. A composite external fixator frame made of CF-reinforced epoxy matrix has been designed, in order to address concerns with current metallic external fixator frames. This composite frame has been used clinically for treating multiple trauma patients with pelvic diastasis, in order to reduce the intrapelvic volume and stabilize the pelvis. Casting materials or plaster bandages are generally used to form splints, casts, or braces. The casting material essentially is a composite material made of woven cotton fabrics (woven gauze) and Plaster of Paris matrix (calcium sulfate). Other reinforcements include fabrics of glass and polyester fibers. Recently, casts made of glass or polyester fiber fabrics, and water-activated polyurethanes are gaining much interest. An ideal cast material should be easy to handle, lightweight, conformable to anatomical shape, strong, stiff, waterproof, radiolucent, and easy to remove. Moreover, it should be permeable to ventilation without which the patient's skin may be scorched or weakened.

In the internal fixation approach, the bone fragments are held together by different ways using implants. The most common types of internal fixation are plates, screws, wires, and nails or rods used inside the body to support the bone directly. Some of the fixation devices are shown in Figure 9.9. Plates are like internal splints that hold the fractured ends of bone together. The plates

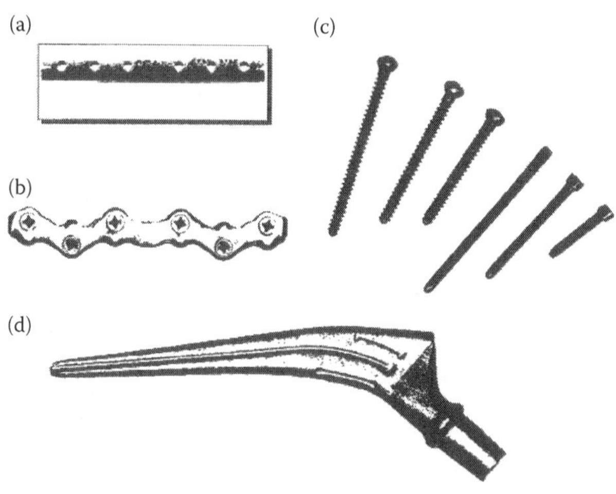

FIGURE 9.9
Examples of medical devices made of composite biomaterials. (a, b) Bone plates made of CF/epoxy and CF/PEEK, respectively, (c) bone screws made of CF/PEEK, and (d) a hip joint stem made of CF/PEEK. (Reprinted from Ramakrishna, S. et al., *Comp. Sci. Tech.*, 61, 1189, 2001. With permission from Elsevier.)

are fixed over the fractured site and are screwed in place. Bone plates may be left in place or removed after bone healing is completed. Bone screws are used for internal fixation more often than any other type of implant. Although the bone screw is a simple device, there are several designs based on how the screw will be used. It can be used alone to hold a fracture, as well as with plates, rods, or nails. Bone screws may be designed for a specific type of fracture. Like bone plate, screws may be left in place, or removed after the bone healing is completed. Materials used for the manufacture of bone plates and screws are discussed in subsection 9.4.1.1. Wires are often used as sutures or threads to "sew" the bones back together. They can be used in conjunction with other forms of internal fixation to hold bones together. They can also be used alone to treat fractures of small bones, such as those found in the hand or foot. In some fractures of the long bones, the best way to align the bone ends is by inserting a rod or nail through the hollow center of the bone that normally contains some marrow. They may be left in the bone after healing is completed. Pins, screws, and rods are also used to construct external fixators, such as frames and rings. Although they are outside the body, the screws and pins go through the skin and muscle to connect to the bone. In this way, they differ from casts and splints, which rely solely on external support.

Conventional fixation implants are made of stainless steel, Co-Cr, or Ti alloys. The surgeon's experience and the type of fracture will judge the bone fracture treatment method. Surgical wires and pins are the simplest implants used to hold the small fragments of bones together. For example, wires are used to reattach the greater trochanter, which is often detached during total hip joint replacement. They are also used to provide additional stability in long oblique or spiral fractures of long bones (femur, humerus, radius, ulna, tibia, and fibula). The most widely used bone screws are cortical bone screws (with smaller threads) and cancellous screws (with larger threads). They are used either to directly fasten bone fragments together or to attach a plate to the fractured bone. However, proper implant design and surgical technique must be utilized to ensure the desired biomechanical outcome of the fixation and to avoid additional tissue trauma and devascularization at the fracture site. The role of composite biomaterials for the development of bone plates and screws are summarized in the following section.

9.4.1.1 Bone Plates and Screws

Plate and screw fixation is the most popular method for rigid internal fixation of the fractured bone. The function of bone plate and screw construct depends on the stability requirements of a particular fracture. Plate-screw constructs can act as load-bearing implants in conjunction with bone grafts, depending on fracture reduction and fragment interference. The plates are typically placed across a fracture with the help of screws in order to neutralize the effect of bending, rotational, and other axial forces on the fracture site.

The bone plates are mostly made of stainless steel, Cr-Co, and Ti alloys. The rigid fixation is designed to provide high axial pressures (also known as dynamic compression) in the fragments of the bone, which facilitate primary bone healing without the formation of external callus. This method allows the exercise of joints near the fracture site just after the operation. After complete bone healing has been obtained by the plate fixation, normally it takes from one to two years after the operation, the plate and screws are removed. However, the rigid fixation is not free from complications which results in bone atrophy beneath the plate. There is a possibility of refracture of bone after the removal of the plates due to bone atrophy. This is attributed to the stress-shielding effect. It may be noted that the modulus of stainless steel (210–230 GPa) is much higher than the 10–18 GPa modulus of the bone. The stiffness mismatch results in a situation where the plate transmits the majority of the stress, and the bone directly beneath the plate experiences less stress even after the fracture has been repaired. The bone underneath the plate adapts to the low stress and becomes less dense and weak. Therefore, the strength of the healed bone is low. Consequently, there is a possibility of bone refracture upon removal of the fixation plate. The stress-shielding effect is more pronounced with the stainless-steel plates than the Ti-alloy plates. It may be noted that the modulus of stainless steel (230 GPa) is higher than that of Ti alloy (110 GPa). This example suggests that "less rigid fixation plates" diminish the stress-shielding problem and it is desirable to use plates whose mechanical properties are close to those of the bone.

As an alternative approach, polymer composite materials are nowadays gaining much interest for use in the fabrication of bone plates, owing to their high strength and bone-like modulus. A typical composite bone plate made of CF/epoxy and CF/PEEK is shown in Figure 9.9a and b, respectively. The polymer composite bone plates may be grouped into nonresorbable, partially resorbable, and fully resorbable bone plates. The nonresorbable composite plates are made of either thermoset polymer composites or thermoplastic composite materials. CF/epoxy and GF/epoxy are a few notable examples of nonresorbable thermoset composites. Some researchers expressed concern over the toxic effects of monomers in partially cured epoxy composite materials (Peluso et al. 1991); hence, research activity on these materials gradually decreased as the technology for making good quality thermoplastic composites made available. CF/PMMA, CF/PE, and CF/PEEK are a few notable examples of nonresorbable thermoplastic composite bone plates. Unlike the thermoset composites, the thermoplastic composites are considered free from the complications associated with unused monomers. Moreover, similar to metal alloy plates, thermoplastic composite plates can be bent or contoured with heating to the shape of the bone at the time of surgery. Currently, there is insufficient data on the long-term *in vivo* behavior of nonresorbable thermoplastic composite materials. Among various materials investigated, the CF/PEEK is reportedly biocompatible and has good resistance to hydrolysis and radiation degradation. Other promising properties include high strength, fatigue resistance, and biological inertness with no mutagenicity or carcinogenicity. These features ultimately lead to minimal tissue responses to polymer composite bone plates.

As another kind of fixation device, bone screws have been developed using various polymer composite biomaterials. There are two types of materials used for the manufacture of bone screws, namely, nonresorbable and resorbable materials. CF/carbon and CF/PEEK are notable examples of nonresorbable types of materials used for the manufacture of bone screws (see Figure 9.9c). A combination of polymer composite plates and screws overcomes the corrosion problem faced by the metal plates and screws. The nonresorbable polymer composite materials are designed to be stable in *in vivo* conditions with no change in the plate stiffness with implantation time. As bone healing progresses, it is desirable that the bone is subjected to a gradual increase of stress, thus reducing the stress-shielding effect. In other words, the stress on the plate should decrease with time, whereas the stress on the bone should increase. This is only possible if the plate loses rigidity in the *in vivo* environment. The nonresorbable polymer composites do not display this desired characteristic. To meet this need, researchers introduced resorbable polymers for bone plate and screw applications. Polylactide (PLA), poly(glycolic acid) (PGA), and their copolymers are good examples of resorbable types of materials used for the manufacture of bone screws and plates. Choueka et al. (1995) proposed fully resorbable composites by reinforcing resorbable matrices with resorbable fibers (poly(L-lactic acid) (PLLA) fibers and calcium phosphate-based glass fibers). One of the advantages often cited for resorbable composite prostheses is that they need not be removed with a second operative procedure, as is recommended with metallic or nonresorbable composite implants. The maximum mechanical property of resorbable materials continues to be a limitation and hence they are limited to only applications where the loads are moderate. In order to improve mechanical properties, the resorbable polymers are reinforced with variety of nonresorbable materials, including CFs. Due to the nonresorbable nature of the reinforcements used, these composites are called partially resorbable composites. According to Zimmerman et al. (1987), the CF/PLA composite possessed superior mechanical properties. However, they lost mechanical properties too rapidly in *in vivo* environments because of delamination. Further work is necessary to tailor the composite materials such that the resorption of the plate and the healing rate of the bone are synchronized.

9.4.2 Joint Replacements

Joints are formed by the ends of two or more bones connected by tissue called cartilage, which enable the movement of the body and its parts. Healthy cartilage serves as a protective cushion, allowing smooth, low-friction movement of the joint. If the cartilage becomes damaged by disease or injury, the tissues around the joint become inflamed, causing pain. With time, the cartilage wears away, allowing the rough edges of bone to rub against each other, causing more pain. When only some of the joint is damaged, a surgeon may be able to repair or replace just the damaged parts. When the entire joint is damaged, a total joint replacement is carried out. To replace a total hip or knee joint, a surgeon removes the diseased or damaged parts and inserts artificial parts, called prostheses or implants. These prostheses are considered medical devices. There are certain issues and regulations, as governed by the U.S. food and drug administration (FDA), regarding the use of these devices for clinical uses. The most common reason for having a hip or knee replaced is osteoarthritis disease. Osteoarthritis is one of the common causes for joint degeneration and sometimes hypertrophic changes in the bone and cartilage of joints in middle-aged people. This is associated with progressive wearing down of opposing joint surfaces with consequent distortion of joint position. Joints also become damaged upon exposure to severe mechanical or metabolic injury.

Over the years, a number of artificial joints have been designed to replace or augment many joints in the body. Unlike those used to treat bone fractures, the artificial joints are placed permanently in the body. The extensive bone and cartilage removed during implantation makes this procedure irreversible. Considering the extent of loading, the complexity of joint function, and the severity of the physiological environment, joint replacement is one of the most demanding of all the implant applications in the body. The most commonly used artificial joints are total hip replacement (THR) and total knee replacement (TKR). The following section addresses the role of composite biomaterials in THR applications.

9.4.2.1 Total Hip Replacement

Joint replacement surgery has revolutionized the treatment of arthritis of the hip, particularly in the older person. The hip joint is a ball and socket, which allows a wide range of motion. A typical hip joint consists of a cup-type acetabular component, and a femoral component whose head is designed to fit into the acetabular cup, thus enabling joint articulations. The shaft of the femoral component (also called femoral stem) is tapered such that it can be fixed into a reamed medullary canal of the femur. The bones of the hip joint are covered by cartilage that protects the bones while allowing easy motion. Surrounding the hip joint is the synovial lining, which produces a lubricant. Tough fibers, called ligaments, connect the bones of the joint and hold them in place, while adding strength and elasticity for movement. Muscles and tendons also play an important role in keeping the hip joint stable. However, many circumstances, in particular osteoarthritis, call for hip replacement. In THR, the surgeon cuts away the ball part of the joint, replacing it with a ball attached to a stem that is wedged into a hollowed-out space in the thigh bone. Damaged cartilage and bone are removed from the socket and a cup-like component is inserted into the socket.

Today, advanced techniques and technologies have revolutionized hip replacements, allowing more patients with arthritis to consider treatments at an earlier stage than they had in the past. Several types of THRs are designed by changing the material and geometry of acetabular cups and femoral stems, and fixation methods. Conventional THRs use stainless steel, Co-Cr, and Ti alloys for the femoral shaft and neck, and Co-Cr alloy or ceramics, such as alumina and zirconia materials, for the head or ball. Earlier designs of acetabular cups were made of Co-Cr alloy. An effort to minimize friction and eliminate metallic wear on particles led Charnley, in the early 1960s, to use polymers for the acetabular component. He first implanted the stainless-steel femoral component with a mating acetabular component made of polytetrafluoroethylene (PTFE). PTFE was selected for a number of reasons. It has a high thermal stability, it is hydrophobic, stable in most types of chemical environments, and is generally considered to be inert in the body. It does not adhere to other materials. It has the lowest coefficient of friction of all solids. However, clinical studies involving PTFE acetabular cups in the THR prostheses showed unacceptably high wear and distortion. The wear debris resulted in extensive tissue reaction and even formation of granuloma. This is attributed to its low compressive stiffness and strength, and increased wear under high stresses during sliding. PTFE is no longer used in such load-bearing applications. Subsequently, acetabular cups made of ultrahigh molecular weight polyethylene (UHMWPE) were developed and found to be successful. The UHMWPE cups are usually supported with a metal backing. Some reported data suggest that creep deformation, plastic distortion, and high wear or erosion of UHMWPE is possible. Although the short-term function of UHMWPE acetabular cups is satisfactory, their long-term performance has been a concern for many years. To improve creep resistance, stiffness, and strength, researchers proposed reinforcing UHMWPE with CFs (Sclippa and Piekarski 1973) or UHMWPE fibers (Deng and Shalaby 1997). Deng and Shalaby (1997) found no appreciable difference in the wear properties of reinforced and unreinforced UHMWPE. With opposite results reported in the literature, the effect of CFs on the wear characteristics of the UHMWPE is a controversial subject. In recent years, certain designs use a dense alumina or zirconia ball and a matching acetabular cup made of similar materials mainly because of the potential advantages of ceramic materials in terms of high hardness and compressive strength, low coefficient of friction, low wear rate, and good biological acceptance of wear particles.

Although THRs are widely used, one of the major unsolved problems in this important application has been the mismatch of stiffness of the femur bone and the prosthesis. As previously mentioned, most of the hip joint stems are made from metal alloys, which are isotropic and at least five to six times stiffer than bone. It has been acknowledged that the metallic stems due to stiffness mismatch induce unphysiological stresses in the bone, thereby affecting its remodeling process. Fortunately, the advanced polymer composites can offer strength comparable to metals, and also more flexibility than metals. Strength of composite stems can be changed without affecting stiffness and vice versa. Moreover, they also offer the potential to tailor implant properties by selecting material ingredients and spatially controlling ingredient composition and configuration, which is useful in reducing the development of high stress regions. This allows one to control engineering properties, such as strength and modulus, according to the performance requirements of the prosthesis. A prosthesis made of polymer composite with spatially or locally varying mechanical properties along the boundary of the prosthesis, results in a more uniform and efficient transfer of stress from the stem to the bone. This may lead to better bone remodeling and longer implant service life. Akay and Aslan (1996) designed injection molded CF/PEEK composite stems (see Figure 9.9d), which possess a mechanical behavior similar to that of the femur. Animal studies indicated that CF/PEEK composite elicits minimal response from muscular tissue. Both *in vivo* and *in vitro* aging studies confirmed the mechanical stability of CF/PEEK up to six months (it may be noted that this period is short and further long-term testing is needed). Finite element analyses and *in vitro* measurements indicated that compared to conventional metallic stems, more favorable stresses and deformations could be generated in the femur using composite stems. Overall, the success of joint replacement has not only caused a greatly increased use of the technique, but has also provoked great interest in ways to avoid or solve the very real problems that still occur in some patients. The vast majority of patients proceed through this surgery without complication. It is ideally suited for the older individual, but in some circumstances it is appropriate for younger patients, and good long-term results can be expected.

9.4.3 Bone Graft Materials

Bone grafting is a surgical method that repairs or replaces the defective bones into healthy bones with the aid of materials or substances either from the patient's own body or from synthetic sources. The materials used for bone grafting are known as bone graft materials. They are widely used in orthopedic surgery, plastic surgery, oral and maxillofacial surgery, and dental surgery. It should be noted that bone is the second most transplanted tissue in humans. Bone graft materials not only fill defective gaps, but also eventually provide mechanical and structural support; thereby enhancing bone tissue growth. By this method, bone defect-healing time is reduced and new bone formation strengthens the defective area by bridging implanted bone graft materials with host tissues. There are a variety of bone grafting methodologies practiced, which include autografting, allografting, xenografting, and alloplastic or synthetic bone grafting, but each vary with their own advantages and disadvantages (Murugan and Ramakrishna 2006). The selection of the method of grafting to use is purely dependent on the nature and complication of the bone defects as well as the choice of available bone graft materials and, of course, the key decision depends on the surgeon's own experience.

Autografting is a class of method in which bone tissue is transplanted from one site to another site of the same individual. The concept is basically the patient's own bone collected from a donor site and transplanted to another site of the same body that requires bone regeneration. It is commonly harvested from the patient's iliac crest in the form of cancellous bone. Allografting is another kind of bone grafting method, which can be defined as tissue transplantation between individuals of the same species, but of nonidentical genetic composition. The materials used as allografts are mostly cancellous, cortical, or a combination of both. Bone banks stock this type of graft materials, which are usually harvested from cadavers. Typically, they are frozen or freeze-dried bones. Xenografting is a method of transplanting tissue from one species to another; bone from animal to human, for example. Bone banks usually stock abundant quantities of xenografts because of their easy harvesting compared to bone from human. Currently, multiple xenografts are being processed, which includes frozen calf bone, freeze-dried calf bone, decalcified ox bone, deproteinized bovine bone, and anorganic bone. As an alternative to these three types of bone grafts, synthetic substances are gaining much interest in use as bone graft materials. A surgical method that uses synthetic substances to repair or regenerate defective bone tissue is known as alloplastic or synthetic bone grafting. The synthetic substances used in bone grafting are called synthetic bone graft materials. Over the past four decades, a variety of synthetic bone graft materials have been developed, which are commonly made of ceramics (e.g., HA), polymers (e.g., PE), and their composites.

A variety of composite biomaterials have been developed for bone grafting applications. In this section, some of the widely used composite materials for bone grafting applications are discussed, including HDPE/HA, PLGA/HA, and collagen/HA. In the 1980s, Bonfield and group introduced the bone analog concept and developed bioactive composites based on HA and HDPE. It has been demonstrated that it has the capability of promoting extensive bone-bonding functions upon implantation. Later, it was commercialized under the name HAPAX™ after a thorough clinical test. Unfortunately, it is not a good biodegradable material, which limits its wider usage in clinical medicine. It is primarily used in middle ear implantation. Simultaneously, bioresorbable composites were developed and investigated as bone graft materials. For example, Laurencin et al. (1996) developed a composite containing HA and PLGA and demonstrated its cellular-compatibility suitable for bone grafting applications. It was found that the composite highly supported osteoblast proliferation, differentiation, and deposition of calcium phosphate minerals. Our group has also explored the possibility of utilizing HA, both at micro and nanolevel, in conjunction with natural (e.g., chitosan) and synthetic polymers (e.g., GMA) in the form of composites suitable for bone grafting and bone drug delivery (Murugan et al. 1998, 2002, 2004). Preliminary results suggest that this type of composite biomaterials may be a better choice for hard tissue applications.

It may be noted that most of the above composites differ from host bone either compositionally or structurally. These features are highly essential for the appreciation of better functionary of biomaterials with host tissue upon implantation. Of particular interest in this context is the combination of HA with collagen (a structural protein of the biological system) into a bioactive bone analog composite form, which appears a natural choice for bone grafting. A composite based on HA and collagen has been developed and investigated (TenHuisen et al. 1995). It shows great promise because of their resemblance to natural bone in terms of chemical composition and functional characteristics. The uniqueness of this composite lies in its spatial orientation between HA and collagen macromolecules. These unique spatial relationships in which they are organized seem to be the source of mechanical strength of the composite. Further, they found that the composite is highly biocompatible, osteoconductive, and suggested that it might be osteoinductive as well. The overall results suggested that the HA/collagen could act as a good bioactive composite for bone grafting applications. The case study evaluations of some of the bone graft materials are discussed in Chapter 9.

9.4.4 Dental Applications

Composite biomaterials are also widely used in dental filling and restoration. Dental treatment is one of the most frequent medical treatments performed on human beings. Dental treatment ranges from filling cavities (also called dental caries) to replacing fractured or decayed teeth. A large variety of materials are used in the dental treatments, such as cavity lining, cavity filling, luting, endodontic, crown and bridge, prosthetic, preventive, orthodontic, and periodontal treatment of teeth. For the benefit of readers, basic aspects of teeth are briefly described, followed by the role of composite biomaterials in dental treatments. Teeth come under the category of hard tissue. All teeth are made of two portions, crown and root, which are demarcated by the gingiva (gum). The root is placed in a socket called alveolus in the maxillary (upper) or mandibular (lower) bones. Teeth possess a thin (<1 mm) surface layer of highly mineralized (90%) dental enamel. The calcium salts of enamel are arranged as fine prisms running perpendicular to the surface. Underlying and supporting this is dentine, a less mineralized (70%) tissue that contains fine liquid-filled tubules running through to the pulp chamber. The pulp chamber carries the nerve and extends up through the root to the center of the tooth. In place of enamel, the surface of the root portion of tooth is covered by cementum, a mineralized tissue similar to bone. Teeth are nonhomogenous, anisotropic, and unsymmetrical. The structure of teeth is also amazing, since human teeth must resist or withstand various amounts and types (compression, flexural, torsion, and their mixed versions) of forces exerted during mastication or chewing and other teeth contacts that occur in a life time.

9.4.4.1 Dental Restorative Materials

Dental restorative materials, as the name suggests, are used to fill tooth cavities (caries) and sometimes to mask discoloration (veneering) or to correct contour and alignment deficiencies. Dental restorations can be classified into two types. Direct restorations are done by inserting filling material directly into the tooth. Indirect restorations are fabricated outside the mouth. Amalgam, gold, alumina, zirconia, acrylic resins, and silicate cements are commonly used for restoring decayed teeth. Amalgam and gold are mainly used in the restoration of posterior teeth, and not preferred for anterior teeth for cosmetic reasons. Moreover, there is concern over the long-term toxicity of silver–mercury amalgam fillings. Acrylic resins and silicate cements have been used for anterior teeth. However, they exhibit poor mechanical properties, which lead to short service life and clinical failures. Dental composite resins, which are translucent with a refractive index matching that of the enamel, have virtually replaced these materials and are very commonly used to restore posterior teeth as well as anterior teeth. Dental composite resin comprises of bisphenol A glycidyl methacrylate (BIS-GMA) as the matrix polymer and quartz, barium glass, and colloidal silica as fillers. BIS-GMA is derived from the reaction of bis (4-hydroxyphenol) and glycidylmethacrylate. Low viscosity liquids, such as triethylene glycol dimethacrylate, are used to lower the viscosity, and inhibitors such as BHT (butylated trioxytoluene, or 2,4,6-tri-tert-butylphenol) are used to prevent premature polymerization. Polymerization can be initiated by a thermochemical initiator such as benzoyl peroxide, or by a photochemical initiator (benzoin alkyl ether) that generates free radicals when subjected to ultraviolet light from a lamp used by the dentist. In other types of composites, a urethane dimethacrylate resin is used rather than BIS-GMA. The filler particle concentration varies from 33 to 78% by weight and size varies from 0.05 to 50 μm. The glass fillers reduce the shrinkage upon polymerization of the resin, and also the coefficient of thermal expansion mismatch between the composite resin and the teeth. They impart high stiffness and strength, and good wear resistance to the dental composite resins. Strong bonding between the fillers and resin can be achieved using silane-coupling agents.

Key requirements for a successful restorative material include: sufficiently low viscosity to enable it to fill the cavity completely; controllable polymerization; coefficient of thermal expansion similar to the dentine/enamel, otherwise the stresses due to the mismatch are thought to contribute to leakage of saliva and bacteria at the interface margins; low shrinkage; and good resistance to creep, wear, and water absorption. When the dental composites are used as a posterior restorative material, their radio-opacity is very important. The detection of caries under a non radio-opaque composite is virtually impossible, and would allow the caries process to continue undetected for far too long. It is not clear what the optimum radio-opacity for composite is, since excessive radio-opacity can potentially mask caries lying behind the restoration. Nevertheless, the composite should be at least as radio-opaque as the enamel. Active research is being pursued around the world to develop high performance dental composite resins.

Dental restoration could also be achieved by the use of silicate-based cements. These cements form when phosphoric acid displaces metal ions from the glass made from alumina silica and other metal oxides. These are known as glass ionomers and have been in use for many years in dentistry. The setting of these cements is facilitated by the use of polymeric acids, which also undergo ionic reactions with calcium phosphate apatites. The glass ionomers are brittle and investigations are still in progress to develop composites of glass ionomers with other materials (e.g., organic resins) in order to improve wear resistance and toughness suitable for restorative applications.

9.4.4.2 Dental Post

Dental post is a rod-like material widely used in a defective tooth to adequately retain a filling or restoration during root canal therapy, which provides retention for a "coping" that replaces lost tooth structure and retains core and crown (see Figure 9.10). The dental post is normally inserted in the root canal and fixed in position using dental cement. It provides a retentive support to the core and crown assembly, and also distributes the forces of mastication to the supporting structures: the root, periodontal ligament, and surrounding bone. Sometimes pins are used either alone or in combination with the post to provide retention to the core material. The core replaces the

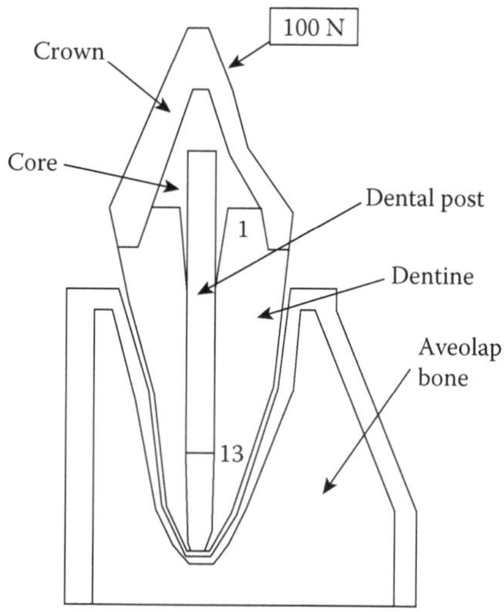

FIGURE 9.10
A schematic of dental post restored tooth. (Adapted from Ramakrishna, S. et al., *An introduction to biocomposites,* Imperial College Press, Singapore, 2004.)

coronal tooth structure that has been lost because of caries and previous restorations. It provides a base that has sufficient bulk and retention for the final restoration, the crown. Cores are usually formed from dental composite resins or amalgam or may be cast in precious or nonprecious alloys in combination with the metal post. Traditionally, dental posts made of stainless steel, Ni-Cr, Au-Pt, or Ti alloys are used based on the assumption that the post should be rigid. Failures reported include corrosion of posts, bending or fracture of posts, loss of retention, core fracture, and root fracture. In recent years, this basic tenet has been strongly questioned and it has been suggested that the modulus mismatch between the post and the dentine should be reduced so as to minimize the occurrence of root fractures (root fracture frequency is 2–4%) and failure of restorations. Later, newer dental posts made of zirconia, short glass fiber reinforced polyester, and unidirectional CF-reinforced epoxy composite posts were introduced. These new posts are adequately rigid and resistant to corrosion and fatigue. A finite element study by Cailleteau et al. (1992) indicated that a post-restored model resulted in a decreased level of stress along the coronal facial portion of the root surface, which peaked abruptly near the apical end of the post (labels 1 and 13 in Figure 9.10 indicate coronal and apical ends, respectively). These findings contradict the belief that conventional posts strengthen the tooth by evenly distributing the external forces acting on the tooth.

It is believed that an ideal dental post should have varying stiffness along its length. Specifically, the coronal end of the post should have higher stiffness for better retention and rigidity of the core, and the apical end of the post should have lower stiffness matching that of the dentine, in order to overcome root fractures due to stress concentration. In other words, it is desirable to have a post with varying stiffness. A post with varying stiffness but no change in the cross-sectional geometry along its length is only possible by using functionally graded composite materials. Ramakrishna et al. (1998) designed and developed a functionally graded dental post using braided CF/epoxy composite technology. It has a high stiffness in the coronal region and this stiffness gradually reduces to a value comparable to the stiffness of dentine at the apical end. In addition to overcoming the root fracture, the graded stiffness post decreases the chances of the post loosening from the dentine by means of eliminating stress concentration in the dentine, and reducing post/dentine interfacial shear stresses. This clearly suggests that innovations in composites design and fabrication lead to better prostheses with improved performance.

9.4.4.3 Dental Arch Wires and Brackets

Dental arch wires are used to correct the alignment of teeth, which is facilitated by bonding orthodontic brackets onto the teeth. An arch wire is placed through the brackets and retained in position using a ligature, a small plastic piece. By changing the tension in the arch wire, the alignment of the teeth is adjusted. The bracket acts as a focal point for the delivery of forces to the tooth generated from wire. It is important for a bracket to have high strength and stiffness to prevent distortion during tooth movement. This technique is also used to splint the traumatized teeth. Traditionally, the arch wires were made of stainless steel and Ni-Ti alloys. Later, polymer-based composite materials were proposed for manufacturing arch wires. GF/PC, GF/nylon, GF/PP, and GF/PMMA are a few notable examples. The stated advantages of using composite arch wires include aesthetics, easy forming in the clinic, and the possibility of varying stiffness without changing component dimensions.

The commonly used biomaterials in the manufacture of dental brackets are stainless steel, polycrystalline alumina, and single crystal alumina. Brackets made from metal alloys show high strength and stiffness, but suffer from poor aesthetics. The ceramic brackets have improved aesthetics, but they are bulkier than the metal alloy brackets. Furthermore, ceramic is abrasive to tooth enamel, and this has, therefore, limited the use of ceramic brackets to upper teeth. Some patients are hypersensitive to metals (Ni, Cr, and Co). It has been reported that these patients' immune system responds with vigorous foreign body allergic reactions causing dermatitis. Use of metallic restorations or braces is not recommended for metal sensitive patients. As an alternative, polymer composite brackets have been developed. Due to their inferior mechanical properties, compared to metal brackets, they are not very successful. There is, therefore, a great need to develop suitable polymer composite dental brackets and, globally, research is progressing in this direction.

9.5 Evolution of Nanocomposite Biomaterials

As previously mentioned, the development and applications of composite biomaterials in human systems dates far back. It may be noted that the HA/collagen system seems to be a better choice for hard tissue applications, owing to its chemical composition and structural similarity with natural bone. It is worth mentioning that most of the HA/collagen composite biomaterials are conventionally processed by anchoring HA particulates into the matrix of collagen. By this method, it is quite difficult to obtain a uniform or a homogeneous composite material similar to natural bone. Further, most of the HA used in this process are of sintered and large-size crystallites, which is in contrast to the natural bone apatite; therefore, it may take a longer time to remodel into bone tissue upon implantation. In addition, some of the composites processed by this method exhibit very poor mechanical properties, probably owing to the lack of a strong interfacial bonding between their constituents. As previously mentioned, this type of composite material truly mimics natural bone in terms of composition, but differs structurally owing to the grain size and form of the reinforcing agent, which might impede the interfacial bonding between their constituents; thus, it may lose osteointegration considerably upon implantation. There is a chance of improving the osteointegration by reducing the grain size of the reinforcing agent or by activating the nucleation of ultrafine apatite growth onto the matrix, which may lead to enhanced mechanical strength and osteointegration with improved biological and biochemical affinity to the host tissues. It is also anticipated that high fracture toughness could be conferred by controlling the extent of interfacial bonding between their constituents. Collectively, it should be noted that conventional composites have been processed with microsize inclusions (also called microcomposites); consequently, it is quite difficult to achieve appropriate interfacial bonding between the constituents. Recently, with advances in nanoscience and nanotechnology, nanocomposites are gaining much interest and are perceived to be beneficial in many aspects as bone grafts over microcomposites. The following sections describe their impact and recently developed processing methodologies with suitable illustrations.

9.6 Nanocomposites: A New Class of Nanobiomaterials

The term "nanocomposite" can be defined as a heterogeneous combination of two or more materials in which at least one of the materials should be on a nanometer length scale. Nanocomposites play a pivotal role in a variety of biomedical applications as a new and versatile class of biomaterials, which are widely used in hard tissue repair and regeneration. Although microcomposite biomaterials enable to provide good performance with host tissues, recently, nanocomposites have been proved to function better than microcomposites, owing to their amazing characteristics, including larger surface area and superior mechanical strength. In addition, most biological systems begin with nanoscale mechanism. For example, bone is a fabulous nanocomposite, precisely evolved by nature's proficiency in using nanoscale hierarchical assembly with key ingredients of HA and collagen; thereby, researchers are trying to emulate such a process for making nanocomposite biomaterials as synthetic bone graft materials. The bone grafts made of HA and collagen demonstrated high osteoconductive and, perhaps, less osteoinductive potential on implantation. Accordingly, choosing HA and collagen as precursors to design nanocomposite bone grafts is perfect and competent, that can also be utilized as a carrier system for the delivery of osteoinductive and osteogenic factors. The current research trend on the HA-based nanocomposite biomaterials in bone applications is given in Table 9.1 (Murugan and Ramakrishna 2005). The compiled data reveal that the HA-polymer nanocomposites are still in infant stage and require much more experimental evidences to support their efficiency for bone grafting. It is interesting to note that recent years

TABLE 9.1

Current Trends in HA-Based Nanocomposite Systems

Nanocomposite Systems	Methods	Experimental Studies Performed		
		Materials Characterization	*In vitro* Cell Culture	*In vivo* Animal Study
HA/collagen	Precipitation	+	–	–
HA/collagen	Biomimetics	+	+	–
HA/collagen	Biomimetics	+	–	+
HA/collagen	Biomimetics	+	+	+
HA/collagen/PLA	Biomimetics	+	+	+
HA/collagen/alginate	Biomimetics	+	+	–
HA/chitosan	Precipitation	+	–	–
HA/gelatin	Biomimetics	+	–	–
HA/silk fibroin	Mechanochemical	+	–	–
HA/PCL	Solvent casting	+	–	–
HA/PLA	Solvent casting	+	–	–
HA/PEG/PBT	Precipitation	+	–	–
HA/PHMA	Biomimetics	+	–	–
HA/polyanhydride	Photo polymerization	+	–	–
HA/PHEMA	Biomimetics	+	–	–
HA/PAA	*In situ* polymerization	+	–	–

Source: Reprinted from Murugan, R. and Ramakrishna, S., *Comp. Sci. Tech.*, 65, 2385, 2005. With permission from Elsevier.

have clearly shown a considerable upsurge in the number of publications concerning HA-polymer nanocomposite systems, which is a good sign for the tremendous growth of this fascinating nanocomposite field.

As HA/collagen nanocomposites are perceived to be more beneficial for various hard tissue applications than their monolithic counterparts, there is a great need to address their processing methodologies and their performance strategies both *in vitro* and *in vivo*. They can generally be processed through three distinct ways: (i) conventional methods, (ii) biomimetic self-assembly; and (iii) tissue engineering approach, which are described below in detail, illustrated with suitable examples.

9.7 Conventional Nanocomposites

Nanocomposites can be made, conventionally, by blending or mixing a heterogeneous combination of two or more materials, differing in morphology or composition, in which at least one of the materials should be on nanoscale. Blending is a technique used to produce a composite product with specific characteristics by combining at least two materials. Although it is not a new concept, it has a gained considerable interest in the past few years. It is well known that custom blending of multiple materials with different characteristics leads to composites with tailor-made distinct properties, but it is quite difficult to have control over homogeneity and uniformity of the secondary or reinforcing phases. The composites are made from preformed components by a process that organizes them in a matrix with particular arrangement in which integration of the components is often a top-down approach; thereby retention of a true nanostructure might be quite complicated. The top-down procedure begins with a macroscopic material that incorporates many nanoscale components into them, leading to nanocomposite. Although there is a possibility of direct mixing of nanoscale components in the process of preparing a nanocomposite, controlling their size and structure is quite intricate.

Very few studies have reported the processing of nanocomposites by blending nano-HA with collagen phases at required compositions (Tampieri et al. 2003). In brief, the nano-HA was synthesized with a routine precipitation method using aqueous solutions of $Ca(OH)_2$ and H_3PO_4 at 40°C–50°C and then it was gently mixed with collagen solution that was dissolved in acetic acid at room temperature and then freeze-dried. The nanocomposite was analyzed and found to be made up of bundles of collagen fibers embedded with nanocrystals of HA in a sponge-like structure. However, the crystallite sizes are not uniform, often aggregated, and randomly distributed into the fibrous matrix; thus, no structural uniformity is observed that is close to natural bone. Further, there is no sign of chemical interaction between the HA and collagen phases, which is probably due to the lack of suitable interfacial bonding between those phases during the conventional mixing process, which is in contrast to the way in which the native collagen is biomineralized. There is also a possibility of migration of particles around the implanted sites if their constituents are not homogeneous or uniformly intact within the matrix, which further gives medical complications with surrounding tissues. Therefore, the nanocomposites having homogeneous distribution of HA particles with controllable size in the matrix of collagen are of great importance and required for their better functionality on implantation. This type of processing method is not preferred for making high performance nanocomposites if anticipate structural and compositional strategy of the natural bone. In order to enhance the interfacial bonding, an advanced processing strategy is required. It is always appreciated to nucleate HA crystallites into the matrix of collagen in a controlled fashion as the nature does while building bone structure, which is perceived to be beneficial to enhance the properties of nanocomposites. Based on the experimental results of several studied, it is possible to make promising nanocomposites with an interfacial bonding between their constituents using a biomimetic approach, which eventually provides micro/nanostructures with controlled nucleation similar to natural bone; thus, they are expected to perform well in hard tissue applications. The following section describes biomimetically derived nanocomposite biomaterials in more detail.

9.8 Biomimetic Nanocomposites

A novel way of processing nanocomposite biomaterials using strategies found in nature have recently received much attention and are perceived to be more beneficial than conventionally processed nanocomposite biomaterials. The term biomimetic can be defined as a microstructural processing technique that either mimics or inspires the biological mechanism, in part or whole, for the design of an accurate and specific system. It is derived from the Greek words, bios meaning life and mimesis meaning imitation. It is also called by several distinct names, such as bionics, biognosis, bioinspired, and biomimicry. Biomineralized bone matrix is a good example of the biomimetic processing of nanocomposite biomaterials. A basic understanding of the mechanism involved in biological mineralization would yield much information about how nature achieves such an elegant process, which is also helpful in the design of exquisite nanocomposite bone grafting materials. The biological process generates highly ordered minerals with hybrid composition, complex texture, and ultrafine crystallites through hierarchical self-assembly.

Biomimetic involves the bottom-up approach, which begins by designing and synthesizing molecules that have the ability to self-assemble or self-organize spontaneously into higher order of microscale or macroscale structures. The smallest building blocks of bone are precisely built at the nanoscale architecture using nanocrystals of HA embedded with fibrous collagen matrix. A key step in the biomimetic strategy is to achieve a controlled nucleation and crystal growth of apatite phase onto collagen matrix, as schematically illustrated in Figure 1.8. This process partly mimics the biological phenomenon and demonstrates a better system for bone regeneration with enhanced osteoconductivity than a pure HA and a pure collagen. So, it is believed that making nanocomposite biomaterials with certain features of natural bone either compositionally or structurally using biomimetic self-assembly may replicate nature's process. A biomimetic nanocomposite was developed by self-assembling HA nanocrystals onto collagen fibers (Roveri et al. 2003). The direct nucleation of HA nanocrystals onto collagen fibers was performed by starting from an aqueous suspension of $Ca(OH)_2$ and H_3PO_4 together with a collagen solution of pH 9–10 at 25°C. The obtained composite product was freeze-dried at −40°C and then gradually warmed to 35°C for 36 h. It was noticed that the nanocrystals of HA elegantly aligned with their *c*-axis preferentially oriented along the collagen fibers, which indicates a close interaction between HA and collagen phases. As this process mimics biomineralization of the natural bone to a certain extent, it is suggested that the HA/collagen nanocomposite can be used for bone repair in orthopedic and maxillofacial surgeries. A similar bone-like nanocomposite consisting of HA and collagen, by a self-organization mechanism using $Ca(OH)_2$, H_3PO_4 and porcine atelocollagen as starting materials was developed by Kikuchi et al. (2001) and their *in vitro* performance was evaluated in beagle dogs. The composite elegantly self-organized into a nanostructure quite similar to natural bone, which might have occurred through a chemical interaction between HA and collagen. The length of self-assembled fiber bundles was found to be 20 μm, and each bundle consisted of many collagen fibrils of 300 nm in length embedded with blade-like HA nanocrystals of 50 nm in size. They found that increasing the degree of self-assembling eventually increases the bending strength of the composite and suggest that the high mechanical strength can be attained by optimizing the self-assembling mechanism between HA and collagen. The *in vivo* performance of this nanocomposite was evaluated in beagle dogs by creating an artificial bone defect. The results of the animal study proved the excellent biocompatibility, osteocompatibility, and bioactivity of the composite with surrounding tissues and stimulated the formation of new bone growth with Haversian system (see Figure 9.11). Further, it enhanced the rate of the bone-healing process compared with conventional biomaterials within a short period, which might have resulted from its nanostructural and compositional similarity with natural bone tissue; thus, it can be considered a good bone graft. This kind of composite can readily be incorporated into bone metabolism rather than being a permanent

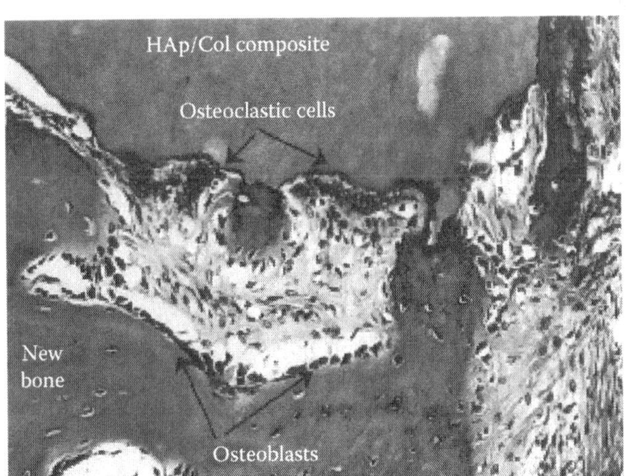

FIGURE 9.11
Biocompatibility of a biomimetic HA/collagen nanocomposite system. (Reprinted from Kikuchi, M. et al., *Biomaterials*, 22, 1705, 2001. With permission from Elsevier.)

implant. Accordingly, the biomimetic processing of composites is perceived to be highly beneficial over conventional processing methods. Although the biomimetic process is still in its infancy, based on the progress in the development of biomimetically self-assembled nanocomposite biomaterials, there is a bright future for creating a new generation of bone graft biomaterials with improved toughness and structural analogy to natural bone tissues.

9.9 Tissue-Engineered Nanocomposites

Although nanocomposites without living cells, as previously mentioned, are considered good biomaterials and provide good performance with the host tissues, particularly in hard tissue applications, it should be noted that some of them are still failing to stimulate several complex biological functions necessary for tissue formation. Since only living cells could ultimately generate a new tissue, a unique approach is to develop nanobiomaterials that are cell responsive upon implantation. The prime concept of tissue engineering is to isolate a small biopsy of specific cells from a patient, to allow them to culture on a perfect scaffold, to transplant the cell-engineered scaffold into the defective site of the patient's body where tissue regeneration is required, and to guide or direct new tissue formation. The ability to satisfy these criteria is largely dependent on three key factors: (i) the cells that create tissue, (ii) the scaffold that gives structural support to cells, and (iii) cell–matrix (scaffold) interactions that direct the tissue growth.

In this section, we address the impact of nanocomposites in tissue engineering applications as scaffolding materials. A tissue engineering approach to treat bone defects must involve the use of osteoconductive scaffold with osteogenic cells and osteoinductive or growth factors, which may create a true bone graft. Figure 9.12 shows a design strategy of tissue-engineered nanocomposite biomaterial with all those factors suitable for bone reconstructive or regenerative applications. As HA is an osteoconductive agent, it can be used as a scaffold matrix for bone tissue engineering. However, it does not possess osteoinduction ability and its biodegradability is also relatively slow. To circumvent these drawbacks, biodegradable polymers can be employed to make a composite in conjunction with HA and osteogenic potential cells. Many investigators prefer to use nano-HA and collagen as precursors to make such nanocomposite grafts because they are the basic ingredients of the natural bone tissue; thereby, they are expected to match the physicochemical, mechanical, and biological features of the natural bone. They are also anticipated to enhance cellular adhesion and bone tissue formation while possessing adequate mechanical strength. Some of the tissue-engineered HA and its nanocomposite biomaterials are listed in Table 9.2 (Murugan and Ramakrishna 2005) and some of their impacts are briefly described below.

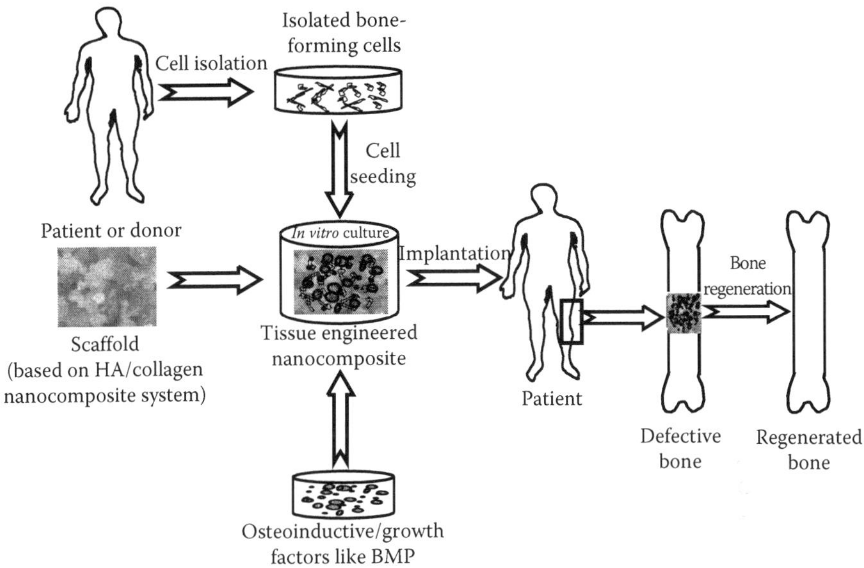

FIGURE 9.12
Design strategy of a tissue-engineered nanocomposite system suitable for bone applications.

TABLE 9.2
Tissue-Engineered HA-Based Nanocomposite Systems

Nanocomposite Systems	Cells/Growth Factors Studied
Nano-HA/collagen	Mesenchymal cells
Nano-HA/collagen	rhBMP-2
Nano-HA/collagen	rhBMP-2/osteoblasts
Nano-HA/collagen	ChS
Nano-HA/collagen/PLA	rhBMP-2
Nano-HA/collagen/PLA	Osteoblasts
Nano-HA/collagen/alginate	Fibroblasts/osteoblasts

Source: Reprinted from Murugan, R. and Ramakrishna, S., *Comp. Sci. Tech.*, 65, 2385, 2005. With permission from Elsevier.

A tissue-engineered HA/collagen nanocomposite matrix seems to be the most promising system for bone reconstructive or regenerative applications. Such a matrix was developed mimicking the composition as well as the microstructure of the natural bone tissue suitable for bone tissue engineering (Du et al. 1999). It was noticed that the mineralized collagen matrix showed a preferential orientation similar to a process that occurred during biological mineralization. Here, collagen matrix serves as a template for HA nucleation and growth. The merit of this system lies not only in its structural reliability, but also on the size-controlled nucleation of the crystal growth with low crystallinity similar to natural bone minerals. The efficacy of this matrix for bone tissue engineering was evaluated with osteogenic potential cells. The osteogenic cells/nanocomposite scaffolds were developed by organ culture technique as well as by conventional method and their *in vitro* cellular functions were investigated. It was noticed that the scaffolds supported well the cellular growth and the related functions, leading to new bone formation. Based on the experimental results, this bone-resembling nanocomposite could be used as a promising system for engineering bone tissues. Later, a three-dimensional (3D) bone-resembling nanocomposite matrix using nano-HA/collagen/osteoblast was developed in conjunction with poly(lactic acid) (Liao et al. 2004a and 2004b). This system highly supports cellular adhesion, proliferation, and migration. Interestingly, the cells penetrated deep into the matrix to about 200–400 μm within a short period (12 days), probably owing to its composition and structural similarity to natural bone; thus, it can be used as a promising scaffold for bone tissue engineering. Its *in vivo* efficacy was also evaluated in a rabbit as a model animal, by implanting in a 15-mm segmental defect. This system was incorporated with rhBMP-2 growth factor for the stimulation of faster bone growth. The biocompatibility, bioactivity, and mechanical reliability of the matrix are well appreciated. The segmental defect integrated after 12 weeks postimplantation, thus its remodeling ability is extremely well; therefore, it can be used as a promising scaffold for bone tissue repair. These experimental examples suggest the suitability of nanocomposite biomaterials for hard tissue reconstructive applications.

9.10 Nanocomposites for Growth Factor Delivery

Growth factors are potent endogenous proteins that regulate a variety of cellular functions involved in the regeneration of tissue (e.g., bone), including adhesion, differentiation, proliferation, and migration. Growth factors have the ability to enhance or impede the segregation or function of other growth factors and also have the ability to promote vascularization. Bone tissue contains a cocktail of growth factors responsible for osteogenesis. These include bone morphogenetic proteins (BMPs), transforming growth factor beta (TGF-β), insulin-like growth factors (IGFs), platelet-derived growth factors (PDGFs), fibroblast growth factors (FGFs), and epidermal growth factors (EGFs). Among them, BMPs differ from other types of growth factors because they are highly osteoinductive, meaning that these proteins have the ability to provide the primordial signal for the differentiation of mesenchymal stem cells into osteogenic cells (osteoblasts). Figure 9.13 illustrates the typical mechanism of action of BMPs observed in endochondral bone formation (Termaat et al. 2005). The sequence of events occurring during osteogenesis include recruitment and proliferation of monocytes and mesenchymal cells, differentiation of these cells into chondrocytes, hypertrophy of

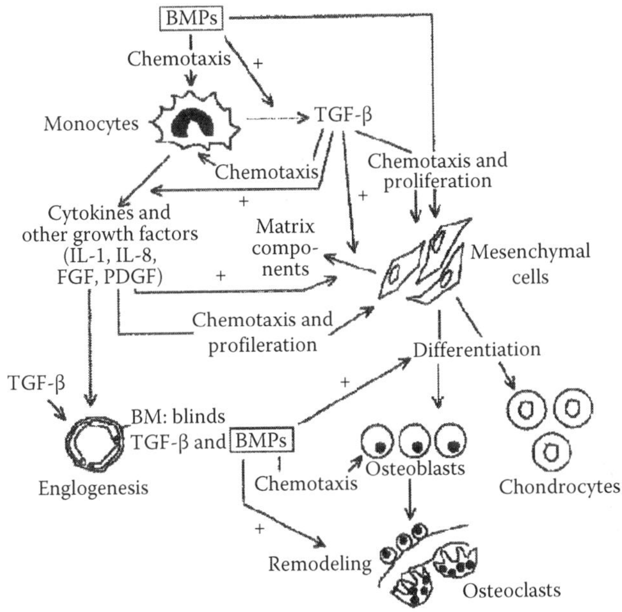

FIGURE 9.13
Key mechanism of action of BMPs in bone repair process. (Adapted from Termaat, M. F. et al., *J. Bone Joint Surg. Am.*, 87, 1367, 2005.)

chondrocytes and calcification of the cartilage matrix, vascular invasion with associated osteoblast differentiation and subsequent tissue formation, and finally remodeling of the newly formed bone and bone marrow formation.

In 1965, Urist discovered that the demineralized bone matrix (DBM) was able to promote new bone tissue formation in bone defective sites (Urist, 1965). It was found, after systematic investigations, that the proteins intact within the matrix were responsible for bone formation, owing to their osteoinductive ability. These proteins were later named BMPs. In the late 1980s, it was found that not a single protein, but a group of proteins in the bone matrix was responsible for osteoinduction. Since then, several BMPs have been identified and characterized, which are designated as BMP-1 to BMP-16, according to their molecular structure. Although the majority of the BMPs are adequate for promoting osteogenesis, BMP-2 plays an important role in the early stage of the differentiation of mesenchymal stem cells to preosteoblasts, while most of the other BMPs promote terminal differentiation of these preosteoblasts to osteoblasts. BMP-2 is therefore considered as a very powerful stimulant for bone formation. Upon confirmation of clinical safety and other issues, the FDA recently approved recombinant human BMP-2 (rhBMP-2) for human use in spinal fusion surgery. Although BMP may represent an integral component in the future of bone tissue engineering, problems potentially exist with the types of carriers currently in use.

Carriers for the delivery of BMPs are used to increase retention of these factors at defective sites for a sufficient period of time to allow regenerating tissue-forming cells to migrate to the defective area and to proliferate and differentiate. Carriers can also serve as a matrix for cell infiltration, while maintaining a space or volume in which repaired tissue formation can occur. Therefore, selection of carrier matrix is of great importance for the effective delivery of BMPs. Currently, several biomaterials are used to deliver BMPs and they can be grouped into three categories: ceramics (e.g., HA and TCP), polymers (e.g., collagen and PLA), and their composites (e.g., HA/collagen and HA/PLA). Among them, collagen and HA are often used because they are key ingredients of natural bone, osteoconductive, and readily bind to host tissues. However, from a materials point of view, HA is the most stable phase and, on the other hand, collagen is the most resorbable phase, which impedes the optimal level of a material's stability required for the release of proteins upon implantation. An ideal delivery system would allow a slow release of the BMP, of biological and immunologically interest, often required to be bioresorbable, and supportive of cell proliferation and angiogenesis. It would also possess enough rigidity to withstand deforming forces until absorbed. Finally, it would be easily processed, handled, stored, and sterilized. It is worth mentioning that the crude extract of BMP is hydrophobic, but as the protein is purified, it becomes more hydrophilic. The implantation of purified, hydrophilic BMPs promotes their dispersion shortly after implantation and before osteoinduction can occur. To prevent the dispersion and to deliver the BMPs to the desired sites, they are normally complexed to carriers that allow a slow release. In this case, the stable phase of bioactive HA combined with the resorbable phase of collagen in a composite form can be used to optimize the benefits of each of these materials for BMP delivery. In addition, the bone bonding property of HA can help to form new bone tissue even after degradation of collagen.

The advances in the fields of biomaterials and nanotechnology recently led to the development of a new generation carrier system, called nanocomposites, with enhanced properties. This kind of nanocomposite carrier system, made of HA and collagen, mimics the physical, molecular, and mechanical properties of the bone extracellular matrix (ECM). The system not only serves as a carrier matrix, but also facilitates protein adsorption, cell activity, and bone tissue formation. Here, we provide two examples that use nano composites as a carrier matrix for the delivery of BMPs. Recently, a HA/collagen nanocomposite system, in which HA nanocrystals and collagen fibers are aligned like natural bone by a self-organization mechanism between HA and collagen *in vitro,* was synthesized and used as a carrier for the delivery of rhBMP-2 (Itoh et al. 2005). The mechanical reliability of this system corroborated well with the strength of autogeneous cancellous bone. HA/collagen nanocomposite implants adsorbing 0 or 400 μg/mL of rhBMP-2 were implanted into bone defects of tibiae in three beagle dogs. As a control, bone defects of 20 mm remained in two beagle dogs and the dogs were allowed to walk using an Ilizarov external skeletal fixator. The *in vivo* findings suggest that the implants induce bone remodeling units and are a superior carrier of rhBMP-2 due to the stimulation of early callus and new bone formation. The authors suggested that the system can be used for anterior fusion of the cervical spine as well as inlay grafting bone defects in weight-bearing sites. Sun et al. (2004) developed a nanocomposite bone graft system made of nano-HA and collagen in conjunction with rhBMP-2. It was used as a graft extender and enhancer on lumbar intertransverse fusion in rabbits. This system was found to be nonimmunogenic, biodegradable, highly effective in osteoconduction and osteoinduction, ready for rapid vascularization and mesenchymal cell invasion, adaptive to various shapes of bone defects, and can provide mechanical support when needed. The authors suggested that the HA/collagen nanocomposite system is an effective carrier for BMP and is a good substitute for autograft bones. These experimental examples clearly indicate that nanocomposites, in particular the HA/collagen system, can be used in growth factor delivery.

9.11 Summary

Nanocomposites are a new and versatile class of nanobiomaterials for many biomedical applications, owing to their enhanced functional characteristics. The experimental data indicate that composite biomaterials are extensively used for biomedical applications, in particular hard tissue repair and regeneration, over the decades, but the use of nanocomposite biomaterials is at an early stage and still growing. Although the *in vitro* and *in vivo* evidences strongly support the use of nanocomposites in hard tissue applications, it further requires complete clinical studies to be declared as a potentially ideal biomaterial.

Glossary

Biomimetics: The development of synthetic systems based on information gained from biological systems (e.g., biomineralization).

Cell: Fundamental, structural, and functional unit of all living beings that is composed of an outer membrane enclosing protoplasm and nucleus.

Cellular biomaterials: The biomaterials that are intact living cells.

Collagen: A fibrous protein with a triple-helical structure that functions to hold tissues together.

Composite: A heterogeneous combination of two or more materials.

Compressive modulus: Ratio of compressive stress to compressive strain below the proportional limit.

Compressive strength: Maximum load sustained by a test specimen in a compressive test divided by the original area of the specimen.

Growth factors: A heterogeneous group of substances whose general purpose is to enhance the rate of healing, e.g., BMP.

Hardness: The ability of the surface of an implant to withstand forces, which is directly related to strength.

Hard tissue: The general term for calcified structures of our body, such as bone and tooth.

Implant: Any medical device made from single- or multiphase materials intended for human health care.

Modulus: One of several measures of strain vs. applied stress (e.g., Young's modulus).

Monolithic: Made from a single material.

Nano: A unit prefix meaning one billionth (1/1,000,000,000).

Nanocomposite: A heterogeneous combination of two or more materials in which one should be in the order of nanometer scale.

Nanomaterials: Materials composed of particles having nanometric tolerances; a nanometer is equal to 10^{-9} m.

Scaffold: A temporary structural construct or matrix used to support the cells for accommodation during tissue fabrication.

Stem cells: Undifferentiated cells that develop specialized cells, which are located in the bone marrow.

Strain: The change in size or shape of a body as a result of applied force.

Stress: An internal force that resists a load, expressed in force per unit area.

Stress-shield effect: Prolonged reduction of stress on a bone, which may weaken and make it prone to fracture. This process can be reversed if the natural state of stress can be restored to its original state.

Surface area: The total area of exposed surface of an object.

Tissue: A collection of similar cells and their surrounding intercellular substances.

Tissue engineering: Development and manipulation of laboratory-grown molecules, cells, tissues, and organs for repair or replacement of the defective body parts.

Toughness: The amount of energy absorbed by a material before breakage.

EXERCISES

9.1 What is composite biomaterial? Give examples.

9.2 Classify the composite biomaterials according to their reinforcing agents with suitable examples.

9.3 Name the different types of composite biomaterials with respect to their biological performances.

9.4 Describe the terms bioinert, bioactive, and bioresorbable materials and give examples for each type.
9.5 What are the biomedical applications of composite biomaterials?
9.6 What kind of materials can be used for load-bearing applications and why?
9.7 What is bone grafting and what are their types? Give some examples of bone graft materials.
9.8 What are the biomaterials used for dental applications?
9.9 Define nanocomposite biomaterials and give examples.
9.10 Describe various methods of processing the nanocomposite system.

References

Akay, M. and N. Aslan. 1996. Numerical and experimental stress analysis of a polymeric composite hip joint prostheses. *J. Biomed. Mater. Res.* 31:167.

Bonfield, W. et al. 1981. Hydroxyapatite reinforced polyethylene: A mechanically compatible implant material for bone replacement. *Biomaterials* 2:185.

Cailleteau, J. G., M. R. Rieger, and J. Ed Akin. 1992. A comparison of intracanal stresses in a post-restored tooth utilizing the finite element method. *J. Endodontics* 18:540.

Choueka, J. et al. 1995. Effect of annealing temperature on the degradation of reinforcing fibers for absorbable implants. *J. Biomed. Mater. Res.* 29:1309.

Deng, M. and S. W. Shalaby. 1997. Properties of self-reinforced ultra-fine molecular weight polyethylene composites. *Biomaterials* 18:645.

Di Silvio, L., M. J. Dalby, and W. Bonfield. 2002. Osteoblast behaviour on HA/PE composite surfaces with different HA volumes. *Biomaterials* 23:101.

Du, C. et al. 1999. Three-dimensional nano-HAp/collagen matrix loading with osteogenic cells in organ culture. *J. Biomed. Mater. Res.* 44:407.

Itoh, S. et al. 2005. Development of a novel biomaterial, hydroxyapatite/collagen composite for medical use. *Biomed. Mater. Eng.* 15:29.

Kikuchi, M. et al. 2001. Self-organization mechanism in a bone-like hydroxyapatite/collagen nanocomposite synthesized in vitro and its biological reaction in vivo. *Biomaterials* 22:1705.

Laurencin, C. T. et al. 1996. Tissue engineered bone-regeneration using degradable polymers: The formation of mineralized matrices. *Bone* 91:S93.

Liao, S. S., F. Z. Cui, and X. D. Zhu. 2004a. Osteoblasts adherence and migration through three-dimensional porous mineralized collagen based composite: nHAC/PLA. *J. Bioactive Compat. Polym.* 19:117.

Liao, S. S. et al. 2004b. Hierarchically biomimetic bone scaffold materials: Nano HA/collagen/PLA composite. *J. Biomed. Mater. Res. Appl. Biomater.* 69B:158.

Mano, J. F. et al. 2004. Bioinert, biodegradable and injectable polymeric matrix composites for hard tissue replacement: State of the art and recent developments. *Comp. Sci. Tech.*, 64:789.

Murugan, R. and S. Ramakrishna. 2004a. Bioresorbable composite bone paste using polysaccharide based nano hydroxyapatite. *Biomaterials* 25:3829.

———. 2004b. Coupling of therapeutic molecules onto surface modified coralline hydroxyapatite. *Biomaterials* 25:3073.

———. 2005. Development of nanocomposites for bone grafting. *Comp. Sci. Tech.* 65:2385.

———. 2006. Nanoengineered biomimetic bone-building blocks. In *Handbook of molecular building blocks for nanotechnology*, ed. G. A. Mansoori, T. F. George, L. Assoufid, and G. Zhang, 301. Germany: Springer-Verlag.

Murugan, R. and K. P. Rao. 1998. Synthesis and characterization of bioactive chitosan bonded bone cement for hard tissue replacement. In *Proceedings of IUPAC Macromolecules*, ed. K. S. V. Srinivasan, 638. New Delhi: Allied Publishers.

———. 2002a. Biodegradable coralline hydroxyapatite composite gel using natural alginate. *Bioceramics* 15:407a.

———. 2002b. Controlled release of antibiotic from surface modified coralline hydroxyapatite. *Trends Biomater. Artif. Organs* 16:43.

Peluso, G. et al. 1991. Rat peritoneal immune response to carbon fiber reinforced epoxy composite implants. *Biomaterials* 12:231.

Ramakrishna, S. et al. 1998. Fiber reinforced composite product with graded stiffness. Singapore Patent Application No. 9800874-1.

———. 2001. Biomedical applications of polymer-composite materials: A review. *Comp. Sci. Tech.* 61:1189.

———. 2004. *An Introduction to biocomposites*. Singapore: Imperial College Press.

Roveri, N. et al. 2003. Biologically inspired growth of hydroxyapatite nanocrystals inside self-assembled collagen fibers. *Mater. Sci. Eng.* C23:441.

Sclippa, E. and K. Piekarski. 1973. Carbon fiber reinforced polyethylene for possible orthopedic uses. *J. Biomed. Mater. Res.* 7:59.

Sousa, R. A. et al. 2003. Processing and properties of bone-analogue biodegradable and bioinert polymeric composites. *Comp. Sci. Tech.* 63:389.

Sun, T. S. et al. 2004. Effect of nano-hydroxyapatite/collagen composite and bone morphogenetic protein-2 on lumbar intertransverse fusion in rabbits. *Chin. J. Traumatol.* 7:18.

Tampieri, A. et al. 2003. Biologically inspired synthesis of bone-like composite: Self-assembled collagen fibers/hydroxyapatite nanocrystals. *J. Biomed. Mater. Res.* 67A:618.

TenHuisen, K. S. et al. 1995. Formation and properties of a synthetic bone composite: Hydroxyapatite-collagen. *J. Biomed. Mater. Res.* 29:803.

Termaat, M. F. et al. 2005. Bone morphogenetic proteins: Development and clinical efficacy in the treatment of fractures and bone defects. *J. Bone Joint Surg. Am.* 87:1367.

Urist, M. R. 1965. Bone: Formation by autoinduction. *Science* 150:893.

Zimmerman, M., J. R. Parsons, and H. Alexander. 1987. The design and analysis of a laminated partially degradable composite bone plate for fracture fixation. *J. Biomed. Mater. Res. Appl. Biomater.* 21A:345.

10

Nanobiomaterials for Tissue Regeneration

10.1 Introduction

Tissue or organ failure, resulting from traumatic or nontraumatic destruction, gives rise to a major health problem that directly affects the quality and length of a patient's life. These circumstances often call for surgical treatments to repair, replace, maintain, or augment the functions of the affected tissue or organ, using some additional functional components to facilitate the patient's quality of life. They have been traditionally treated with the help of tissue or organ procured from a donor site, as mentioned in Section 1.1. It may be noted that over eight million surgical procedures to treat tissue and organ failures are performed annually in the USA alone. Over 80,000 patients are still awaiting tissue and organ transplantations. In this regard, a potential solution is needed to overcome the limitations of traditional tissue transplantation methods and, at the same time, to increase the accessibility and long-time survivability of the tissue implants.

The search for alternative approaches has resulted in the emergence of the concept of tissue engineering, whereby tissue or organ failure is addressed by using synthetic materials cultured with appropriate cells harvested from a patient or donor and then implanted in the patient's body where tissue regeneration is required. The synthetic materials used for this purpose are generally called biomaterials. Biomaterials have the advantage of eliminating the surgical process of procuring tissues or organs encountered in the traditional graft procedures, and eliminating the chance of graft rejection or transmission of infectious diseases. In addition, availability, reproducibility, and cost-effectiveness make biomaterials more suitable for tissue engineering applications. Although biomaterials have been used in human health-care systems for more than 50 years, the medical community still faces many problematic cases due to the biomaterials' failure before fulfilling their intended functions. There are many reasons for the failure of biomaterials, but one of the prime factors is related to lack of sufficient tissue regeneration around the biomaterials immediately after implantation, which occurs mainly due to the poor surface interaction of biomaterials with the host tissue.

In this concern, it is essential to design biomaterials with superior surface properties (e.g., surface area and surface roughness) to facilitate favorable host–tissue interactions for their long-term survivability, and to enhance tissue regeneration. High surface area is one of the key properties of biomaterials, which influences cell adhesion and cell density. Surface roughness is another key determinant factor for the occurrence of sufficient host–tissue interactions. It has been hypothesized that cell–matrix interactions are governed by surface properties and their imperative interactions are found to occur within 1 nm of the implant surface (Kesemo and Lausmaa 1986). Apart from surface chemistry, it is also worth mentioning that the cells live in a complex mixture of pores, ridges, and fibers of extracellular matrix (ECM) in a micro and nanofeatured environment. This is because cells attach, organize, and grow well around fibers with diameters smaller than those of the cells. Therefore, designing a biomimetic micro and nanoenvironment favorable for desired cellular behaviors, such as adhesion, migration, proliferation, and differentiation, is key to the success of tissue engineering. This information eventually led to the concept of nanobiomaterials for tissue engineering applications.

10.2 Concept of Tissue Engineering

Tissue engineering is one of the emerging fields of biomedical engineering, which applies the principles and methods of engineering and life sciences toward the development of viable substitutes capable of repairing or regenerating the functions of damaged tissue that fails to heal spontaneously. Tissue repair is a process, which involves the usual inflammatory cell cascade, followed by matrix deposition and then a remodeling process, which attempts to regenerate the damaged tissue into healthy tissue. By contrast, tissue regeneration involves gradual replacement of damaged tissue with identical healthy tissue. The major advantage of the tissue engineering approach is that tissues can be perfectly reconstructed in such a way that they match exactly the patient's requirements and can be transplanted into the patient's body with minimal surgical intervention, which eventually conquers several limitations encountered in conventional tissue transplantations.

The prime concept of tissue engineering is to harvest a small biopsy of specific cells from the donor site, seed them on a scaffold in order to culture a specific tissue, and transplant the cultured tissue into the defective site of the patient's body that needs tissue regeneration. The ability to satisfy these criteria is largely dependent on three key factors: (i) the cells that create tissue, (ii) the scaffold that gives structural support to cells, and (iii) cell–matrix (scaffold) interactions that direct the tissue growth (see Figure 9.12). Among them, cells are the prime determinant factor for the success of tissue engineering because they are the basic unit of all life. There are different types of cells that could be used for tissue reconstruction, and they are commonly categorized as mature cells (nonstem) and stem cells. Although the use of mature cells dates far back, they are generally differentiated cells, which give rise to a low rate of proliferation. As an alternative, stem cellsare gaining much recognition owing to their ability to overcome many of the limitations of mature cells. The potential of stem cells is briefly discussed in Section 10.3 with experimental examples. Scaffold is another important determinant factor for the success of tissue engineering, which basically provides a structural support for the cells to grow in the three-dimensional (3D) space into a specific tissue. The success of the scaffold typically depends on the quality of the starting material and the fabrication methodology, which are discussed in detail in Sections 10.4 and 10.5, respectively. Cell–matrix (scaffold) interactions are another key determinant factor for the success of tissue engineering because it greatly influences tissue growth. As previously mentioned, cell–matrix interactions are governed by surface properties and their imperative interactions are found to occur within 1 nm of the implant surface. Furthermore, the growth of new tissue depends on the way the seeded cells interact with the scaffold. In this regard, cell seeding density must be optimized to enhance the cell–matrix interactions. On the other hand, several growth factors and biological molecules are also involved in the cell–matrix interactions.

10.3 The Promise of Stem Cells

A key factor in the tissue engineering approach for repair or regeneration of defective tissue is the use of an appropriate cell source. Currently, there is a variety of cells available corresponding to specific tissues. Although mature cells dates back a successful history and still remain an important source for tissue engineering, rapid advances are being made in identifying new cell types that have the capacity to transform into a specific cell type that may be required to produce appropriate tissue. Stem cells have recently been recognized as a promising alternative to mature cells, owing to their enormous potential in generating a spectrum of tissues with adequate functions. With the advances in cell biology, several well-characterized, tissue-specific stem cells are currently available for tissue engineering.

Stem cells, by definition, are immature or undifferentiated cells that are capable of both self-renewal and differentiation into more specialized types of cells in response to appropriate signals. The tissues that can now be engineered using stem cells comprise a diverse range, from epithelial surfaces to skeletal tissues. This ability allows them to act as a good repair system for the defective tissue or organ in the body. Stem cells are generally classified into three types: totipotent (e.g., zygote), pluripotent (e.g., embryonic stem cells), and multipotent (e.g., mesenchymal stem cells). The totipotent stem cells are capable of producing any type of cells/tissues. The pluripotent stem cells are capable of producing most cells/tissues, while multipotent stem cells produce a limited number of cells/tissues with specific functions. Stem cells are also categorized into embryonic or adult cells according to their source of origin. Embryonic stem cells, as their name suggests, are derived from the early stage of the embryo development. Although embryonic stem cell research is thought to have much greater potential than adult stem cells, several ethical and legal controversies still exist concerning their use for humans. Besides, some important clinical and safety issues also hinder their use to a certain extent. On the other hand, adult stem cells have considerable biological and clinical interests. Basically, these are undifferentiated cells found in differentiated adult tissues. They are also called somatic stem cells. The potential advantage of using adult stem cells is that the patient's own cells could be easily isolated, expanded in culture with appropriate functions, and then transplanted into the patient's body where tissue regeneration is required. By this approach, there is no chance of immune rejection and certain ethical and legal issues can also be conquered. These cells are typically harvested from bone marrow. The bone marrow chiefly constitutes two distinct stem cells: (i) hematopoietic stem cells (HSCs), which are responsible for the formation of blood cells; and (ii) mesenchymal stem cells (MSCs), which are responsible for the formation of bone cells. The basics and efficacy of MSCs for tissue engineering are briefly discussed in the following section.

10.3.1 Mesenchymal Stem Cells

Mesenchymal stem cell transplantation is considered a promising method to improve a variety of tissue functions of mesenchymal origin. MSCs are one of the well-characterized populations of stem cells residing in a variety of adult mesenchymal tissues; thereby they are well adopted for tissue engineering with considerable interests and subsequently for clinical practice. These cells were first recognized by Friedenstein and group in the 1960s, wherein they noticed that an adherent, fibroblast-like cell population could have the ability to regenerate the essentials of normal bone (Friedenstein et al. 1968). It is worth pointing out that the early investigations using these cells were mainly focused on bone tissue engineering. Nowadays, these cells are being applied to a variety of tissue engineering, including cartilage, myocardium, liver, nerve, spinal cord, and dermal tissues. The advantages of using MSCs are that they can be easily harvested from the donor site and cultured into a spectrum of tissue-specific phenotypes of mesenchymal origin, such as bone, cartilage, muscle, marrow stroma, and tendon (see Figure 10.1) (Caplan and Bruder 2001). These features attracted the attention of the biomedical community toward stem cell-based therapy, in particular MSCs. The list of tissues with the potential to be engineered is growing progressively

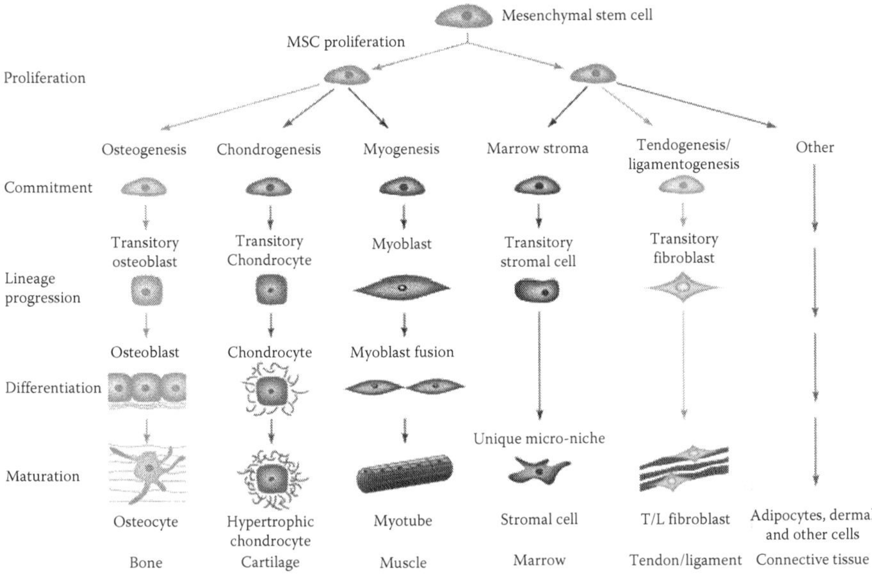

FIGURE 10.1
A schematic of the mesengenic process, showing stepwise cellular transitions from the putative mesenchymal stem cell to highly differentiated phenotypes. (Reprinted from Caplan, A. I. and Bruder, S. P., *Trends Mol. Med.*, 7, 259, 2001. With permission from Elsevier.)

in recent days because of the advances in stem cell biology and sophisticated characterization techniques, which indicates the prospects for future MSC-based tissue engineering.

Numerous investigations have reported the effective delivery of MSCs using scaffolds made of polymers, ceramics, and their composites. Recently, Li et al. (2005) reported the ability of MSCs to differentiate into chondrocytic phenotype, a cartilage-specific tissue. First, they fabricated the nanoporous biodegradable polymer scaffolds using poly(ε-caprolactone) (PCL) by the electrospinning method, and then *in vitro* assessment of chondrogenesis, in the presence of transforming growth factor-β (TGF-β), was examined. The results indicated that the MSCs are capable of giving rise to chondrocytes and also stimulate the synthesis of cartilage-associated ECM proteins throughout the scaffold. Therefore, they suggested that the electrospun PCL scaffold is a practical carrier system for MSCs transplantation in tissue engineering-based cartilage repair. Another interesting study, reported by Yoshimoto et al. (2003), demonstrated the ability of MSCs to differentiate into osteoblastic phenotype. To facilitate this, the authors manufactured the nanofeatured PCL scaffolds by electrospinning and their ability of MSCs differentiation was studied under *in vitro* cell culture condition. They found that the scaffolds provided a suitable environment to stimulate the MSCs to differentiate into osteoblastic phenotype, a bone-specific tissue. Furthermore, the scaffolds supported in synthesizing ECM of type I collagen throughout the matrix, which is a good sign of mineralized tissue formation; therefore, the authors suggested that the PCL scaffold may be a potential candidate for bone tissue engineering. This experimental information suggests that most of the cells are anchorage-dependent and will not survive if delivered without a suitable scaffold. Processing a perfect scaffold with all the qualities similar to natural ECM is therefore of great importance for tissue engineering.

10.4 Nanobiomaterials: A New Generation Scaffolding Material

Recent progress in nanoscience and nanotechnology has greatly increased the success rate of nanobiomaterials as a scaffolding material in tissue engineering. Scaffold, by definition, is a temporary supporting structure for growing cells and tissues. It is also called synthetic ECM, which plays a significant role in supporting the cells to accommodate. These cells then undergo proliferation, migration, and differentiation in 3D, eventually leading to the formation of a specific tissue with appropriate functions. Numerous studies reported the prospects of nanobiomaterials as tissue scaffolds. Nanobiomaterials generally refers to biomaterials with a basic structural unit less than 100 nm (nanostructured), crystalline solids with a grain size less than 100 nm (nanocrystals), ultrafine powders with an average particle size less than 100 nm (nanopowders), and extremely small fibers with a diameter less than 100 nm (nanofibers). A nanometer is a billionth of a meter (10^{-9} m). It is worth mentioning that all hard and soft tissues of our body contain plenty of cells living in ECM at the nanoscale hierarchical structure elegantly designed by Mother Nature. For example, bone tissue can be considered as an assembly of various levels of hierarchical structural units designed on many length scales, ranging from macro to nano, using essential organic and inorganic components, to facilitate the multiple functions required for tissue formation. The nano or microfeatured environment of the ECM is critical for the proper functioning of cells and tissues. The cells can attach and organize well around the nanobiomaterials compared to their microscale counterparts because of their typical surface properties. The fact is that nanobiomaterials have an increased number of atoms and crystal grains at their surfaces, and possess higher surface area to volume ratio compared to conventional microscale biomaterials, which makes the surface of the nanobiomaterials more reactive to cultured cells (during *in vitro*) and to host tissue (during *in vivo*), and thus greatly enhance the cell–matrix interactions, leading to faster tissue regeneration. In this regard, the rate of tissue regeneration will be greater for nanobiomaterials compared to conventional biomaterials. The nanobiomaterials are therefore perceived to be beneficial for tissue engineering applications as a new generation scaffolding material. To facilitate these measures, the scaffold should possess some essential characteristics, which are discussed in the following section.

10.5 Characteristics of a Scaffold

The structural and behavioral characteristics of the tissue scaffold are critical to ensure normal cell activities and performance of the cultured tissues. An ideal scaffold for tissue engineering should possess all the qualities of a natural ECM and should function in the same way as that of ECM under physiological conditions. However, there is no clear guideline that defines the so-called ideal scaffold. It should be noted that the characteristics of a scaffold vary, corresponding to the tissue types where the scaffold is to be applied. For example, a scaffold for engineering bone tissues requires osteoconductive features, but it is not required for engineering nerve or dermal tissues. Some of the basic characteristics of a perfect scaffold for generalized tissue engineering applications are given in Table 10.1. Any scaffold, irrespective of applications, should be biocompatible, meaning that it should not provoke any rejection, inflammation, or immune responses. The scaffold should provide a 3D template with interconnected porous architecture for the maximum loading of cells, tissue ingrowth, and transportation of nutrients and oxygen. It should be able to facilitate several biochemical and biological processes, in synthesizing specific proteins, required for healthy tissue growth in the bodily environment. It is worth pointing out that the majority of tissue engineering applications require scaffolds that are biodegradable, but the rate of degradation must match the rate of tissue regeneration. The scaffold should be mechanically strong to withstand hemodynamic and other biological forces during *in vivo*, otherwise it may hinder tissue formation. In addition, the scaffold should have high surface area to facilitate better cell adhesion and interaction with each other, and should also have surface roughness similar to that of natural tissues for the occurrence of enhanced host–tissue interactions. The scaffold should also be vascular supportive because cells will not survive without an adequate blood supply. Finally, the scaffold should be stable during storage, and must be sterilizable, in order to avoid toxic contaminations, without compromising any structural or other related properties. The pragmatic success of a tissue scaffold is not only dependent on the above measures, but is also dependent on appropriate communication between the cells, tissues, and the host system as a whole.

TABLE 10.1

Characteristics of Tissue Scaffold

Characteristics	General Remarks
Biocompatible	Biologically compatible to host tissue, i.e., should not provoke any rejection, inflammation, or immune responses.
Biodegradable	The rate of degradation must perfectly match the rate of tissue regeneration and the degraded product(s) should not harm the living tissues.
Vascular supportive	Should provide channels for blood supply for fast and healthy tissue regeneration.
Nontoxic	Should not evoke toxicity to tissues.
Nonimmunogenic	Should not evoke immunogenic response to tissues.
Noncorrosive	Should not corrode at physiological pH and at body temperature.
Porosity with interconnected pores	To maximize the space for cellular adhesion, growth, ECM secretion, revascularization, adequate nutrition, and oxygen supply without compromising mechanical strength.
3D Structure	To assist cellular ingrowth and transport of nutrition and oxygen.
High surface area to volume ratio	To accommodate high density cells.
Surface modifiable	To functionalize chemical or biomolecular groups to improve tissue adhesion.
Adequate mechanical strength	To withstand hemodynamic and other biological forces *in vivo*.
Sterilizable	To avoid toxic contamination.

10.6 Types of Scaffolding Materials

The materials used for the manufacture of a scaffold play a key role in supporting the growth of cells, which are cultured on the scaffold. In this regard, the selection of materials is of great importance for the success of tissue engineering. Based on the facts discussed in the introduction, nanobiomaterials are perceived to be more beneficial than their microscale counterparts, owing to their superior surface characteristics. A variety of biomaterials have been investigated as scaffolding materials for tissue engineering applications, including metals, ceramics, polymers, and composites thereof. Each type of material has its own distinct properties that can be advantageous for specific tissue engineering. The choice of materials depends on the type of tissue to be reconstructed. For example, metals and ceramics are widely used for manufacturing scaffolds for hard tissue applications, while polymers are used for soft tissue applications, and composites are considerably used for both applications because of their mechanical properties (see Table 1.6). This information helps the clinicians to choose the right material for a specific application. In the following sections, we focus our attention on the widely used nanobiomaterials, in particular ceramic and polymeric nanobiomaterials, for tissue engineering applications.

10.6.1 Ceramic Nanobiomaterials

As mentioned in Chapter 7, ceramics represent a class of nanobiomaterials, which is widely used as a scaffolding material in hard tissue repair and regeneration (e.g., bone). The ceramics used in tissue engineering can be classified into three major groups corresponding to their ability to interact with host tissue: (i) bioinert (e.g., alumina and zirconia), (ii) bioactive (e.g., HA and bioglass), and (iii) bioresorbable (e.g., tricalcium phosphate). For bone tissue engineering, it is desirable if the scaffolding material mimics the natural bone in chemical composition and phase structure, to facilitate better osteointegration and other related functions. In this regard, HA, $Ca_{10}(PO_4)_6(OH)_2$, may be considered a good choice of scaffolding material. HA possesses most of the qualities required for hard tissue engineering. The basic chemical composition, structure, preparation methods, and characterization techniques are discussed in detail in Chapter 5 with experimental examples.

10.6.2 Polymeric Nanobiomaterials

As mentioned in Chapter 8, polymers represent the largest class of biomaterials. Polymers in the form of nanofibers are considered as a unique class of scaffolding material and are in demand for a variety of tissue engineering applications compared to other types of nanobiomaterials, owing to their functional properties, design flexibility, and surface modifiability. The polymer nanofibers used for this purpose are commonly called polymeric nanobiomaterials. A nanofiber generally refers to a fiber having a diameter size in the range of 1–100 nm. Although the polymer nanofibers have many desirable characteristics, they tend to possess low mechanical strength (e.g., low stiffness) compared to nanophase metals and ceramics; thus, they are often used in soft tissue reconstructions, but are also used in hard tissue reconstructions in conjunction with nanophase ceramics. Polymers used in tissue engineering can be grouped into (i) naturally derived and (ii) synthetic polymers. The naturally derived polymers are biodegradable. Collagen, gelatin, and chitosan are a few notable examples. The synthetic polymers can be either biodegradable or nonbiodegradable. Poly(lactic acid) (PLA), poly(glycolic acid) (PGA), and poly(lactic-co-glycolic acid) (PLGA) are notable examples of biodegradable polymers, and poly(ethylene) (PE), poly(ethylene terephthalate) (PET), and poly(tetrafluoroethylene) (PTFE) are notable examples of nonbiodegradable polymers. In most circumstances, biodegradable polymers, either from natural or from synthetic origin, are considered a good choice for tissue engineering rather than nonbiodegradable polymers. However, degraded products from the biodegradable polymers must be nontoxic and should not elicit any foreign body reaction.

10.7 Scaffold Designing using Nanobiomaterials

Designing scaffolds with structural features similar to natural ECM is essential for tissue engineering. Numerous studies have been conducted in processing tissue scaffolds quite similar to natural ECM in the authors' laboratory (Yang et al. 2004, 2005; Murugan and Ramakrishna 2006). These scaffolds possess high surface area, high aspect ratio, high porosity, small pore size, and low density. These features are essential for the improvement of cell adhesion, which is a significant issue in the initial stage of tissue engineering because cell migration, proliferation, and differentiation functions typically depend on cell adhesion. Although tissue scaffolds can be manufactured by multiple methods, only a few methods have the ability to produce scaffolds with nanofibrous structure, which include self-assembly, phase separation, and electrospinning. The processing methods and characterization techniques of nanofibrous scaffolds are discussed in detail in Chapter 8.

10.8 Tissue-Engineered Ceramic Nanobiomaterials

To produce tissue-engineered nanobiomaterials composed of ceramic materials and cells, it is necessary to understand the influence of these materials on cellular behavior and function. For cells cultured onto ceramic scaffolds, cell behavior and function depends on the characteristics of the scaffolding material. Cell interactions with these scaffolds are generally studied using cell culture methods. Cells in culture are generally plated over the surface of ceramic nanobiomaterials and the extent of cell adhesion and spreading on the surface can be measured. A variety of cell culture methods exist to assess cellular behavior, which are cultured onto ceramic scaffolds, and the differences between these methods are critically important for better interpretation of cellular interactions. In this section, some of the widely used ceramic nanobiomaterials and cell culture methods are discussed. Among the ceramic nanobiomaterials, nano-HA has considerable interest in tissue engineering, owing to its excellent cell compatibility and bioactivity. A number of studies have reported *in vitro* and *in vivo* assessments of the biological responses to nano-HA. A few notable examples of the tissue-engineered HA-based nanobiomaterials are listed in Table 10.2 (Murugan and Ramakrishna 2005). Recently, Huang et al. (2004) reported

TABLE 10.2

A List of Examples of Tissue Scaffolds Made of Ceramic-Based Nanobiomaterials

Tissue Scaffolds	Cells Studied
Nano-HA	Osteoblast-like cells Mesenchymal stem cells
Nano-HA	Osteoblast cells
Nano-HA/collagen	Mesenchymal cells
Nano-HA/collagen	Osteoblast cells
Nano-HA/collagen/PLA	Osteoblast cells

Source: Reprinted from Murugan, R. and Ramakrishna, S., *Comp. Sci. Tech.*, 65, 2385, 2005b. With permission from Elsevier.

the *in vitro* assessment of the biological response to nano-HA. They prepared the nano-HA by a precipitation reaction, and the nano-HA suspension was subsequently electrosprayed onto glass substrates using a novel processing route to maintain nanocrystals of HA. The *in vitro* cell compatibility of nano-HA was studied with human osteoblast-like cells and the results are shown in Figure 10.2. It can be seen from Figure 10.2a, that the prepared HA particles are in the nanometer size range (50–80 nm in length), and no secondary phase is observed as evidenced by x-ray diffraction analysis (see Figure 10.2b), which confirms the phase purity of nano-HA. The results of *in vitro* cell culture studies confirmed the ability of nano-HA to support cell adhesion and growth. The cells were able to attach to the nano-HA surfaces and maintain their osteoblastic morphology with visible filapodia attached to nano-HA particles (see Figure 10.2c). There were large areas of confluent cells after seven days of culture and fiber-like ECM was produced (see Figure 10.2d), which provides evidence for better cell–matrix interactions.

The *in vitro* response of sol-gel-derived nano-HA with human MSCs was investigated in order to confirm their biocompatibility and bioactivity (Manso et al. 2002). The *in vitro* results showed that human MSCs adhered to nano-HA and exhibited better proliferation signals on their surface. Evidence of proliferation of MSCs was observed with a tendency to spread onto the surface as if forming groups, thus supporting not only biocompatibility, but also enhanced bioactivity of the material. This behavior is considered important, since it simulates on an artificial surface several steps of the cell-cycle occurring in a tissue environment, without the need for an interfacial protein scaffold. The authors concluded that these surfaces interact with the MSCs in a manner that might be useful for tissue engineers to design scaffolds as an alternate to biological ECM. Porous biomaterials are of great interest in tissue engineering, as cells and tissues invade into pores for their extensive growth, and also help the transportation of nutrient and oxygen supply to the cells. In addition, the pores provide a mechanical interlock, thereby leading to a firmer fixation of the biomaterials upon implantation. As bone tissue grows well into

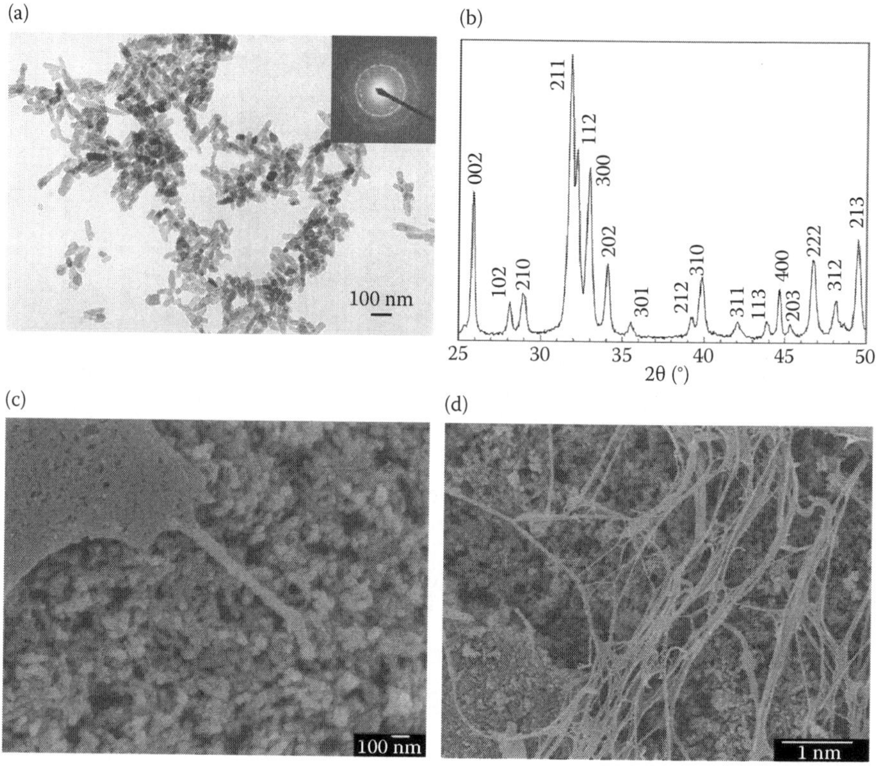

FIGURE 10.2
Characteristic results of nano-HA produced by wet chemical method (a) transmission electron micrograph and selected area of diffraction pattern (inset) of nano-HA, (b) x-ray diffraction pattern of nano-HA, and scanning electron micrographs showing (c) the attachment of human osteoblast-like cells onto nano-HA, and (d) ECM produced by the cells onto nano-HA-sprayed glass substrate. (From Huang, J. et al., *J. Mater. Sci. Mater. Med.*, 15, 41, 2004. With permission from Springer Science+Business Media.)

the pores, it is expected to increase the strength of the implanted biomaterial. The *in vitro* studies on the enhanced functions of osteoblasts (bone-forming cells) on ceramic nanobiomaterials have been reported (Webster et al. 2000). The authors extensively studied select functions of osteoblasts on nano-HA (with grain size of 67 nm) and conventional HA (with grain size of 179 nm) using *in vitro* cellular models. Osteoblasts were seeded onto the HA substrates and cultured under standard cell culture conditions. The results of cell culture studies provided evidence of increased osteoblast proliferation onto nano-HA when compared to conventional HA and to reference substrate (borosilicate glass). Although the osteoblast proliferation trend was similar on nanophase and conventional HA after one day of culture, it was significantly greater on nano-HA after three and five days of culture, which indicates that the nanophase provides a highly adhesive substrate to facilitate better cell adhesion and long-term cell growth. The results further provided evidence of enhanced long-term functions, in particular synthesis of alkaline phosphatase and concentration of calcium in the ECM, of osteoblasts cultured on nano-HA than on conventional HA.

It is worth indicating that although the nano-HA serves as an excellent bone tissue scaffold, it behaves as a typical brittle material; therefore, it is only used in certain bone tissue repair applications. In order to improve reliability, it is necessary to introduce some biocompatible reinforcement agents or matrix materials. However, introduction of foreign materials may decrease the reliability of HA; thus, choosing the reinforcement agents or matrix materials is of great importance. Composite of nano-HA with collagen is perceived to be beneficial in improving the reliability of nano-HA, and, at the same time, both are the key components of natural bone tissue. Osteogenic cell-engineered HA/collagen nanocomposite scaffold structures were developed using culture techniques as well as conventional methods, and their *in vitro* cellular functions were studied (Du et al. 1999). It was noticed that the scaffolds well supported the cellular growth and related functions, leading to new bone formation. Later, a 3D bone-resembling nanocomposite matrix using nano-HA/collagen/osteoblasts was developed in conjunction with PLA (Liao et al. 2004). This system supported cellular adhesion, proliferation, and migration. Interestingly, the cells penetrated deep into the matrix to about 200–400 μm within a short period (12 days), probably owing to its composition and structural similarity to natural bone tissue; thereby providing a promising scaffold for bone tissue engineering. In this light, ceramic nanobiomaterials clearly represent a unique and promising class of scaffolding material for tissue engineering applications, but limited to hard tissue repair and regeneration.

10.9 Tissue-Engineered Polymeric Nanobiomaterials

Among the polymeric nanobiomaterials, FDA-approved biodegradable polymers are of considerable interest in tissue engineering. A few notable examples of the tissue-engineered polymeric nanobiomaterials are listed in Table 10.3 (Murugan and Ramakrishna 2006). As previously mentioned, to produce tissue-engineered nanobiomaterials composed of polymers and cells, it is necessary to understand the influence of these materials on cellular behavior and function. For cells cultured onto polymer scaffolds, cell behavior and function depends on the characteristics of the scaffolding material. Cell interactions with these scaffolds are generally studied using cell culture techniques. Cells in culture are generally plated over a polymeric scaffold surface and the extent of cell adhesion and spreading on the surface can be measured. Since many investigators use

TABLE 10.3

Some of the Biodegradable Polymers for Tissue Engineering Applications, Differentiated with Respect to their Fiber Orientation

		Types of Fiber Orientation		
Biodegradable Polymers	**Solvents**	**Random**	**Aligned**	**Applications**
Synthetic polymers				
Poly(L-lactic acid)	Mixture of dichloromethane and dimethylformamide	✓	✓	Neural tissue engineering
Poly(glycolic acid)	Hexafluoro-2- propanol	✓	✓	Tissue scaffolds
Poly(lactide-co-glycolide)	Hexafluoro-2-propanol	✓	✓	Cardiac tissue engineering
Poly(caprolactone)	Mixture of methylene chloride and dimethylformamide	✓	–	Cartilage/bone tissue engineering
Poly(urethane)	Mixture of tetrahydrofuran and dimethylformamide	✓	–	Wound dressing
Naturally derived polymers				
Collagen	Hexafluoro-2-propanol	✓	✓	Tissue scaffolds
Gelatin	Trifluoroethanol	✓	–	–
Chitosan	Acetic acid	✓	–	–
Chitin	Hexafluoro-2-propanol	✓	–	Wound dressing

Source: From Murugan, R. and Ramakrishna, S., *Tiss. Eng.*, 13, 1845, 2007. With permission from Mary Ann Liebert, Inc., publishers.

many different cell culture techniques to assess cellular behavior with polymeric matrices, some of the widely are discussed in this section. Matthews et al. (2002) processed the collagen nanofibrous scaffolds and *in vitro* cellular compatibility was studied using smooth muscle cells (SMCs). The results suggest that the scaffold has excellent biocompatibility, cellular compatibility, and are capable of promoting cell ingrowth and related functions (see Figure 10.3a). This study thus demonstrated the feasibility of using collagen as a good tissue scaffold. Yang et al. (2005) processed the poly(L-lactic acid) (PLLA) nanofibrous scaffolds, with randomly oriented fibers, and the *in vitro* cellular compatibility was studied using neural stem cells. The results suggest that the scaffold has excellent biocompatibility, cellular compatibility, and is highly supportive to cell differentiation and related functions. The results further indicate that most of the cells have a bipolar shape with extended neurites and the neurite outgrowth is randomly spread over the scaffold (see Figure 10.3b), which implies a good sign for cell–matrix interactions under *in vitro* cell culture conditions.

Yang et al. (2005) also reported the feasibility of processing PLLA nanofibrous scaffolds with well-aligned fibers and the *in vitro* cellular compatibility was studied using neural stem cells. They observed the influence of fiber orientation on the cell growth. A representative phase contrast light microscopy image of a cell-cultured scaffold is shown in Figure 10.3c. The results indicated that cells were well attached to the scaffold and showed an extensive neurite-like outgrowth, which is a good sign of their differentiation. Interestingly, the results revealed that the cells elongated and their neurites outgrew along the direction of the fiber orientation, which shows the significance of spatial orientation of the fibers on cellular growth behavior. To observe the expression of the cytoskeleton proteins of neural stem cells as well as the relationship between the cytoskeleton proteins and fiber orientation of the scaffolds, a laser scanning confocal microscopy (LSCM) observation was performed and a representative micrograph is shown in Figure 10.3d. It can be seen from the results that the cells exhibited a classical contact guidance by growing parallel to the fibers. It is also noticed that the majority of the differentiated cells show bipolar shape with two extended neurites, which emerged from the regions of the somas, parallel to aligned fibers and were symmetrically distributed around the soma. However, some exceptional cases were also noticed (indicated by arrow). Although neurite outgrowth was not affected by the fiber orientation during the initial period, they all turned through large angles in order to grow in the direction of fiber orientation, which implies the significance of fiber orientation in directing cell growth. The collective information thus obtained from the above experimental examples provided evidence for the enhanced performance of polymeric nanobiomaterials for tissue engineering applications.

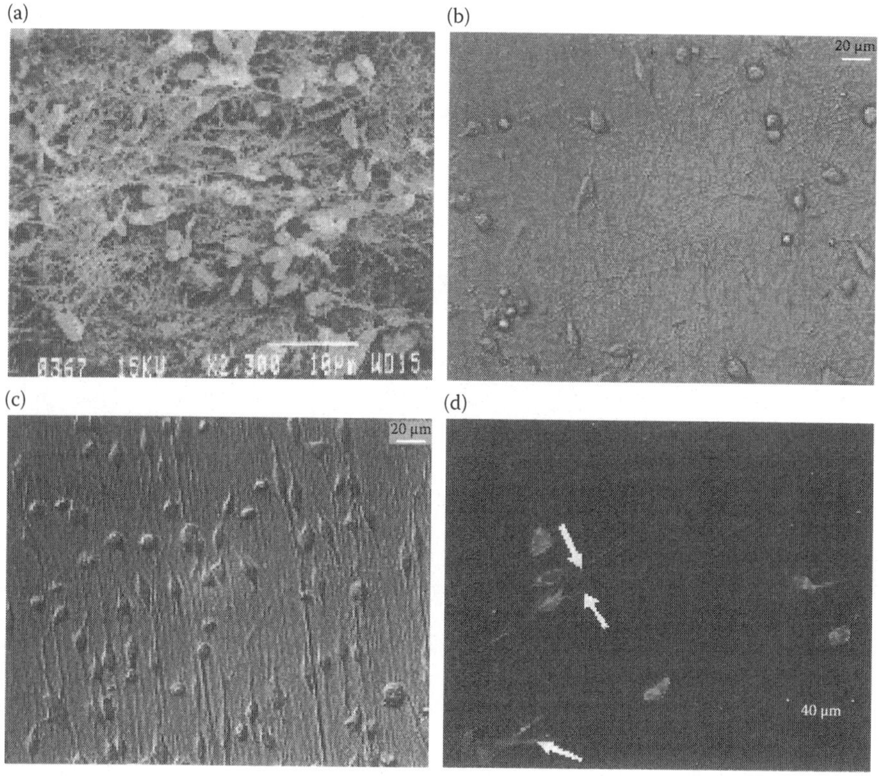

FIGURE 10.3
SEM micrographs showing cell–matrix interactions within the electrospun nanofibrous scaffolds made of (a) collagen (From Matthews, J. A. et al., *Biomacromolecules,* 3, 232, 2002), (b) randomly oriented poly(L-lactide) nanofibers, and (c, d) well-aligned poly(L-lactide) nanofibers, evaluated in the authors' laboratory. (Reprinted from Yang, F. et al., *Biomaterials,* 26, 2603, 2005. With permission from Elsevier.)

10.10 Patterning of Biomaterials for Cell Engineering

Control of cell position, growth, and subsequent function is a fundamental focus in the development of a new generation of biomaterials for use in cell and tissue engineering. As far as we know, surface chemistry and topography (surface structure) of biomaterials greatly influence cell behaviors, such as adhesion, migration, orientation, guidance, differentiation, proliferation, protein synthesis and segregation, and gene expression, essential for tissue formation. Designing biomaterials suitable for regulating such functions is, therefore, of great importance for a variety of biological and biomedical applications, including tissue engineering. As discussed earlier, tissue engineering aims to repair or regenerate the complex tissue functions of the defective tissue with the help of synthetic (biomaterials) and living (cells) components by integrating them in appropriate conditions that support the cells to organize and assemble into a functional tissue. In this regard, adhesion and controlled spreading of the cells onto the biomaterials is a critical prerequisite for the success of engineering physiologically functional tissues. This step primarily depends on the surface properties of the biomaterials, because host cells, tissues, and other essential biological substances first contact the material's surface, both *in vitro* and *in vivo*, when a material comes in contact with the biologic environment. Therefore, one of the key challenges is to design surface-active biomaterials favorable for cells and other essential biomolecules, by modulating surface chemistry and/or topography. Recent investigations also suggest that cells respond strongly to a nanofeatured environment in terms of increased cell adhesion, differentiation, proliferation, cytoskeleton development, and gene expression, because of their unique surface functional characteristics. For example, Dalby et al. (2002a) demonstrated increased, long-term cell adhesion (endothelial cells) and subsequent cellular responses onto nanotopographical surfaces (islands of 13 nm height) formed by the polymer demixing method (phase separation). The group investigated the endothelial cell behavior on nanotopographical surfaces with different heights of nano-islands (13, 35, and 95 nm) and revealed that, although cells respond to all nanosurfaces, a decrease in the height of the islands rapidly increases certain cell behavior, such as initial cell adhesion, long-term cell adhesion, and well-defined cytoskeleton development (see Figure. 10.4). In another study,

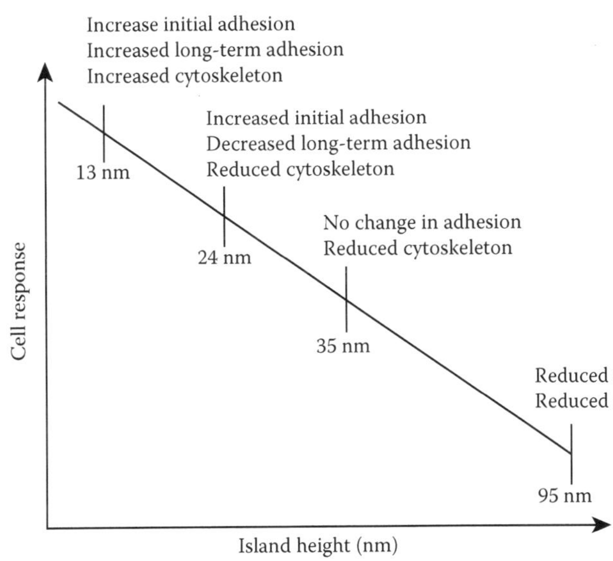

FIGURE 10.4
Drawing depicting the relationship between PS/PBrS (polystyrene and poly(4-bromostyrene) island size and fibroblast response. (Reprinted from Dalby, M. J. et al., *Biomaterials*, 23, 2945, 2002a. With permission from Elsevier.)

Yang et al. (2005) reported that nanoscale fibrous biomaterial (i.e., PLLA) promotes neural cell adhesion and differentiation better than microscale ones, which leads to the formation of faster neurite outgrowth and other cellular processes. These studies, in addition to others, clearly indicate the impact of nanofeatures in dictating cell behaviors; which leads to the concept of surface patterning of biomaterials in discrete steps, ranging from nano to micro, for use in cell/tissue engineering as well as to study the fundamental aspects of cell biology.

Patterning of surfaces can be done by a variety of methods using micro- and nanofabrication technologies. Most of these methods were originally adapted from the microelectronics field, where they are used for the fabrication of integrated circuits and other miniature electronic components. From a biomaterials point of view, patterning can be broadly grouped into two categories: chemical and topographical. In general, cell adhesion can be modulated by chemical patterning and cell behavior can be controlled by topographical patterning. The following sections discuss in detail these patterning methods and how they can be adapted to produce spatially oriented structures and their cellular responses.

10.10.1 Chemical Patterning

Chemical patterning refers to the use of substrates with patterns of chemical species. Patterning of self-assembled monolayers (SAMs) of chemical species is a good example of chemical patterning. SAMs are versatile molecular assemblies generally used to modify the properties of biomaterial surfaces with enhanced functionalities suitable for many demanding applications, in particular cell/tissue engineering, because SAMs are also known to strongly influence cell attachment. A wide variety of techniques have been developed in the last few years for the patterning of SAMs, including the conventional method of photolithography and the unconventional method of microcontact printing (μCP). All these techniques were primarily applied to produce micro or nanopatterned surfaces suitable for controlled cell adhesion or protein adsorption. Although the photolithographic technique is highly used for producing complex and accurate pattern networks with high resolution, it has certain disadvantages to widen their usage. For example, this technique can only be applied to pattern certain materials that are photosensitive and most of the chemicals used in this technique are toxic or incompatible with cells and other biomolecules. This technique typically requires expensive instrumentation and clean-room facilities for the production of photomask and spin-coating of photoresist, essential for patterning, which makes this technique more expensive. This technique can be applied only for patterning planar surfaces and it is poorly suited for patterning 3D substrates, which are highly important for engineering physiologically functional tissues. These limitations stimulated the development of μCP. The details of the methodology and processing steps involved in this technique are described in the following section with experimental examples.

10.10.1.1 Patterning by Microcontact Printing

Microcontact printing is a popular technique in soft lithography because of its simplicity, flexibility, and ability to pattern many biomaterials, in particular tissue-culture substrates, with features of sizes down to 1 μm without using any expensive equipment or a special laboratory facility (e.g., class 100 or class 1000). In addition, importantly, this versatile technique can be extended to pattern nonplanar surfaces (3D assembly), unlike the conventional photolithography method, where it is not feasible and the material to be patterned need not be photosensitive. Figure 10.5 shows a schematic illustration of the major processing steps involved in the pattern formation

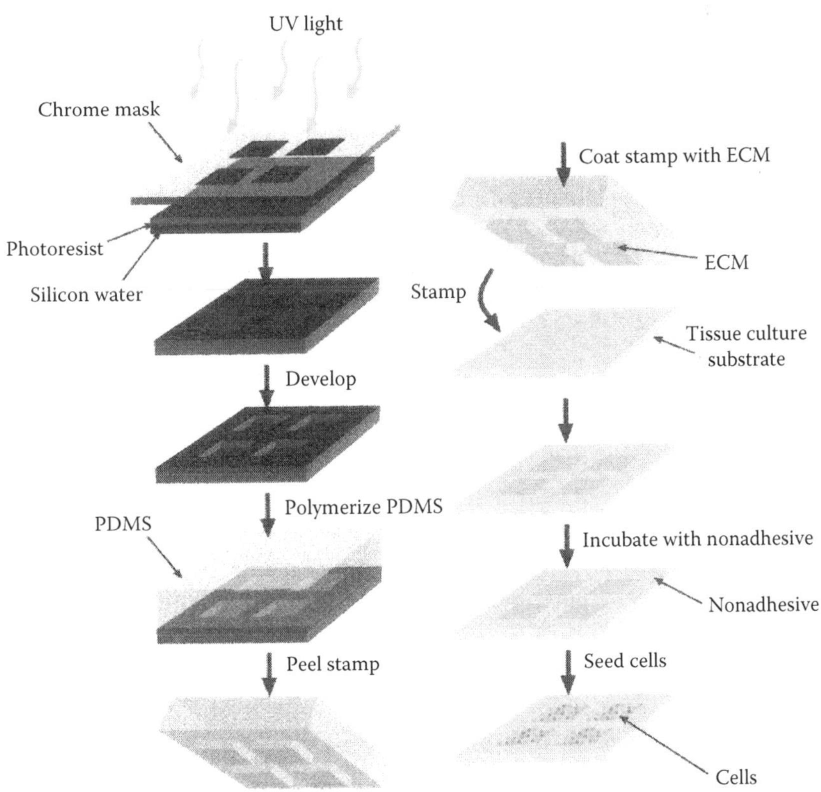

FIGURE 10.5
Schematic of micropatterning process. PDMS stamps are generated by photolithography (left column) and, using these stamps, ECM proteins are printed onto tissue-culture substrates upon which cells are seeded (right column). (Reprinted from Wendy, F. L. and Christopher, S. C., *Mater. Today*, 8, 28, 2005. With permission from Elsevier.)

using μCP (Wendy and Christopher 2005). This method is based on the use of an elastomeric stamp to print a pattern of material of interest (e.g., ECM proteins) on a solid substrate with the help of molecular self-assembly. There are three major components associated with this technique, namely, master, stamp, and ink. The master is a solid material (e.g., silicon), often created by a standard photolithography with desired geometry and with high-resolution features specific to applications. The stamp is a soft elastomeric material, often created by casting an elastomeric material (e.g., polydimethylsiloxane (PDMS), $(H_3C)(SiO(CH_3)_2)_nSi(CH_3)_3)$ over a predesigned master. The "ink" is nothing more than a functional material chosen to pattern on the substrate material. In the patterning process, the stamp is first inked with a solution made of materials of interest and then the stamp is brought into contact with the surface of the substrate material, letting the stamp and the substrate remain undisturbed for a period of time, which ultimately yields the geometrical pattern of the stamp onto the substrate material. Note that, prior to μCP, the stamp is allowed oxygen plasma treatment to oxidize the outer surface of the stamp, facilitating surface hydrophilization, which could eventually assist the adsorption of the ink to the stamp's surface. The surface only at the regions of the stamp in contact with the substrate is deposited in the form of SAMs with features of a few micrometers to nanometers in size. The unstamped regions are backfilled with another material of interest (e.g., non cell-adhesive compounds) in the form of SAMs to ensure that the cells grow only on the cell adhesive regions. In this way, the substrate could be imprinted with multiple SAM surfaces. The resultant patterned surface could be used to study the fundamental aspects of cell behaviors in both small- and large-scale cell cultures. This technique may also be useful for the fabrication of sheets of cells in defined patterns and shapes for use in tissue engineering.

Recently, Vogt et al. (2004) demonstrated the impact of micropatterned protein surfaces, made by μCP, on neuronal polarity determination. The pattern structures used in this study had meshes of 50×100 μm with somal adhesion sites of 22 μm in diameter and lines of 4 μm in width (see Figure 10.6). One line emerging from a somal adhesion node was always continuous (for axonal outgrowth), while three were interrupted (for dendritic outgrowth). They used three types of patterns with different gap sizes on the interrupted lines. The patterns were evaluated for their suitability in cortical neuronal culture and their polarity was studied with respect to the magnitude of the patterned surfaces. Figure 10.7 shows an optical micrograph of cortical neurons cultured onto the patterned surface. As seen from the figure, cell bodies adhered to the node points of the pattern with high fidelity, while neurite extension occurred along both types of lines. After several days in culture, the formation of geometrically defined networks could be observed similarly as on uninterrupted patterns. The authors have also investigated the orientation of axons and dendrites in the patterned network through double patch-clamp measurement (current clamp mode). For this, action

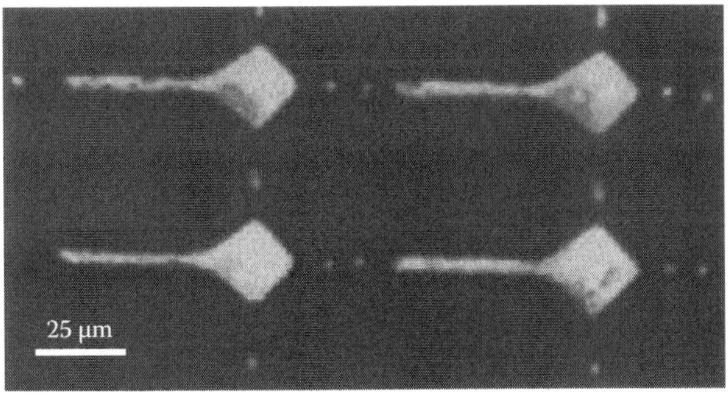

FIGURE 10.6
Optical micrograph of well-defined protein patterns against an uncoated polystyrene background. The picture was taken after stamping with an inking solution containing the fluorescent dye sulforhodamine to allow visualization. (Reprinted from Vogt, A. K. et al., *J. Neurosci. Methods,* 134, 191, 2004. With permission from Elsevier.)

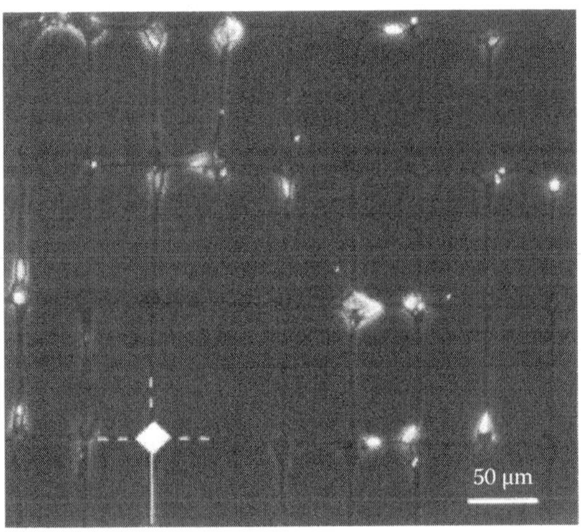

FIGURE 10.7
Optical micrograph showing a network of cortical neurons grown on protein pattern on day 12. (Reprinted from Vogt, A. K. et al., *J. Neurosci. Methods,* 134, 191, 2004. With permission from Elsevier.)

potentials were evoked in one cell at a time, while the effect on the other cell was monitored without applying stimuli. A typical recording of two synaptically coupled cells is shown in Figure 10.8 (solid line denotes stimulated cell and dotted line denotes unstimulated cell), which shows evidence for the synaptic formation. This kind of patterned system may have tremendous potential in designing artificial neuronal cell networks as well as in neural tissue engineering.

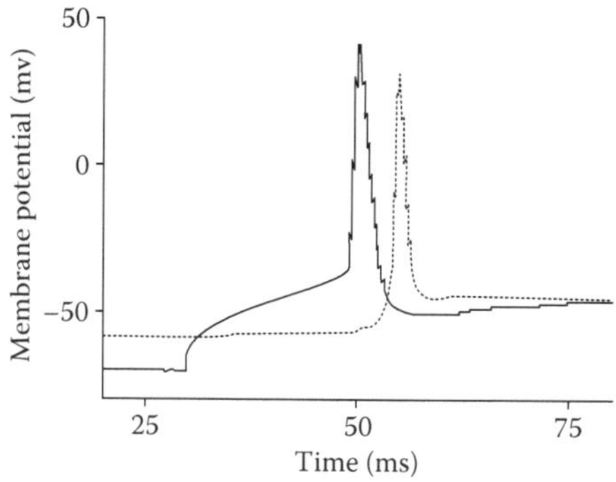

FIGURE 10.8
Double patch-clamp measurements for the detection of synapses. An action potential was elicited through a depolarizing current pulse in one cell, while the effect on the other cell was monitored without applying a stimulus. In this example, the postsynaptic potential was large enough to trigger a postsynaptic action potential (solid line: stimulated cell, dotted line: unstimulated cell). (Reprinted from Vogt, A. K. et al., *J. Neurosci. Methods,* 134, 191, 2004. With permission from Elsevier.)

10.10.2 Topographical Patterning

Topographical patterning refers to the use of substrates with patterns of texture by modulating their shape (e.g., grooves or ridges) and size with features in the range of a few microns to nanometers. Patterning of texture is nothing more than a physical modification of the surface in an ordered manner. The cells have been found to strongly respond to the surface features of the biomaterials where they are cultured, both *in vitro* and *in vivo.* For example, fibroblasts sense the substrate's topography using filopodia present as thin extensions on the cell lamellae or emanating directly from the cell body (Dalby et al. 2002b). Once a suitable site for adhesion is sensed, other cellular activities, such as focal adhesions, stress fibers, and microtubules, are developed, which stabilize the contact between cells and surfaces. The success of any biomaterials depends on the interaction of host cells/tissues with their surfaces. Therefore, designing biomaterials' topography suitable to enhance cellular responses is a good option and essential to organize cells and subsequent tissue growth for cell/tissue engineering applications and is also important in developmental biology to study the cell behaviors, cell–substrate interactions, and cell–cell communications.

Currently, there are many techniques employed for patterning biomaterial surfaces with nanoscale topographical features to investigate cell–surface interactions, essential for cells and tissue engineering. Among them, electron beam lithography, phase separation, self-assembly, nanocontact printing, colloidal lithography (CL), and nanoimprint lithography (NL), are notable examples. The ability to implement these nanofabrication technologies in a manner that is cost effective, high throughput, and scalable for commercial production of cellular substrates is still a challenging task and requires continued efforts. Although electron beam lithography can be used to produce patterned surfaces with nanoscale features, this method is somewhat expensive and time consuming. In addition, speed of this technique is too slow for patterning of large areas, but to study the cell responses to nanotopographical features often require surfaces patterned over large areas. Phase separation is a simple method and could be employed to pattern large areas, but controlling size and surface geometry is poor. Self-assembly and contact printing are a good choice, as discussed in the earlier sections, for producing nanostructures. Lithographic techniques, particularly CL and NIL, are recent developments and show great promise in patterning surfaces with the desired nanoscale topography, with features less than 100 nm in resolution, in a convenient, rapid, and inexpensive manner. In the following section, the methodology of NIL in patterning biomaterial surfaces and their cellular responses, are described in detail with experimental examples.

10.10.2.1 Nanoimprint Lithography

Nanoimprint lithography is a simple and potential technique for patterning surfaces with topographical features less than 100 nm in size. In addition, it is possible to control the spatial distribution of chemical species on the structured surface. This technique can be applied to pattern 2D or 3D nanotopography of different geometry on a wide range of biomaterial substrates suitable for cell and tissue engineering, where the anchorage-dependent cells are cultured. This versatile patterning technique, in principle, replicates topographical patterns by means of applied pressure and temperature in which a rigid master (e.g., silicon) with nanostructure features is imprinted (pressed) into a polymer resist (e.g., poly(methyl methacrylate); PMMA), resulting in a relief replica of the master on the substrate's surface. There are two basic steps involved in this technique. The first is the imprint step in which a master (also called "mold") with custom-made nanotopography is pressed into a polymer resist (usually in the form of a thin film) layered on a substrate material, followed by removal of the master. This step duplicates the nanotopography of the master on the polymer resist. During the process, the polymer resist needs to be heated to a temperature above its glass transition (Tg), because the resist becomes a viscous liquid state at this temperature that facilitates the polymer to flow and mold easily into the shape of the master. For example, to transfer the pattern from a rigid master into a PMMA resist requires about 110°C. PMMA shows an excellent material as a resist for NIL, because it has a small thermal expansion coefficient of about 5×10^{-5} per °C and a small pressure shrinkage coefficient of about 3.8×10^{-7} per psi. Note that the topography of the master can be designed with a desired geometry by photolithography and reactive ion etching (RIE), for example. The second step is the pattern transfer, where an anisotropic etching process (i.e., RIE) is used to remove the residual resist in the compressed area. This step transfers the thickness contrast pattern into the entire resist, leaving polymer patterns on the substrate material. Note that the NIL processing is fundamentally different from stamping (μCP) using a monolayer of self-assembled molecules because it is more like a physical process than a chemical process.

Recently, Yim et al. (2005) created nanopatterned silicon substrate using polymer thin film made of PMMA, comprising gratings with 350 nm line width, 700 nm pitch, and 350 nm depth, by NIL and the efficacy of the nanopatterned system in regulating cell behaviors was studied. The surface topography of the substrates used in this study is shown in Figure 10.9. The gratings were about 350 nm wide on both the nanoimprinted PMMA (Figure 10.9a and b) and the replica PDMS sample (Figure 10.9c). The surface topography was maintained, even with a coating of collagen (type I bovine collagen) on the PDMS (see Figure 10.9d). To evaluate the cellular responses to patterned surfaces, SMCs were plated on these substrates and their morphology and concomitant orientation were studied, with respect to their elongation and alignment. The cell culture results show that the patterned surface with nanotopographical features can effectively direct cell orientation and their functions (see Figure 10.10). The cells cultured on the surface with nanogratings adapted with an elongated morphology and were

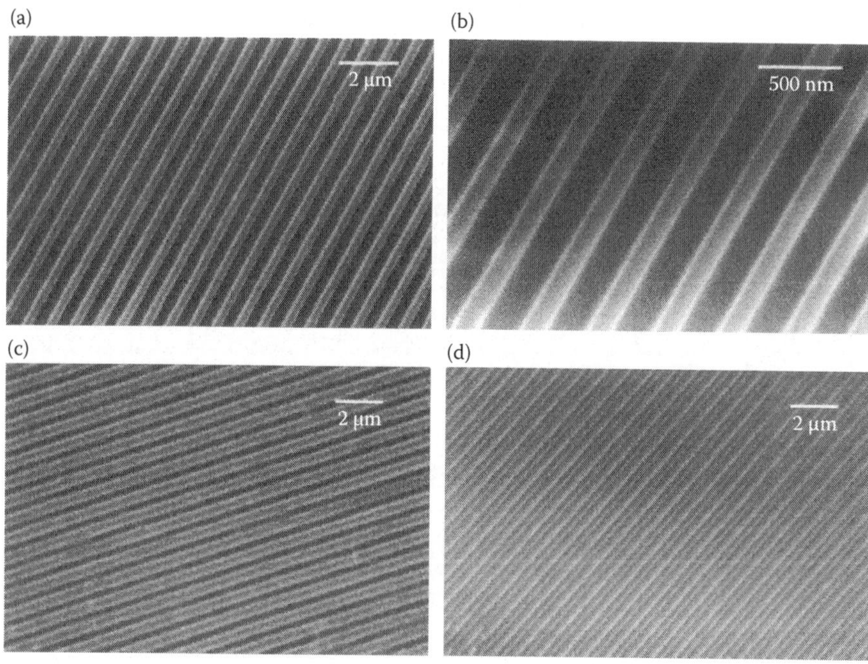

FIGURE 10.9
SEM micrographs of (a, b) nanoimprinted gratings on PMMA coating on SiO_2 wafer, (c) PDMS nanopatterned by replica molding, and (d) collagen-coated PDMS with nanopattern. Bar = 2 μm for a, c and d, bar = 500 nm for B. (Reprinted from Yim, E. K. F. et al., *Biomaterials*, 26, 5405, 2005. With permission from Elsevier.)

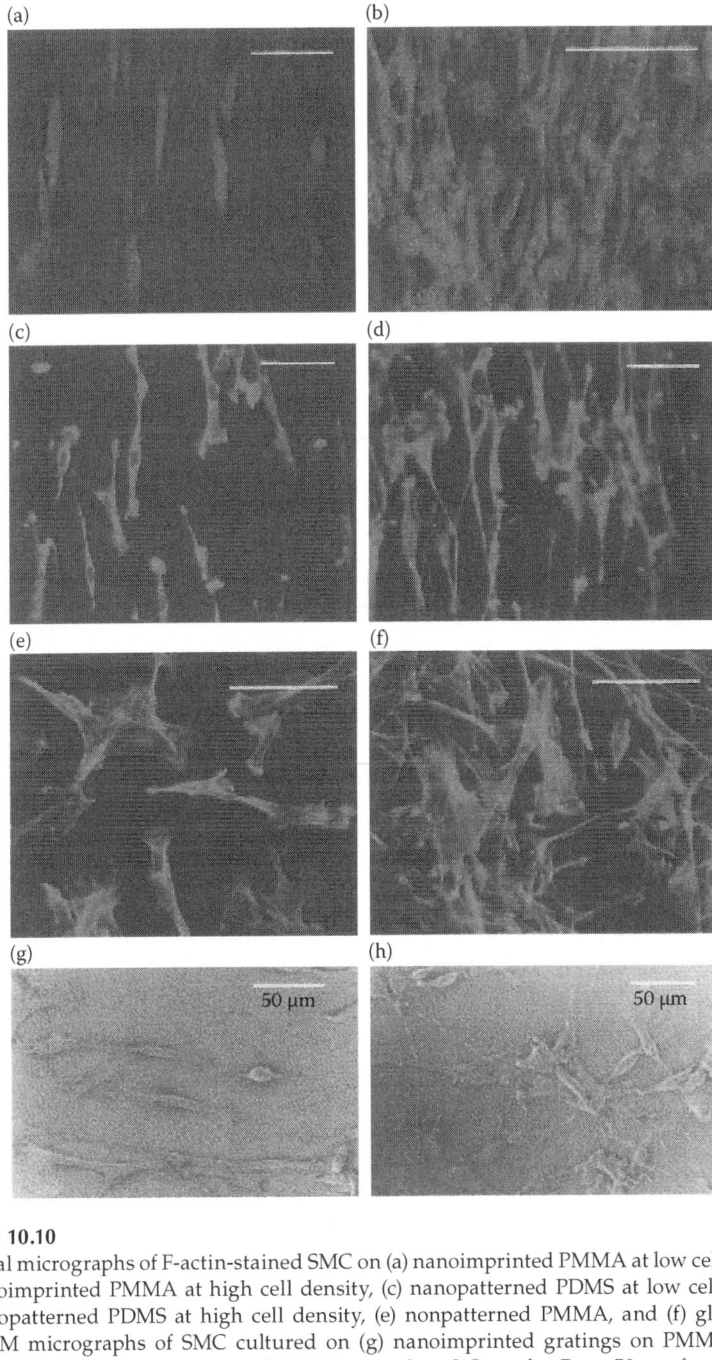

FIGURE 10.10
Confocal micrographs of F-actin-stained SMC on (a) nanoimprinted PMMA at low cell density, (b) nanoimprinted PMMA at high cell density, (c) nanopatterned PDMS at low cell density, (d) nanopatterned PDMS at high cell density, (e) nonpatterned PMMA, and (f) glass cover slip. SEM micrographs of SMC cultured on (g) nanoimprinted gratings on PMMA coated on SiO_2 wafer, and (h) nonpatterned PMMA coated on SiO_2 wafer. Bar = 50 μm for all except (b) bar = 100 μm. (Reprinted from Yim, E. K. F. et al., *Biomaterials*, 26, 5405, 2005. With permission from Elsevier.)

mostly parallel to one another. By contrast, SMC cultured on unpatterned surfaces showed neither elongation nor orientation at both low and high cell densities. The cells were significantly elongated on the nanopatterned grating surfaces compared to nonpatterned surfaces. The elongated morphology and alignment, which resemble the natural state of SMCs *in vivo*, suggest that nanopatterned surfaces would be a more favorable substrate for the study of cell–substrate interactions. The authors suggested that the NIL has great potential in producing structures for studying cell physiology in response to nanotopography and in developing medical devices with nanoscale features. These experimental examples clearly demonstrate the impact of patterned biomaterial surfaces to regulate cell behavior essential for tissue development.

10.11 Tissue-Engineered Products: The Artificial Skin and Cartilage

The aim of this section is to introduce a few tissue-engineered products that have either been clinically used or are rapidly approaching clinical use for tissue repair. The final stage in the development of a tissue-engineered substitute is the application of this technology to clinical needs. To date, tissue-engineered skin and cartilage are the only products commercially available for use in human applications, and are briefly presented in this section.

For skin repair, a wide variety of materials have been proposed and clinically tested. Globally, a variety of skin substitutes have been introduced onto the market. Integra® is the most widely used synthetic skin substitute in the treatment of burns, which consists of cross-linked bovine collagen and glycosaminoglycans, coated on one side with a porous silicone membrane in order to allow migration of the patient's own endothelial cells and fibroblasts. Apligraf® is the most sophisticated commercially available skin substitute, derived by combining a gel of bovine collagen (type I) with allogeneic fibroblasts and keratinocytes. It is one of the most expensive products and is available in a ready-to-use form with a five-day shelf life. Likewise, a variety of tissue-engineered skin products are commercially available for clinical uses and some are given in Figure 10.11 (Jones et al. 2002). The case study evaluations of synthetic skin substitute products are discussed in Section 10.2 in detail.

For cartilage repair, only a few tissue-engineered products have recently been introduced onto the market. At present, most of the currently available tissue-engineered cartilage products target cartilage defects in the knee joints, which are highlighted below, with reference to their respective

Trade name	Schematic representation	Layers	Cost	Cost per cm^2
Biobrane™ (Dow Hickam/Bertek Pharmaceuticals, Sugar Land, TX).	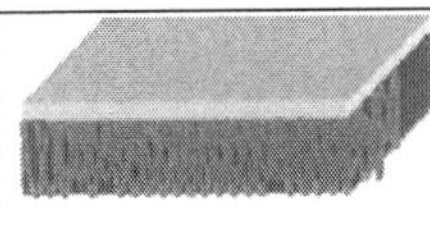	1. Silicone 2. Nylon mesh 3. Collagen	5 × 5 cm £12.00	£0.48
Transcyte® (Advanced Tissue Sciences, Inc. La Jolla, CA, USA)	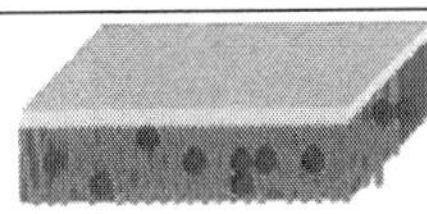	1. Silicone 2. Nylon mesh 3. Collagen seeded with neonatal fibroblasts	13 × 9 cm £921.15	£7.87
Apligraf® (Organogenesis Inc, Canton, MA and Novartis Pharmaceuticals Corporation, East Hanover, NJ)	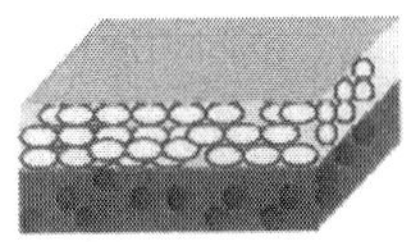	1. Neonatal keratinocytes 2. Collagen seeded with neonatal fibroblasts	7.5 cm diam disc £626.00	£14.20
Dermagraft® (Advanced Tissue Sciences, Inc, La Jolla, CA, USA)	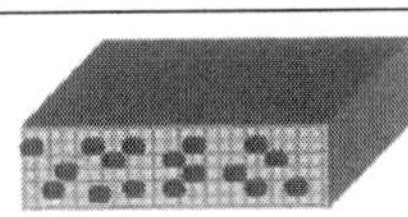	1. Polyglycolic acid (Dexon™) or polyglactin-910 (Vicryl™) seeded with neonatal fibroblasts	5 × 7.5 cm £267.80	£7.14
Integra® (Integra Life Science Corporation, Plainsboro, NJ)	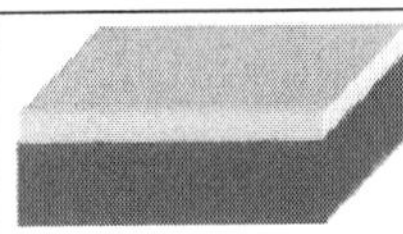	1. Silicone 2. Collagen and glycosaminoglycan	10 × 25 cm £830.00	£3.32
Alloderm® (Lifecell, Woodlands, TX)		1. Acellular de-epithelialised cadaver dermis	4 × 12 cm £283.00	£5.90
Epicel™ (Genzyme Tissue Repair Corporation, Cambridge, MA.)	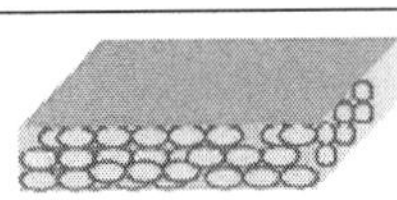	1. Cultured autologous keratinocytes	Not yet licensed in U.K.	
Laserskin™ (Fidia Advanced Biopolymers, Italy) also marketed as Vivoderm™ by ER Squibb and Sons Inc.	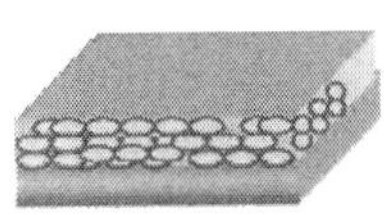	1. Cultured autologous keratinocytes 2. Hyaluronic acid with laser perforations	Not yet licensed in U.K.	
Cadaveric allograft (from not for profit skin banks)	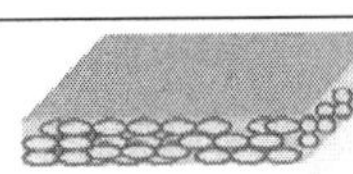	• Cryopreserved in order to retain viability • Lyophilised • Glycerolised	Similar price for all three various sizes	£0.60

FIGURE 10.11
Some of the commercially available skin substitutes. (Reprinted from Jones, I., Currie, L., and Martin, R., *Br. J. Plast. Surg.*, 55, 185, 2002. With permission from Elsevier.)

company profiles. One of the first tissue-engineered products available for clinical use is Carticel®, developed by Genzyme Biosurgery (USA). Carticel® uses autologous cultured chondrocytes for the repair of cartilage defects in the femoral condyle (medial, lateral, or trochlea), due to acute or repetitive trauma in patients who have had an inadequate response to prior arthroscopic or other surgical repair procedures. Globally, approximately 4000 patients were treated with Carticel® in the period from 1995 to 2000, and results are encouraging. Verigen (Germany) introduced a product called CACI® (collagen-covered autologous chondrocytes implantation) for use in articular cartilage. It has been used successfully in the treatment of numerous patients in Europe and Asia Pacific regions. CaReS®, another kind of tissue-engineered cartilage product, developed by ARS ARTHRO AG (Germany) for damage to the knee, is a 3D mechanically stable transplant based on patient-specific autologous cartilage cells and a collagen matrix. The implant has a solid form and is biomechanically stable, which simplifies implantation, allows for minimally invasive surgical application, and promises early weight bearing and reduced rehabilitation time. BioSeed®-C, developed by BioTissue Technologies GmbH (Germany), is an autologous, 3D chondrocyte graft that is used to treat articular cartilage defects in the femoral condyle, tibia plateau, talus, or acetabulum. Preclinical trials have shown that cells in this 3D environment begin to redifferentiate and thus assume their original form and function. In addition to these products, a large number of companies offer autologous chondrocyte transplants for cartilage repair. The case study evaluations of some of these products are discussed below.

10.12 Case Study

Recent technological advancements in biomaterials and biological sciences have propelled the emergence of novel tissue-engineered products that promise to replace dysfunctional tissues and organs. Tissue-engineered products are synthetic (manmade) and are derived from the right biomaterials by engineering their structure and properties to closely match the tissues to be repaired. These products have functional characteristics required for the regeneration of specific tissues upon implantation. Integra®, an artificial skin substitute, is a notable example. It is a commercial product of Integra Life Sciences, Inc., USA, and holds FDA approval for burn and reconstructive surgery. It is basically a bilayered structural material composed of (i) a thick inner matrix consisting of porous bovine tendon collagen and chondroitin-6-sulfate and (ii) a thin outer membrane made of silicone. The inner layer serves as an ECM to promote cell growth and related function, while the thick outer layer serves as a bacterial barrier. This unique skin substitute provides a temporary scaffold for skin regeneration, allows early wound excision, immediate closure of the wound, allows no scar formation, controls fluid loss, and helps to improve other functional and aesthetic qualities. Here, we emphasize two case studies in which Integra® was used as an artificial skin.

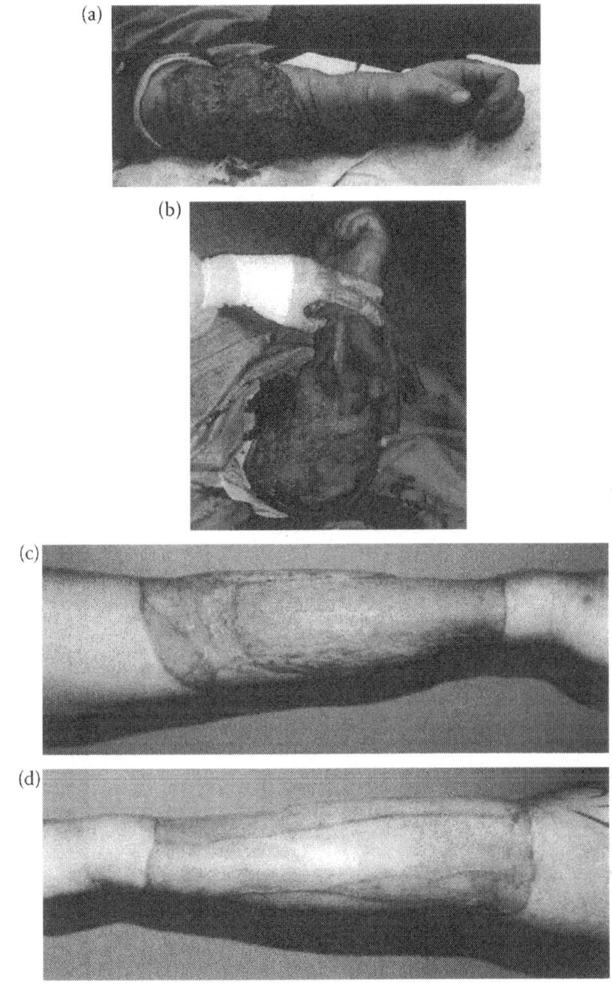

FIGURE 10.12
(a) Radial view of the forearm at the time of the accident, (b) ulnar aspect, showing the severed structures and complete degloving, (c) result after 6 months (radial aspect), and (d) result after 6 months (ulnar aspect). (Reprinted from Wolter, T. P., Noah, E. M., and Pallua, N., *Br. Assoc. Plastic Surg.*, 58, 416, 2005. With permission from Elsevier.)

The first case study, reported by Wolter et al. (2005), describes the use of Integra® for the case of a 22-year-old man who suffered an avulsion injury of the left upper extremity including the elbow region, in an industrial accident (Figure 10.12a and b). On physical examination, the patient's avulsed skin flap showed partly compromised skin and there was no sign of fracture. Of course, sensory and motor function of the hand was intact. On surgery, the skin flap was devascularized and completely removed. The defect was then primarily closed with Integra® sheets. On follow-up, except on day 3, no sign of infection was observed throughout the healing period. After 6 months, the patient had good motor function of the arm, pliable skin, and no significant hypertrophic scars. The defective areas appeared to have sufficient new tissues (see Figure 10.12c and d). Overall, the clinical results of this investigation show that the use of Integra® in an upper extremity avulsion injury has resulted in improved functional and aesthetic outcomes. The authors have also claimed that it was the first use of Integra® in degloving or avulsion injury and suggested that Integra® is an alternative for immediate coverage of the region of large avulsion injuries.

In another case study, Noah et al. (2004) reported the case of a 31-year-old woman, who suffered a chemical burn injury to the face caused by sulfuric acid, treated with delayed Integra® reconstruction. On physical examination, full thickness burn areas were found on the forehead, cheeks, and neck. The patient's eyes, the nose, and the mouth area were nearly unaffected (see Figure 10.13a), but the ear cartilage was lost. On surgery, the necrotic tissues were excised in the regions of the cheeks and the neck down to the platyma (see Figure 10.13b), and a temporary coverage was applied with Mepitel™ (Molnlycke Health Care). Three days later, the excised surfaces were covered with fresh cadaver skin and, 1 week later, the excision was completed and 46 pridie drilling holes were made in order to stimulate granulation. Three weeks later, Integra® was applied to the excised wounds and fixed with sutures (see Figure 10.13c). In order to overcome the difficulty of optimal dressing, the authors used an industrial foam to form a helmet-like coverage of the Integra® implant. The foam helmet helps to maintain constant pressure during tissue healing. At 8 months follow-up, the patient's defective area had recovered with a new tissue growth and the aesthetic results were excellent (Figure 10.13d). This investigation demonstrated successful skin reconstruction using Integra®. These two clinical studies thus suggest the safety and efficacy of artificial skin substitutes for the treatment of skin injuries.

10.13 Summary

The experimental examples summarized in this chapter represent some of the developments of nanobiomaterials for tissue engineering applications. Tissue engineering is an emerging multidisciplinary field, comprising several specialties, such as materials science and engineering, nanotechnology, cell biology, and medicine, aimed at developing biological substitutes to restore, maintain, or improve tissue function that fails to heal spontaneously. Although tissue engineering research is being carried out to construct almost all types of tissues of the human body, very few tissue-engineered

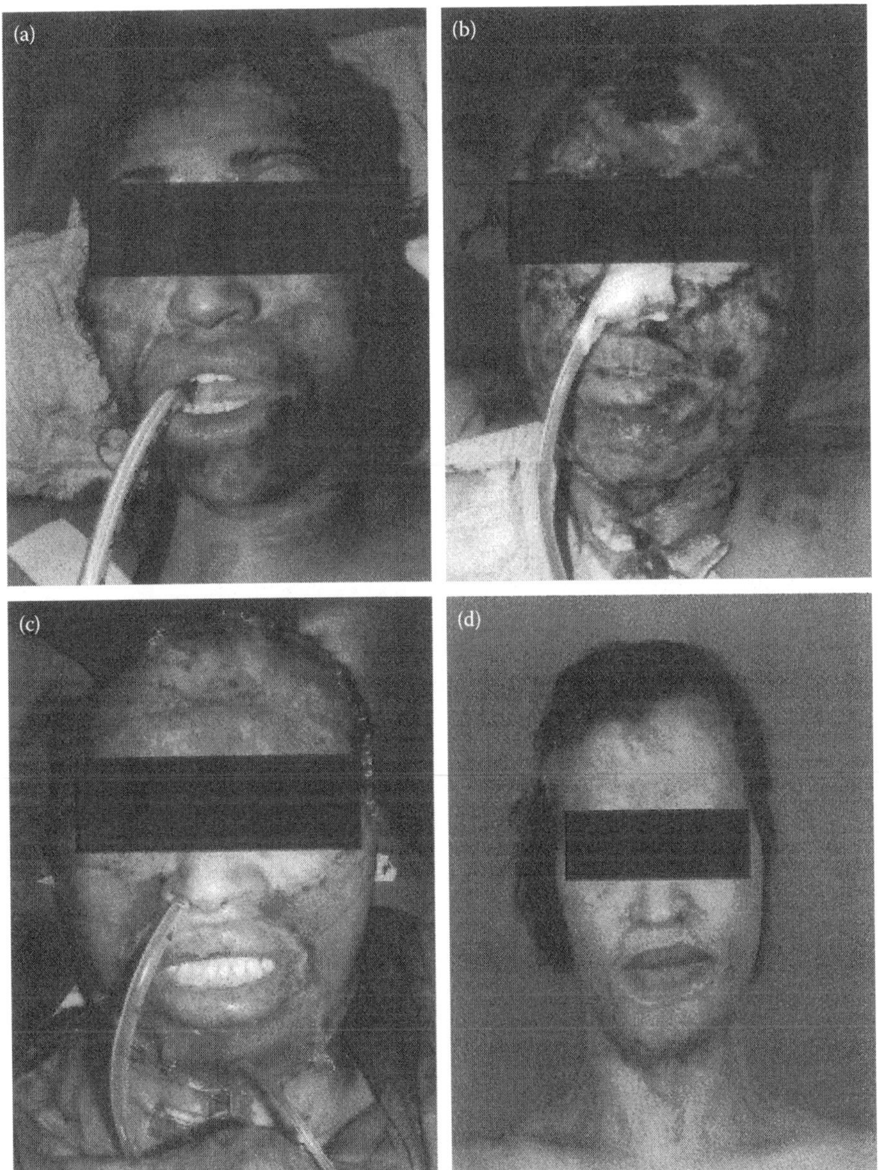

FIGURE 10.13
(a) Full thickness burn areas on forehead, cheeks, and neck, (b) the necrotic tissues were excised immediately in the region of the cheeks up to the fat layer, in the region of the neck up to the platysma, (c) Integra® artificial skin was applied to excised wounds, and (d) results after 8 months. (Reprinted from Noah, E. M. et al., *Burns* 30, 280, 2004. With permission from Elsevier.)

products are currently available for human use, in particular skin and cartilage repair, and some are still under laboratory or clinical trials. However, the tissue engineering approach may also deliver products suitable for other tissue reconstructions in the near future.

Currently, most tissue-engineered products use biomaterials rather than nanobiomaterials, as this field is still in its infancy. Although preliminary investigations seem to support the impact of nanobiomaterials in various tissue engineering applications, significant advancements are necessary to realize their full potential in clinical use. This is an exciting time to be involved in nanobiomaterials in order to formulate them as a clinically ideal system for tissue engineering, with great challenges and also great expectations ahead.

Glossary

Adult stem cell: An undifferentiated cell found in a differentiated tissue, which is able to self-renew and to differentiate into tissue-specific cell types from which it originated.

Allograft: Tissue or organ transplanted from one individual to another of the same species.

Alloplast graft: Any synthetic material substituted to repair or replace defective parts of the body.

Artificial organ: A medical device or implant intended to replace the body organs.

Autograft: Tissue or organ transplanted within the same body.

Bioactivity: Ability of the implant to play a vital role in the metabolic processes of the living body.

Biocompatibility: Ability of the implant to perform with an appropriate host response in a specific application.

Biodegradability: Susceptibility of the implant to be decomposed by a living organism.

Bioinert: No host response to the material.

Biomaterial: Any synthetic material that is biocompatible to the tissues and to the body upon implantation. It can be metal, ceramic, polymer, and a composite of each.

Biomineralization: A conversion process of organic substances to inorganic derivatives by living organisms, especially microorganisms.

Biopsy: Removal of a small portion of tissue, usually for the purpose of making a diagnosis.

Bone: A rigid, yet dynamic connective tissue consisting of calcium phosphate-based minerals embedded with collagen fibers in conjunction with osteogenic cellular elements.

Bone marrow stromal cell: A kind of stem cell found in bone marrow that has the ability to generate bone, cartilage, and other connective tissues.

Cell: Fundamental, structural, and functional unit of all living beings that is composed of an outer membrane enclosing protoplasm and nucleus.

Collagen: A fibrous structural protein that functions to hold tissues together.

Composite: A heterogeneous combination of two or more materials.

Corrosion: A chemical or electrochemical degradation of metals due to surrounding environmental factors.

Differentiation: A process whereby an unspecialized cell acquires the features of a specialized cell.

Electrospinning: A fiber processing technique, which utilizes electrostatic forces to produce extremely fine fibers ranging from a few micrometers to nanometers in diameter.

Embryonic stem cell: An undifferentiated cell found in an embryo that is able to produce a spectrum of specialized cell/tissue types.

Extracellular matrix: The surrounding material of a cell including ground substances and fibers.

Fiber: The individual strands of material that form a nonwoven construct.

Graft: A transplant.

Growth factors: A heterogeneous group of substances capable of enhancing tissue growth.

Hard tissue: The general term for calcified structures of the body (e.g., bone and tooth).

Hematopoietic stem cells: A stem cell from which all blood cells develop.

Hydroxyapatite: A calcium phosphate-based material with chemical composition $Ca_{10}(PO_4)_6(OH)_2$, rich in bone minerals.

Immunogenic: Capable of stimulating an immune response.

Implant: Any medical device or prosthesis inserted or grafted in the human body.

Implantation: A surgical procedure by which a medical device or prosthesis is placed in the human body, either temporarily or permanently.

***In vitro*:** A biological study performed in the laboratory. In other words, outside the living body.

***In vivo*:** A biological study performed inside the living body.

Mesenchymal stem cell: A cell derived from the immature embryonic connective tissue.

Metabolism: A general term used to designate all biochemical changes that occur to substances within the body by either anabolism or catabolism.

Micro: A unit prefix meaning one millionth (1/1,000,000).

Modulus: One of several measures of strain vs. applied stress (e.g., Young's modulus).

Monolithic: Made from a single material.

Multipotent: The ability of a single stem cell to develop into a small number of cell types of the body, which have a specific function.

Nano: A unit prefix meaning one billionth (1/1,000,000,000).

Nanobiomaterials: Biomaterials composed of particles or grains having nanometric tolerances; a nanometer is equal to 10^{-9} m.

Nontrauma: Any injury or wound caused by disease.

Organ: A differentiated part of an organism adapted for a definite function.

Osteoconduction: An action associated with ingrowth of capillaries and migration of bone-forming cells from the host into 3D matrix.

Pathogen: Any organism that is capable of producing disease.

Phenotype: Observable characteristics of an organism, resulting from the interaction of its genotype with the environment.

Plasticity: Ability of stem cells from one adult tissue to generate the differentiated cell type of another tissue.

Pluripotent: Ability of a single stem cell to develop into many different cell types of the body.

Polymer: A long chain, high molecular weight material consisting of repeated monomer units.

Porosity: A ratio of void volume to total volume expressed in terms of percentage.

Proliferation: Expansion of cell population by continuous division of a single cell into two identical daughter cells.

Prosthesis: A medical device that is capable of replacing the organs or tissues.

Protein: A large biomolecule composed of one or more chains of amino acids in a specific sequence.

Resorption: Dissolution of a substance.

Scaffold: A temporary structural construct or matrix used to support the cells for accommodation during tissue fabrication.

Stem cell: An undifferentiated cell that is capable of producing specialized types of cells.

Stem cell therapy: A treatment in which stem cells are induced to differentiate into specific types of cells/tissues for the purpose of tissue repair.

Surface area: The total area of exposed surface of an object.

Tissue: A collection of similar cells and their surrounding intercellular substances.

Tissue engineering: Development of human tissues or organs in the laboratory from cells removed from the patient or other sources.

Totipotent: Ability of a single stem cell to develop into all types of cells/tissues of the body.

Transplantation: Surgical transfer of tissue or organ from one place to another.

Trauma: Any injury or wound caused by an external force.

Vascular: A medical term pertaining to blood vessel.

Xenograft: Tissue or organ transplanted from one species onto a different species.

EXERCISES

10.1 Why is tissue engineering important?

10.2 Distinguish between tissue repair and tissue regeneration.

10.3 What is a scaffold and what kind of material can be used as a scaffolding system?

10.4 Define and classify stem cells.

10.5 What are the advantages of using mesenchymal stem cells in tissue engineering?

10.6 Do the cells grow *in vitro* without a scaffold?

10.7 What are the advantages of using nanobiomaterials in tissue engineering as a scaffold?

10.8 What is extracellular matrix and what does it contain?

10.9 Describe the key characteristics of tissue scaffold.

10.10 Provide some examples of ceramics and polymers used in tissue engineering.

10.11 List some of the commercially available tissue engineering products and their applications.

10.12 What does the future hold for tissue engineering?

References

Caplan, A. I. and S. P. Bruder. 2001. Mesenchymal stem cells: Building blocks for molecular medicine in the 21st century. *Trends Mol. Med.* 7:259.

Dalby, M. J. et al. 2002a. *In vitro* reaction of endothelial cells to polymer demixed nanotopography. *Biomaterials* 23:2945.

———. 2002b. Polymer demixed nanotopography: Control of fibroblast spreading and proliferation. *Tissue Eng.* 8:1099.

Du, C. et al. 1999. Three-dimensional nano-HAp/collagen matrix loading with osteogenic cells in organ culture. *J. Biomed. Mater. Res.* 44:407.

Friedenstein, A. J., K. V. Petrakova, and A. I. Kurolesova. 1968. Heterotopic transplants of bone marrow. Analysis of precursor cells for osteogenic and haemopoietic tissues. *Transplantation* 6:230.

Huang, J. et al. 2004. In vitro assessment of the biological response to nano-sized hydroxyapatite. *J. Mater. Sci. Mater. Med.* 15:41.

Jones, I., L. Currie, and R. Martin. 2002. A guide to biological skin substitutes. *Br. J. Plast. Surg.* 55:185.

Kesemo, B. and J. Lausmaa. 1986. Surface science aspects on inorganic biomaterials. *CRC Crit. Rev. Biocomp.* 2:335.

Li, W. J. et al. 2005. A three-dimensional nanofibrous scaffold for cartilage tissue engineering using human mesenchymal stem cells. *Biomaterials* 26:599.

Liao, S. S., F. Z. Cui, and X. D. Zhu. 2004. Osteoblasts adherence and migration through three-dimensional porous mineralized collagen based composite: nHAC/PLA. *J. Bioactive Compat. Polym.* 19:117.

Manso, M. et al. 2002. Biological evaluation of aerosol–gel-derived hydroxyapatite coatings with human mesenchymal stem cells. *Biomaterials* 23:3985.

Matthews, J. A. et al. 2002. Electrospinning of collagen nanofibers. *Biomacromolecules* 3:232.

Murugan, R. and S. Ramakrishna. 2004. Nanostructured biomaterials. In *Encyclopedia of nanoscience and nanotechnology*, ed. H. S. Nalwa, 595. Stevenson Ranch, CA: American Scientific Publishers.

———. 2005a. Bioactive nanomaterials in bone grafting and tissue engineering. In *Handbook of nanostructured biomaterials and their applications in nanobiotechnology*, ed. H. S. Nalwa, 141. Stevenson Ranch, CA: American Scientific Publishers.

———. 2005b. Development of nanocomposites for bone grafting. *Comp. Sci. Tech.* 65:2385.

———. 2006. Nanophase biomaterials for tissue engineering. In *Nanotechnologies for tissue, cell and organ engineering*, ed. S. S. R. Challakumar, 216. Stevenson Ranch, CA: American Scientific Publishers.

———. 2007. Design strategies of tissue engineering scaffolds with controlled fiber orientation. *Tiss. Eng.* 13:1845.

Noah, E. M. et al. 2004. A case of successful delayed reconstruction using a collagen based dermal substitute of a chemical burn injury to the face caused by sulphuric acid. *Burns* 30:280.

Vogt, A. K. et al. 2004. Impact of micropatterned surfaces on neuronal polarity. *J. Neurosci. Methods* 134:191.

Webster, T. J. et al. 2000. Enhanced functions of osteoblasts on nanophase ceramics. *Biomaterials* 21:1803.

Wendy, F. L. and S. C. Christopher. 2005. Engineering biomaterials to control cell function. *Mater. Today* 8:28.

Wolter, T. P., E. M. Noah, and N. Pallua. 2005. The use of Integra® in an upper extremity avulsion injury. *Br. Assoc. Plastic Surg.* 58:416.

Yang, F. et al. 2004. Fabrication of nano-structured porous PLLA scaffold intended for nerve tissue engineering. *Biomaterials* 25:1891.

———. 2005. Electrospinning of nano/micro scale poly(L-lactic acid) aligned fibers and their potential in neural tissue engineering. *Biomaterials* 26:2603.

Yim, E. K. F. et al. 2005. Nanopattern-induced changes in morphology and motility of smooth muscle cells. *Biomaterials* 26:5405.

Yoshimoto, H. et al. 2003. A biodegradable nanofiber scaffold by electrospinning and its potential for bone tissue engineering. *Biomaterials* 24:2077.

Index

O

P

Q

R

S

An environmentally friendly book printed and bound in England by www.printondemand-worldwide.com

PEFC Certified

This product is from sustainably managed forests and controlled sources

www.pefc.org

PEFC/16-33-415

MIX

Paper from responsible sources

FSC® C004959

www.fsc.org

This book is made entirely of sustainable materials; FSC paper for the cover and PEFC paper for the text pages.

#0123 - 171013 - C0 - 234/156/20 [22] - CB